1997
YEAR BOOK OF
DERMATOLOGIC SURGERY®

Statement of Purpose

The YEAR BOOK Service

The YEAR BOOK series was devised in 1901 by practicing health professionals who observed that the literature of medicine and related disciplines had become so voluminous that no one individual could read and place in perspective every potential advance in a major specialty. In the final decade of the 20th century, this recognition is more acutely true than it was in 1901.

More than merely a series of books, YEAR BOOK volumes are the tangible results of a unique service designed to accomplish the following:

- to *survey* a wide range of journals of proven value
- to *select* from those journals papers representing significant advances and statements of important clinical principles
- to provide *abstracts* of those articles that are readable, convenient summaries of their key points
- to provide *commentary* about those articles to place them in perspective

These publications grow out of a unique process that calls on the talents of outstanding authorities in clinical and fundamental disciplines, trained literature specialists, and professional writers, all supported by the resources of Mosby, the world's preeminent publisher for the health professions.

The Literature Base

Mosby and its Editors survey more than 1,000 journals published worldwide, covering the full range of the health professions. On an annual basis, the publisher examines usage patterns and polls its expert authorities to add new journals to the literature base and to delete journals that are no longer useful as potential YEAR BOOK sources.

The Literature Survey

The publisher's team of literature specialists, all of whom are trained and experienced health professionals, examines every original, peer-reviewed article in each journal issue. More than 250,000 articles per year are scanned systematically, including title, text, illustrations, tables, and references. Each scan is compared, article by article, to the search strategies that the publisher has developed in consultation with the 270 outside experts who form the pool of YEAR BOOK editors. A given article may be reviewed by any number of editors, from one to a dozen or more, regardless of the discipline for which the paper was originally published. In turn, each editor who receives the article reviews it to determine whether or not the article should be included in the YEAR BOOK. This decision is based on the article's inherent quality, its probable usefulness to readers of that YEAR BOOK, and the editor's goal to represent a balanced picture of a given field in each volume of the YEAR BOOK. In addition, the editor indicates

Table of Contents

Journals Represented

Mosby and its Editors survey more than 1,000 journals for its abstract and commentary publications. From these journals, the Editors select the articles to be abstracted. Journals represented in this YEAR BOOK are listed below.

Aesthetic Plastic Surgery
American Journal of Epidemiology
American Journal of Pathology
American Journal of Surgery
Annals of Plastic Surgery
Annals of Surgery
Archives of Dermatology
Archives of Family Medicine
Archives of Otolaryngology–Head and Neck Surgery
British Journal of Cancer
British Journal of Plastic Surgery
British Journal of Radiology
British Journal of Surgery
Burns
Canadian Journal of Anaesthesia
Canadian Journal of Plastic Surgery
Canadian Medical Association Journal
Cancer
Cancer Research
Dermatologic Surgery
Diabetes Care
Ear, Nose, and Throat Journal (ENT-Ear, Nose, and Throat Journal)
European Journal of Dermatology
European Journal of Plastic Surgery
International Journal of Aesthetic and Restorative Surgery
Journal of Clinical Anesthesia
Journal of Clinical Oncology
Journal of Dermatologic Surgery and Oncology
Journal of Geriatric Dermatology
Journal of Hand Surgery (American)
Journal of Investigative Dermatology
Journal of Laboratory and Clinical Medicine
Journal of Nuclear Medicine
Journal of Surgical Research
Journal of the American Academy of Dermatology
Journal of the American College of Surgeons
Journal of the American Medical Association
Journal of the National Cancer Institute
Journal of the Royal College of Surgeons of Edinburgh
Lancet
Laryngoscope
Nature Medicine
Otolaryngology–Head and Neck Surgery
Plastic and Reconstructive Surgery
Scandinavian Journal of Plastic and Reconstructive Hand Surgery
Transplantation
Western Journal of Medicine

World Journal of Surgery
Wound Repair and Regeneration

STANDARD ABBREVIATIONS

The following terms are abbreviated in this edition: acquired immunodeficiency syndrome (AIDS), cardiopulmonary resuscitation (CPR), central nervous system (CNS), cerebrospinal fluid (CSF), computed tomography (CT), deoxyribonucleic acid (DNA), electrocardiography (ECG), health maintenance organization (HMO), human immunodeficiency virus (HIV), intensive care unit (ICU), intramuscular (IM), intravenous (IV), magnetic resonance (MR) imaging (MRI), and ribonucleic acid (RNA).

NOTE

The YEAR BOOK OF DERMATOLOGIC SURGERY is a literature survey service providing abstracts of articles published in the professional literature. Every effort is made to assure the accuracy of the information presented in these pages. Neither the editors nor the publisher of the YEAR BOOK OF DERMATOLOGIC SURGERY can be responsible for errors in the original materials. The editors' comments are their own opinions. Mention of specific products within this publication does not constitute endorsement.

To facilitate the use of the YEAR BOOK OF DERMATOLOGIC SURGERY, as a reference tool, all illustrations and tables included in this publication are now identified as they appear in the original article. This change is meant to help the reader recognize that any illustration or table appearing in the YEAR BOOK OF DERMATOLOGIC SURGERY may be only one of many in the original article. For this reason, figure and table numbers will often appear to be out of sequence within the YEAR BOOK OF DERMATOLOGIC SURGERY.

Introduction

The YEAR BOOK OF DERMATOLOGIC SURGERY has been a truly significant contribution since its inception 5 years ago with the 1992 edition. As you can see, there has been a change in editors after 5 years and the previous editors are to be applauded for their excellent work and contributions. Personally, I have looked forward to the arrival of each edition to help me continue to improve and update my knowledge and skill. The prior editors, Neil Swanson, M.D., Stuart Salasche, M.D., and Richard G. Glogau, M.D., have provided insight into the world's best literature associated with dermatologic surgery. Each of them is a superb physician, leader, teacher, and friend. Under the leadership of Dr. Swanson, they have done an outstanding job. It is my goal to continue their tradition and uniqueness.

I was honored to be asked by Mosby–Year Book to succeed Neil Swanson, M.D. as Editor-in-Chief of this series. We have assembled a group of associate editors who should continue the fine undertakings of Drs. Salasche and Glogau.

Duane C. Whitaker M.D., Director of Dermatologic Surgery at the University of Iowa has been a leader, teacher, and innovator in dermatologic surgery for a number of years. He continues to be rated as one of our best professors at our yearly cadaver "Superficial Anatomy and Cutaneous Surgery" course. Duane has edited the Oncology chapter in addition to contributing throughout. With the significant advances in melanoma evaluation and therapy (i.e., smaller margins, sentinel node evaluations, and adjunctive interferon), this section is critically important for the dermatologic surgeon. The remaining sections in oncology are of value as most dermatologic surgeons also consider themselves cutaneous oncologists.

Diamondis J. Papadopoulos, M.D. is Co-head of Dermatologic Surgery at Emory University in Atlanta. Dr. Papadopoulos brings youth and enthusiasm (this is not to say that Duane and I are not youthful) and his perspective on cosmetic procedures. He edited the Esthetic Dermatologic Surgery section with assistance from myself. In part because of his Greek heritage, Dr. Papadoupolos has published not only in the United States, but also in the European journals. His frequent contacts throughout this area should bring an added perspective to our publication. Botulinim toxin was incorporated into our practice during this year and there are articles on this as well as those updating liposuction, filler injections, dermabrasions, chemical peels, hair transplantation, sclerotherapy, and aging skin.

In addition to the responsibility of editing their own chapters, each editor has overlapped and supplied material in areas of special interest. With our geographic and practice diversities, the editors each bring strong talents to the YEAR BOOK OF DERMATOLOGIC SURGERY and I am delighted and excited that Drs. Whitaker and Papadoupolos have joined me in this project.

I expect that there will continue to be exciting changes and am pleased to announce that for the 1998 edition we will have a separate section on dermatologic surgical pathology which will be edited by Terry L. Barrett, M.D. Dr. Barrett is currently Director of the Dermatology Residency Program at the Naval Medical Center, San Diego. He is board certified in dermatology, pathology, and dermatopathology and should be a valuable addition to our editorial staff.

The staff at Mosby–Year Book has been excellent and most competent. We appreciate their continued efforts and support in the preparation of this year's YEAR BOOK OF DERMATOLOGIC SURGERY.

Hubert T. Greenway, M.D.

1 Concepts and Techniques

Introduction

Perhaps this was truly the "Year of the Laser." The proliferation of the concept of laser resurfacing propelled a number of articles as well as CME educational courses as dermatologic surgeons sought to master and introduce this technique to their patients and practices. Because of our wealth of experience and knowledge of lasers (as well as the pre- and postoperative care of the skin) this new technology is an easy match. My mentor and friend Leon Goldman, M.D., truly the father of medical lasers, is owed a great debt by each of us. Leon now resides here in San Diego and continues to be active in laser research, teaching, and education. Although there appears to be some controversy regarding which of the different carbon dioxide lasers is "best" for laser resurfacing, it appears that acceptable results can be obtained with different systems. Just as our mentors had various systems for dermabrasion and chemical peeling, so it may be with lasers for facial resurfacing. Patient selection is an important factor.

Advances in our understanding of wound healing and the treatment of scarring continue. Certainly we can surgically remove a hypertrophic scar or keloid; the science and art are to keep it from reforming. Combined modalities may offer advantages.

Improvements in our local anesthesia continue to interest me as we seek to limit any unpleasantness for our patients. However, appropriate technique may be a more important factor. There is certainly "art" to local anesthesia just as there is with surgery.

The Miscellaneous section contains several articles which are provoking and may assist us in our daily or future practice. These include nutrition in elderly patients (for many of us nutrition was not a significant part of our formal training in the past), a primer on angiogenesis, gene transfer, thoughts on interferon in wound contracture, and even an innovative way of assisting liposuction of the breast surgically.

Ethical judgments and medical legal applications affect each of us and the way in which we practice our profession. Even with managed care we must continue to be the patient's advocate. Each patient must be treated as we would wish that our family would be treated. Dr. Frederic Mohs instilled in myself and others "just do what is best for the patient, and then don't worry about whatever else may happen." I suspect these guidelines serve us well as we continue to see both more articles and situations in this area.

Hubert T. Greenway, M.D.

Wound Healing

The Use of Antioxidants in Healing
Martin A (Warner-Lambert Co, Morris Plains, NJ)
Dermatol Surg 22:156–160, 1996   1–1

Introduction.—Antioxidants are important in all phases of the wound healing process. They are needed to neutralize the oxygen species released by neutrophils and other cells during the inflammation phase. They are also essential in the formation of collagen by viable fibroblasts during the proliferative phase. During the remodeling phase, antioxidants are needed to normalize blood coagulation and reduce scarring.

Antioxidants.—The various antioxidants perform different roles in the healing process. Pyruvate can enter cells; it provides intracellular protection of DNA and enhances cellular growth and repair. Vitamin E protects the cell membranes from lipid peroxidation induced by oxygen radicals. Endogenous fatty acids, in the correct ratio of saturated and unsaturated fatty acids, can replace the membrane fatty acids damaged by oxygen radicals, thus improving membrane function, cellular viability, and intracellular transport of pyruvate and reducing the intracellular production of unsaturated fatty acids, which reduces the need for oxygen.

Combined Therapy.—Several studies have shown the beneficial effects of CRT (sodium pyruvate, vitamin E, and fatty acids) on wound healing. In vitro studies have shown that the production of oxygen radicals and associated cellular damage was inhibited in skin and white blood cells exposed to ultraviolet light and toxic chemicals. Animal studies have demonstrated increased wound healing with decreased scarring and reduced size, duration, and severity of herpes simplex viral infection in animals treated with CRT. CRT has also reversed doxorubicin-impaired wound healing in rats and peripheral blood monocyte viability.

Conclusions.—Sodium pyruvate, vitamin E, and fatty acids each facilitate repair of oxygen radical-induced cellular damage by activity on a different part of the cell. The combination has a synergistic effect that may dramatically enhance cellular repair.

▶ Enhanced wound healing continues to entice our thoughts as we seek better results for our patients. Years ago at a missionary hospital in Africa, I was introduced first-hand to the problems of wound healing in malnourished individuals. Our patients today may have more information on nutrition and supplementation than their health care providers, albeit some of it tainted and nonapplicable. The knowledge that a decrease in Vitamin C at the wound site decreases the rate of wound healing as well as the positive effect of topical Vitamin E antioxidant on scarring focuses our attention on the local area. This paper encourages consideration of antioxidants in wound healing.

H.T. Greenway, M.D.

Transforming Growth Factor-β: Activity and Efficacy in Animal Models of Wound Healing
Roberts AB (Natl Cancer Inst, Bethesda, Md)
Wound Rep Reg 3:408–418, 1995   1–2

Purpose.—Wound healing is influenced by several different growth factors, that with the broadest spectrum of action being transforming growth factor-β (TGF-β). The mechanisms of action of TGF-β are becoming clear only with understanding of its multiple isoforms and their differential regulation and autoinduction, its ability to be complexed in "latent" forms and sequestered by the extracellular matrix, its unique receptor signaling pathway, and its specific cellular stimulatory activities. Current knowledge about TGF-β is reviewed, focusing on its ability to improve or accelerate healing.

TGF-β and Wound Healing.—Upon its release from activated platelets, TGF-β can act on and be secreted by any of the various types of cells involved in the healing process. It is distinguished from all other growth factors by its unique set of serine-threonine kinase receptors (Fig 1). Signaling through this pathway mediates TGF-β's stimulation of chemotaxis, fibrogenesis, angiogenesis, and autoinduction of expression (Fig 2).

Many studies have investigated the effects of TGF-β on wound healing in animals, including both basal and impaired tissue repair. Many different vehicles have been used to deliver TGF-β to experimental wounds—prolonged local exposure appears beneficial. Repair may also be enhanced by systemic TGF-β administration as long as 24 hr before wounding. In addition to improved healing of dermal wounds, beneficial effects have been noted at nondermal sites as well, including the bone, intestine, eye, and mouth. Studies of scarring suggest that the TGF-β isoform profile of a healing wound has important effects on wound cellularity and architecture.

Conclusions.—Many different animal studies have shown that TGF-β enhances wound healing, paving the way for its clinical application. The potential uses of TGF-β are limited only by the need to develop appropriate treatment modes and schedules. In the future, TGF-β treatment may be used in the treatment of various chronic, nonhealing wounds and as a preventive treatment for surgical patients, especially those with impaired healing.

▶ This is a nice review article about a very important group of peptides with a wide-ranging presence and biological processes that include angiogenesis, fibrogenesis, and chemotaxis. The three isoforms of TGF-β and their differential regulation and auto induction may have a significant impact on tissue

TABLE 3.—Wound Dressings

Classification	Compositions	Indications	Examples	Advantages	Disadvantages
Films	Polyurethane or co-polyester with adhesive backing	Split skin graft donor sites, acute partial-thickness wounds w/minimal exudate Nondraining primarily closed wounds, superficial burns, IV & catheter sites	Op-site, Bioclusive, Opraflex Tegaderm, Uniflex, Blisterfilm, Visulin, Ensure, Clingfilm, Vioflim, Acuderm, Omiderm, Dermafilm[3]	Transparency allows for wound inspections Reduces frequency of dressing changes Fluid retention Decrease wound pain at donor sites	Fluid retention may lead to excess fluid collection Cost May adhere to some wounds[†] Can be difficult to apply[†] Does not debride wound Generally not ideal for exudative wounds
Hydrocolloids	Contain hydrophilic colloidal particles (quar, karaya, gelactic, carboxymethyl cellulose) bound to polyurethane foam	Acute or chronic partial or full-thickness wounds. Stage I to IV pressure ulcers; friction blisters, stasis ulcers	Cutinova hydro, Ultec, Duoderm, Comfeel Ulcus, Restore, Actiderm, Hydrapad, Granuflex E, Intrasite, Intact, Tegasorb[3]	Debrides wound Absorbs exudate Protection of wound Does not adhere to wounds Easy to apply Reduced frequency of dressing changes Gel creates moist wound healing	Cost Opaque dressing Foul smell of gel may be confused w/infection Gel leakage onto clothing
Hydrogels	Contain 80-99% water. Cross-linked polymer such as polyethyleneoxide, polyvinyl	Acute or chronic partial thickness exudative wounds acute, painful wounds post dermabrasion, laser wounds, chemical peels	Vigilon, Biofilm, Geliperm, Cutinova Gel, Elastogel, Intrasite Gel, Span Gel[3]	Soothing to patient Diminishes wound pain Does not adhere to wound Good for exudative wounds Semitransparent	Nonadhesive; requires additional dressing to secure Cost Must be changed more frequently; every 1-3 days

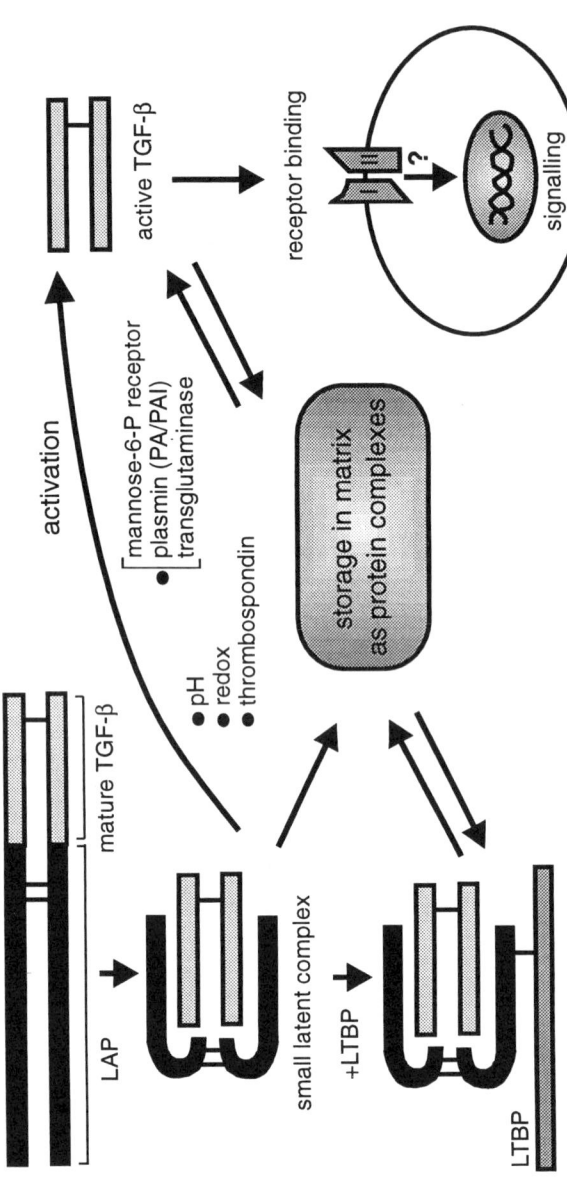

FIGURE 1.—Regulation of latent TGF-β activation is central to its bioavailability. After proteolytic processing to the resultant LAP and mature C-terminal TGF-β, TGF-β is secreted from cells or released from platelets in the form of either a small latent complex consisting of TGF-β in noncovalent association with LAP or a large latent complex formed by the covalent addition of LTBP to LAP, as shown. These complexes can either be activated directly or serve to localize TGF-β to matrix, where it can be stored or activated under appropriate conditions. Depending on the cellular context and environment, different activation mechanisms have been shown to be operative, resulting in exposure of the receptor-binding epitope of TGF-β and subsequent activation of cellular signaling through its serine-threonine kinase receptors (Courtesy of Roberts AB: Transforming growth factor-β: Activity and efficacy in animal models of wound healing. *Wound Rep Reg* 3:408–418, 1995.)

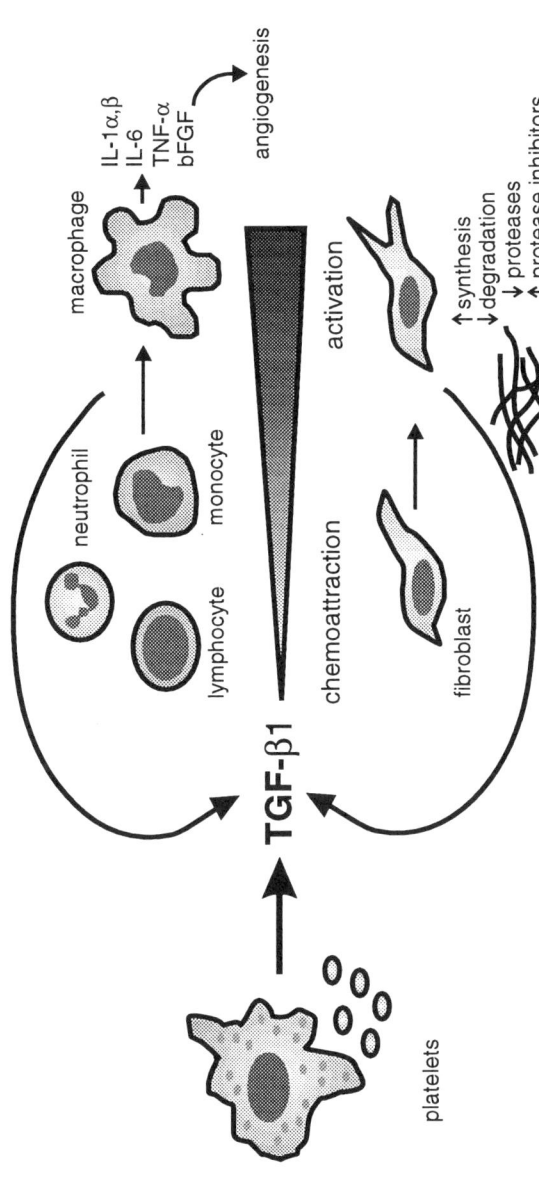

FIGURE 2.—TGF-β integrates the action of several cell types involved in tissue repair. After its release from degranulating platelets, lymphocytes, monocytes, neutrophils, and fibroblasts are chemoattracted by low concentrations of active TGF-β, then activate macrophages to secrete cytokines and fibroblasts to elaborate extracellular matrix. Importantly, each of these cell types is autoinduced or otherwise stimulated to secrete TGF-β, thus extending its action in the repair process. (Courtesy of Roberts AB: Transforming growth factor-β: Activity and efficacy in animal models of wound healing. *Wound Rep Reg* 3:408–418, 1995.)

repair, clotting, and carcinogenesis. Even though approximately 10 years have gone by since its first description, this molecule will eventually play a prominent role in the everyday practice of dermatologic surgery, probably through the development of compounds that affect wound healing. I think we all need to keep a close eye on the future developments and their applications concerning this growth factor.

D.J. Papadopoulos, M.D.

The Effect of Interferon α_{2b} on the Expression of Cytoskeletal Proteins in an In Vitro Model of Wound Contraction
Nedelec B, Shen YJ, Ghahary A, et al (Univ of Alberta, Canada)
J Lab Clin Med 126:474–484, 1995   1–3

Background.—Contraction is a normal element of wound healing occurring in 3 phases: a lag phase, a rapid contraction phase, and a slow contraction phase. However, patients with hypertrophic scarring have excessive wound contraction. The cellular and molecular mechanisms have not been fully elucidated, but it is believed that fibroblasts are central to the wound contraction process. The contractile properties of both normal and hypertrophic scar fibroblasts were investigated at the cellular and molecular levels.

Methods.—Fibroblast cultures were established from paired dermal biopsy specimens from normal and hypertrophic scar samples of 5 patients recovering from burns. Some of these cultured fibroblasts were exposed to serum and some to interferon alfa-2b (IFN alfa-2b) for 144, 96, 48, or 0 hours, then assayed with fibroblast-populated collagen lattices. The collagen cell surface area was measured at 2, 4, 6, 8, 10, 12, 24, 48, and 72 hours, and cell viability was determined. Ribonucleic acid was extracted from 4 paired strains of IFN alfa-2b–treated and untreated normal and hypertrophic fibroblasts, were hybridized with specific radiolabeled cDNA probes, and were examined with Northern blot analysis. The cells in the fibroblast-populated collagen lattices were examined with confocal laser scanning microscopy after rhodamine-labeled phalloidin staining.

Results.—The cell strains treated with IFN alfa-2b had a short lag phase, then a 24-hour rapid contraction phase, with contraction completed at 72 hours. The control fibroblasts from both normal and hypertrophic areas had average reductions of 79% in the gel surface area. These contractile abilities were progressively reduced over time in the IFN alfa-2b fibroblasts, with no significant differences between normal and hypertrophic fibroblasts. The fibroblasts that were exposed to IFN immediately before lattice polymerization showed no contraction reduction or cytotoxic effects. Interferon treatment also resulted in reduced RNA message levels, with specific reduced expression of γ-actin messenger (mRNA) RNA in the hypertrophic cells and of β-actin mRNA in the normal cells, nonstatistically significant reductions in the expression of α-tubulin, but no effect on vimentin or α-actinin expression. Histologic changes also occurred in association with interferon treatment, including a lack of elongation, bipolarity, and unidirectional orientation in the fibroblasts. No significant histologic differences were found between the untreated normal and hypertrophic fibroblasts when examined with confocal laser scanning microscopy.

Conclusions.—There are no differences in the contractile abilities of fibroblasts in normal dermis and hypertrophic scars. Interferon treatment reduces the rate and extent of the phases of contraction in a time-dependent manner without having cytotoxic effects, suggesting that this treatment affects the mechanism of contraction rather than cell attachment. This treatment effect is associated with reduced expression of β- and γ-actin mRNA. The organization of the actin filaments is also changed with IFN treatment, without the characteristic bipolar morphology of contractile cell.

▶ The findings that IFN alfa 2-b is associated with reductions in mRNA for β and γ actin as well as fibroblast alterations document its role in wound contraction and healing. As I reflect on our work with intralesional injections in the treatment of both basal cell carcinoma and squamous cell carcinoma, we saw and do see excellent healing of the treatment site without ulcerations and so on and histologically observed preservation of the normal appendages. Interferon reduction in wound contraction could offer its usefulness as an agent in the prevention of hypertrophic scarring.

H.T. Greenway, M.D.

Transforming Growth Factor β₁ Improves Wound Healing and Random Flap Survival in Normal and Irradiated Rats

Nall AV, Brownlee RE, Colvin CP, et al (Univ of Florida, Gainesville; Chase Cancer Ctr, Philadelphia)
Arch Otolaryngol Head Neck Surg 122:171–177, 1996   1–4

Background.—For patients with head and neck cancer, preoperative irradiation may lead to impaired wound healing. Transforming growth factor β_1 (TGF-β_1) accelerates wound healing in animal studies, but its effects on wound healing and flap survival after chronic irradiation are unknown. The effects of chronic irradiation on wound healing and random flap survival (FV) and the ability of topical TGF-β_1 treatment to improve healing and FV in this situation were studied in rats.

Methods.—Four groups of rats were included in the randomized study. Group-1 animals received no irradiation and no TGF-β_1 treatment, those in group 2 received TGF-β_1 but not radiation, those in group 3 received radiation therapy but no TGF-β_1, and those in group 4 received radiation plus TGF-β_1. Radiation therapy consisted of a 15-Gy dose to the dorsal skin given 4 months before surgery. All animals underwent McFarlane skin flap surgery. Topical TGF-β_1 treatment consisted of a 4-μg dose applied to the flap bed. Wound tensile strength and FV were evaluated 1 week after surgery. Histologic staining for collagen and TGF-β_1 was also performed.

Results.—Tensile strength and FV were nonsignificantly reduced by irradiation. In rats that had and had not undergone irradiation, TGF-β_1 treatment improved tensile strength. Flap survival was also better in the animals receiving TGF-β_1, significantly so in rats receiving both radiation and TGF-β_1. Animals receiving TGF-β_1 had the most mature collagen around wound edges. The results of immunohistochemical staining for TGF-β_1 were similar in the 4 groups.

Conclusions.—Topical TGF-β_1 treatment enhances wound healing and random flap survival in rat skin. This is so both for animals that have and have not been irradiated. The authors call for the development of an animal model of radiation-impaired wound healing in which the optimum dose of TGF-β_1 to enhance wound healing and FV can be determined.

▶ As if to underscore the importance of the previous article comes this article, which describes the relative benefit of using TGF-β1 in a wound-healing model with and without radiation. The authors do mention that the amount of TGF-β1 used to achieve an excellent result needs to be worked out and that extrapolating in human terms regarding cost yields a figure of $200 for one dose of 10 µg. The quantity or the number of applications necessary, again in human terms, is not known at this time. Much work needs to be done, not only with TGF-β1, but -β2 and -β3, which also hold great promise in the area of wound healing.

D.J. Papadopoulos, M.D.

Scar Formation: The Spectral Nature of Fetal and Adult Wound Repair
Ferguson MWJ, Whitby DJ, Shah M, et al (Univ of Manchester, England; New York Univ)
Plast Reconstr Surg 97:854–860, 1996   1–5

Introduction.—Scarring can result in adverse cosmetic, functional, and growth outcomes. A primary goal of plastic surgery is to prevent scarring. There are certain fetal wounds that heal with little or no scarring, and this phenomenon has generated research into the underlying biological mechanisms of fetal wound repair. Results of these studies may have applications for the development of human fetal surgery and the experimental manipulation of adult wound healing to reduce scarring.

Fetal Wounds.—There are numerous histologic, cellular, and molecular differences between fetal and adult wound repair, including the sterile, fluid, warm fetal environment, and the kinetics of the deposition, turnover, and relative composition of wound extracellular matrix molecules. These and other factors must meet 2 criteria to be classified as major causative factors in scar formation: first, reducing levels of these factors should improve or prevent scar formation in adult wound repair, and second, increasing levels should induce or worsen scar formation in fetal wound repair. Most of the differences in healing have not been adequately investigated using these criteria.

Factors in Fetal Wound Scarring.—Studies have shown that gestational age is an important factor in fetal wound scarring in sheep, mice, and rats. It can be safely generalized that skin wounds in early gestation embryos generally heal without scarring, but last gestation fetuses are more likely to heal with adult-like scarring. Studies of wound healing responses should use both short-gestation and long-gestation animal models. Another important factor in scarring is the specific organ that is wounded. Most studies of fetal wound repair have involved the skin. Fetal bones heal more rapidly than adult bones; they heal with what are considered unhealable postnatal defects of 3 times bony width, including periosteum. Different organ systems in the fetus may have different periods of scar-free healing. There are also differences in fetal wound repair in animals, such as rabbits, mice, and sheep. Studies must take into account differences in underlying developmental biology, mode of placentation, and mechanism of molecule transfer from mother to fetus, e.g. via placenta or yolk sac. Researchers must also remember that most laboratory animals are from inbred strains that minimize variations from animal to animal. However, humans are outbred, and sheep, pigs, and opossums are more outbred than laboratory mice and rats. The extent of tissue damage also affects scarring; small wounds heal without scarring, but larger wounds scar. It is likely that different degrees of tissue damage at the same gestational age may heal with or without scarring in fetuses.

Discussion.—Some of what we know about fetal wound repair has been applied in experimental manipulation of adult wound repair. Alteration of the growth factor profile early in wound repair appears to be a major factor in controlling scar formation. It has been hypothesized that wound healing is phylogenetically maximized for rapid healing under dirty conditions to prevent life-threatening septicemia resulting in an extreme response in amount and type of growth factor at the wound site. This massive response floods out the endogenous regenerative potential of the dermis and results in scar formation. Adjusting the balance of the growth factor response early in wound repair results in normal healing, but with significantly reduced scarring. The outlook for therapeutic reduction of human scarring after trauma is very promising. Therapeutic reduction of scarring in adults is discussed in detail.

▶ It will be interesting to see how new technologies will incorporate our improved understanding about wound repair mechanisms into new therapies. As we select those factors that affect wound healing in a positive way, we will, with the help of recombinant technology, probably be in a position to intervene quickly and effectively to improve surgical scars. Based on the information that we currently have, it would be interesting to see what relative concentration of TGF-1, TGF-2 and TGF-3 and PDGF are in blacks who have keloids and those who do not. In doing so, we may be able to develop a predictive marker that will enable us to intervene before keloid formation.

D.J. Papadopoulos, M.D.

Imposition of a Physiologic DC Electric Field Alters the Migratory Response of Human Keratinocytes on Extracellular Matrix Molecules

Sheridan DM, Isseroff RR, Nuccitelli R (Univ of California, Davis)
J Invest Dermatol 106:642–646, 1996   1–6

Introduction.—The migratory response of keratinocytes is influenced by the composition of the underlying matrix. This migration is heightened by substrates of fibronectin and types I and IV collagens and is inhibited by laminin. The migratory patterns of several cell types are altered by direct current (DC) electrical fields as low as 10 mV/mm. The strength of the directed migratory response of motile cells in an electric field, or galvanotaxis, that produces the best in vitro response is nearly identical to that measured near wounds in guinea pig skin in vivo. The effect of the superimposition of a DC electrical field on keratinocytes migrating on extracellular matrix proteins ordinarily encountered in the healing wound was investigated.

Methods.—Cultured human keratinocytes derived from a single primary source of neonatal foreskin epidermis were plated on types I and IV collagen, fibronectin, laminin, and tissue culture plastic matrices. Time-lapse video microscopy was used to monitor the effect of an applied DC electrical field on directional migration over a 2-hour period (Fig 1). The cosine of the angle of migration in relation to anodal–cathodal orientation was calculated so that directionality could be quantitated.

Results.—Migration toward the negative poles was seen on all matrices; in controls (no applied field) migration was random. When the field strength was increased from 100 mV/mm (the physiologic level) to 400 mV/mm, directional response did not significantly increase. The degree of directionality and the average net cell translocation differed significantly according to the substrate being observed. Keratinocytes plated on types I and IV collagens showed the greatest cathodal migration in response to the DC electrical field. In contrast, this response was lowest on the laminin substrate. Cells on fibronectin had an intermediate response.

Conclusion.—Findings show that the imposition of DC electrical fields at strengths similar to those measured at wound edges in vivo result in directed migration of human keratinocytes. The intensity of the response varied and depended on the composition of the underlying substrate. These results may be meaningful for both short-term and long-term wound healing.

▶ This interesting study may have introduced a new variable that may be manipulated to allow for better wound healing. The potential applications are enormous, especially for burns and lower-extremity ulcers. Clearly, much work needs to be done before this sort of information can be applied clinically, but all of us eagerly await further developments.

D.J. Papadopoulos, M.D.

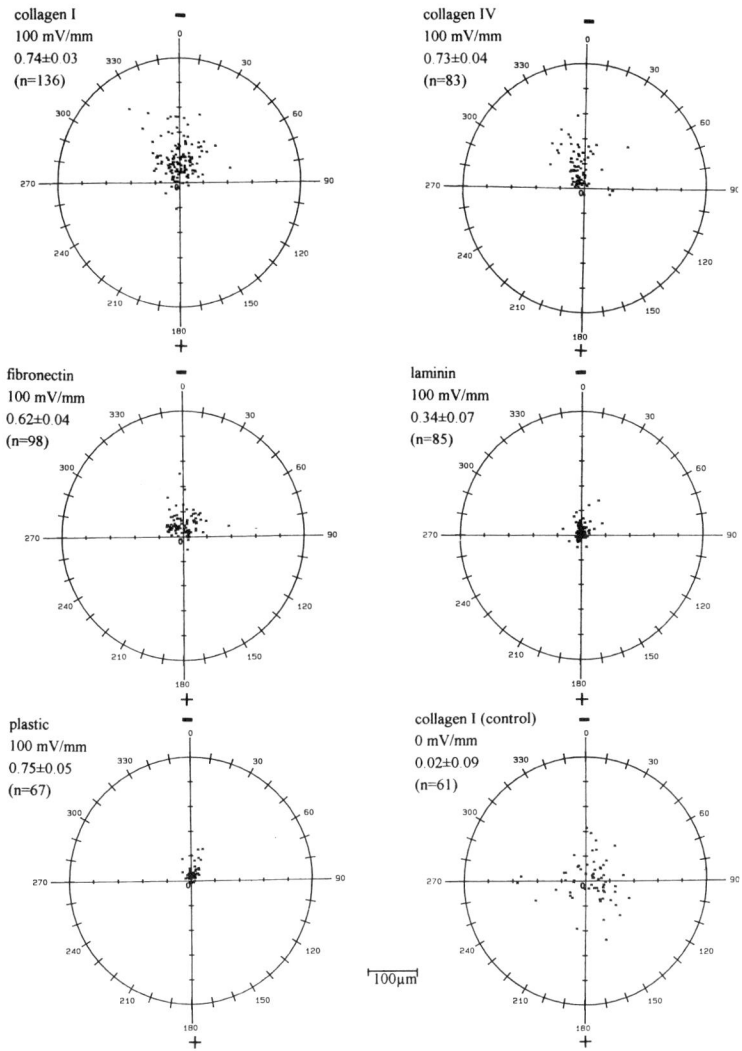

FIGURE 1.—Cellular translocation distribution of human keratinocytes on extracellular matrix substrate after imposition of a direct current electric field. Human keratinocytes were plated on different matrices. Directed migration in an applied electric field was quantified by calculating the average cosine of the angles of migration in relation to the anodal–cathodal orientation. Migration paths were recorded and traced from a video screen. The starting position of each cell is represented by the center of the circle, and the final position was plotted as a single point on the graph (0° indicates cathodal direction; 180° indicates anodal direction). The average cosine of the translocation ± SEM is indicated at the upper left corner of each plot. The *n* value is the number of cells. (Reprinted by permission of Elsevier Science Inc. from Sheridan DM, Isseroff RR, Nuccitelli R: Imposition of a physiologic DC electric field alters the migratory response of human keratinocytes on extracellular matrix molecules. *J Invest Dermatol* 106:642–646, copyright 1996 by the Society for Investigative Dermatology, Inc.)

The Effect of Hyperbaric Oxygen on Different Phases of Healing of Ischaemic Flap Wounds and Incisional Wounds in Skin

Quirinia A, Viidik A (Univ of Aarhus, Denmark)
Br J Plast Surg 48:583–589, 1995   1–7

Background.—Ischemia can impair wound healing and increase vulnerability to wound infection. Because oxygen is a necessary component in the synthesis and maturation of collagen, ischemic wounds have less scar tissue and a greater risk of wound rupture. The effect of treatment with hyperbaric oxygen (HBO) was studied in ischemic and normal-healing wounds.

Methods.—Eighty rats were divided into 8 groups of 10 animals. In each animal, ischemic H-shaped double flap wounds and normal incisional wounds were created. Except for the animals in group 2, the rats were given oxygen treatments in a monoplace chamber for 90 minutes daily for a varying number of days. After 10 or 20 days, the animals were killed and the wounds were removed and tested biomechanically. In addition, the length of surface necrosis was measured.

Results.—In the control group, the normal incisional wounds had significantly greater wound strength than the ischemic flap wounds. Treatment with HBO during the first 3 days resulted in 41% to 57% increases in all stress and strain parameters in the ischemic flap wounds, whereas the biomechanical improvements in wound healing were no longer apparent when HBO treatment was continued until day 9. Treatment given between days 4 and 9 resulted in decreased biomechanical wound strength. There was no effect of HBO treatment on normal incisional wound healing. No differences were found in the length of surface necrosis or wound shrinkage associated with the different treatment schedules.

Conclusions.—Treatment with HBO within the first few days of wound healing can significantly enhance the healing process in ischemic wounds without affecting the healing process in normal incisional wounds.

▶ The use of HBO in dermatologic surgery is extremely limited, as expected for a number of reasons. It must be used early and is not universally available. Treatment during the inflammatory phase appears to be optimal, allowing fibroblast proliferation. The authors note a once-a-day treatment to accomplish this, while noting that angiogenesis is stimulated during the relative hypoxic periods. Perhaps there are other roles for HBO in dermatologic surgery and skin cancer treatment.

H.T. Greenway, M.D.

Wound Closure and Materials

Moist Wound Healing With Occlusive Dressings: A Clinical Review
Kannon GA, Garrett AB (Med College of Virginia, Richmond)
Dermatol Surg 21:583–590, 1995   1–8

Introduction.—In recent decades, occlusive dressings have become the standard for wound care. The many different types of occlusive dressings available enhance wound healing mainly through the prevention of wound desiccation, which leads to quicker re-epithelialization. The various types of occlusive dressings, and the advantages and disadvantages of each, were reviewed.

Moist Wound Healing.—Occlusive dressings ensure moist wound healing and prevent eschar formation and stimulate growth factors, fibroblasts, and keratinocytes, as well as inflammatory and phagocytic activity. It was initially feared that occlusive dressings would lead to increased infection rates, but even when bacterial colonization occurs, wound infection rates are generally lower than with nonocclusive dressings. Occlusive dressings serve as barriers to microbes, as well as to fluid loss and trauma. These dressings are easy to apply, do not have to be changed often, and reduce wound pain.

Types of Occlusive Dressings.—All of the various types of occlusive dressings have advantages and disadvantages (Table 3). Hydrocolloid dressings have been well-studied and are widely used for chronic skin ulcers. They are not well-suited for wounds with heavy exudate that will bleed through the dressing. These wounds are better managed with highly absorbent hydrogels or foams, or with alginates. Alginates may also be used for full-thickness wounds or for postoperative wounds in need of hemostasis. Dry wounds are generally treated with hydrofilms, hydrocolloids, or hydrogels. Hydrogels are useful for dermabrasion, chemical peel, and other painful wounds because they sooth the patient. Films are widely used on IV sites and split-thickness donor sites. Occlusive dressings are not suitable for use on ischemic or clinically infected wounds. Some of these dressings, such as hydrocolloids and cellophane, are used to enhance delivery of topical steroids. Cost is a major disadvantage with the use of occlusive dressings; Biobrane, for example, is too expensive for use in routine dermatologic practice. However, given the reduced need for dressing changes, occlusive dressings can sometimes reduce the overall costs of treatment.

Summary.—Moist wound healing with occlusive dressings has some important advantages in clinical practice, mainly in the promotion of wound re-epithelialization. The various types of occlusive dressing materials are each suited to certain types of wounds.

▶ Occlusive dressings clearly promote wound healing and decrease pain in our patients. Table III lists a variety of "Examples," but I found the "Classification" group to be the most helpful in the organization of my thinking as

Type	Description	Examples	Advantages	Disadvantages
Foams	Either hydrophilic or hydrophobic. Nonocclusive. Usually polyurethane or gel film coated.	Acute or chronic partial thickness exudative wounds that require mechanical debriding	Cutinova Plus, Ulcer Care, Lyofoam, Synthaderm, Allevin, Epigard[3]	Debrides wound Absorbs exudate	Cost Opaque Requires additional dressing May become incorporated into the wound Cannot be used on dry wounds More frequent dressing changes needed
Calcium Alginate	Nonwoven composite of fibers from calcium alginate, a cellulose-like polysaccharide	Partial-thickness wounds with high exudate, choice for full-thickness wounds, Postoperative wounds for hemostasis, stasis ulcers	Sorbsan, Kaltostat[3]	Hemostatic Highly absorbent Good for full-thickness wounds Reduced frequency of dressing changes. Gel creates moist wound healing	Requires secondary dressing Cost Gel may have foul odor Not ideal for dry wounds as may become adherent
Biobrane	Silicone rubber w/nylon and porcine collagen bilaminate	Partial thickness wounds split-thickness graft donor sites, superficial burns	Biobrane[3]	Flexible for irregularly contoured wounds	Difficult to apply Cost May become incorporated into the wound Contains silicone Can impair wound healing in some cases May have higher infection rates

(Continued)

TABLE 2.—Concentrations of Ceftriaxone in Surgical Wound Tissue Measured at the End of Each Operation* and in Fluid From the Surgical Wound

Sample	Concentration		
	A	B	C
Wound tissue (µg/g)	1,282 ± 404	657 ± 320	255 ± 209
Range	830–1,850	355–1,130	95–620
Fluid from the wound† (µg/mL)	859 ± 345	431 ± 279	117 ± 45
Range	420–1,342	145–851	62–173

Data reported as mean ± standard deviation.
*Operation time period range: A = from 40 to 70 minutes; B = from 70 to 120 minutes; C = from 120 to 180 minutes. The fluid was collected and measured 24 hours postoperatively.
(Reprinted by permission of the publisher from Chalkiadakis GE, Gonnianakis C, Tsatsakis A, et al: Preincisional single-dose ceftriaxone for the prophylaxis of surgical wound infection. Am J Surg 170: 353–355, Copyright 1995 by Excerpta Medica Inc.)

and 24 hours after surgery; compared these values with previously reported pharmacokinetic data on IV and IM ceftriaxone injections in healthy volunteers; and assessed the efficacy of intraparietal administration.

Methods and Findings.—Twenty patients undergoing abdominal surgery were included in the study. Preincisional ceftriaxone injection resulted in high concentrations of antibiotic in the wound tissue and fluid. The highest levels in plasma were recorded at 1.5 hours. Plasma levels exceeded the minimal inhibitory levels of most aerobic gram–positive and gram–negative organisms for 24 hours. Exceptions were *Pseudomonas aeruginosa, Acinetobacter* species, and *Streptococcus faecalis*. None of the patients exhibited local or general complications (Tables 1 and 2).

Conclusions.—Preincisional ceftriaxone injection is beneficial in 2 ways. Very high levels of the antibiotic in the wound prevent sepsis, and good serum levels minimize systemic complications for 24 hours.

▶ The wound levels of drug determine the efficacy of antibiotic prophylaxis and these authors from Crete, Greece present a most intriguing way of obtaining appropriate tissue drug levels. This may offer a way to ensure the drug is present at the site of possible bacteria entry at the time of cutaneous surgery and could become as common as the IV usage by our colleagues during their procedures under sedation or general anesthesia. This intrigues me immensely and I hope to provide further results to our readers in the future.

H.T. Greenway, M.D.

Warmed Local Anesthetic Reduces Pain of Infiltration
Fialkov JA, McDougall EP (Univ of Toronto)
Ann Plast Surg 36:11–13, 1996   1–16

Introduction.—The perception of pain has been linked with the perception of temperature. Therefore, it was hypothesized that the pain of anesthetic infiltration could be affected by altering the temperature of the

TABLE 3 (cont.)

N-terface	Monofilament plastic	Immobilizing graft sites, Partial-thickness wounds	N-terface[3]	Transfers exudate to outer membrane Nonadherent to wound	Cost Requires secondary dressing May cause fluid accumulation
Cellophane	Cellulose with glycerine or glycerol plasticizer added.	Split-thickness donor graft sites. Delivery of topical steroids.	Saran Wrap	Readily available Transparent Inexpensive	Difficult to apply Excessive fluid collection under wound Poor tensile strength to dressing

*Exception is Cutinova gel.
†Exception is Omiderm.
(Reprinted by permission of the publisher from Kannon GA, Garrett AB: Moist wound healing with occlusive dressings: A clinical review. *Dermatol Surg* 21:583–590, Copyright 1995 by Elsevier Science Inc.)

I consider my options in different situations. Cost, of course, becomes a significant factor. One of my early uses years ago was for donor sites for split-thickness skin grafts to eliminate pain. Today, our greatest application is on the face after laser resurfacing procedures both for enhanced healing and to decrease pain.

H.T. Greenway, M.D.

Prevention of Hypertrophic Scars by Long-Term Paper Tape Application
Reiffel RS (White Plains Hosp, NY)
Plast Reconstr Surg 96:1715–1718, 1995   1–9

Introduction.—A number of different techniques have been tried to remove hypertrophic scars, with limited success. When a static deforming force is applied to the skin—as with indwelling sutures—the skin eventu-

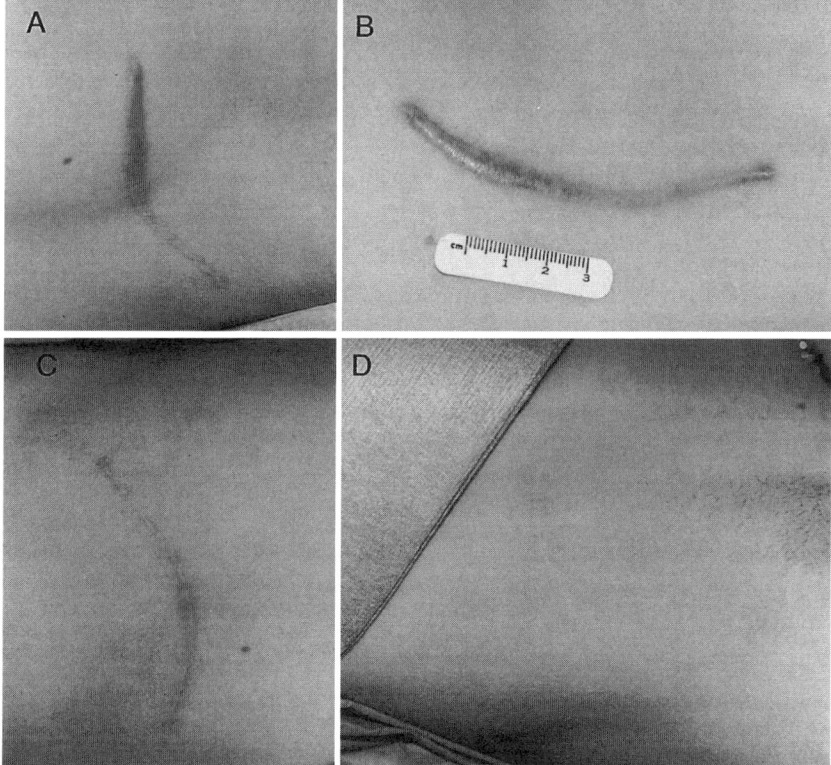

FIGURE 3.—(*Above*) A 25-year-old nurse underwent a rib resection for a thoracic outlet syndrome through a scar extending from her axilla onto her breast. The scar became hypertrophic and pruritic, especially the anterior portion on the breast, widening to 10 mm at 3½ months. (*Below, left*) The scar was revised and paper tape begun at the time of suture removal at 2 weeks. By 2½ months, the scar was soft, flat, and much paler, with no itching; the tape was discontinued. (*Below, right*) Her final examination, at 2½ years, revealed an almost imperceptible scar. (Courtesy of Reiffel RS: Prevention of hypertrophic scars by long-term paper tape application. *Plast Reconstr Surg* 96:1715–1718, 1995.)

ally stretches to eliminate that force. The scar does not start to widen until about 2 weeks after surgery. The use of paper tape to reduce the forces applied to skin wounds in the hope of a reduction in hypertrophic scarring is reviewed.

Experience.—At 2 weeks after surgery, paper tape was placed transversely across the wound in an attempt to control scar widening. Even with daily tape changes, however, this technique did not reduce widening. Further analysis suggested that the process of hypertrophy is stimulated by longitudinal stretching, parallel to the wound's long axis. Patients were instructed to apply paper tape longitudinally over the susceptible wound.

All ointments and skin oil were removed from the skin, and a liquid adhesive was applied, when necessary. A strip of 1-inch paper tape was applied to the normal skin beyond the wound, then pulled as it was laid down on the wound to compress it. The tape was changed every day by the patient for at least 2 months, until the wound became pale and soft. The technique was used on many different sites, including the neck, chest, joints, and breast, with very good results. It was also able to prevent recurrent hypertrophy in wounds that were surgically revised (Fig 3).

Conclusions.—Longitudinal paper taping that starts at 2 weeks after surgery can prevent hypertrophic scarring of skin wounds. This technique appears to relieve longitudinal stretching of wounds that cross relaxed skin tension lines. Even in patients with surgically revised scars, the technique produces a thin, soft, pale scar.

▶ The longitudinal application of tape to prevent hypertrophic scarring is intriguing. Other studies to lend support include those that compare silicone gel sheeting to non-silicone sheeting/tape. The "longitudinal" nature of the application prior to development of the hypertrophic scar, even in re-excisions, is creative and well supported by his photographs. Perhaps we should give this a try and see if we can achieve similar results!

H.T. Greenway, M.D.

The Use of Calcium Alginate Dressings in Deep Hand Burns
Kneafsey B, O'Shaughnessy M, Condon KC (Cork Regional Hosp, Ireland)
Burns 22:40–43, 1996   1–10

Introduction.—Deep burns of the hand present a common surgical challenge. There can be substantial bleeding with difficult hemostasis. Coverage of deep structures may be required. The use of calcium alginate, which has both hemostatic and gel-forming properties, was described in the management of full-thickness burns of the hand.

> *Case Report.*—Man, 29, had full-thickness burns of the dorsum of both hands. The burns were treated with escharotomies with topical silver sulphadiazine cream in polythene gloves and prophylactic antibiotics. Because he had a prosthetic heart valve, his

anticoagulant therapy was changed to heparin, then stopped on day 9, when the burns were excised under tourniquet to the level of the dorsal vessels on 1 hand and the extensor mechanism on the other. The wounds were covered with calcium alginate felt, then a light bulky dressing, and the tourniquet was released. Two days later, the dressings were removed and the alginate gel was washed away with saline. The granulating surface on the left hand was covered with thick sheet grafts taken from the thigh, which took fully within 4 days. A saline-moistened Kaltostat dressing was applied to the exposed extensor tendons of the right hand for 4 days, until granulation tissue had grown. Then sheet grafts were applied after the alginate gel was removed. The patient achieved satisfactory function with intensive physiotherapy. He returned to work 8 months after injury.

Discussion.—Calcium alginate is highly effective in the achievement of hemostasis after burn excision. The gel that results is nonstick, so its removal does not cause repeated bleeding. Typically, a good bed of granulation tissue is grown within 1 to 2 days. Because granulation is encouraged, tendon excision and flap cover may be avoided and a sheet graft may be accomplished early.

▶ Calcium alginate dressing is used much less frequently in dermatologic surgery than the other occlusive dressings discussed elsewhere in this issue. However, there may be occasions where exposed tissue may require granulation before a graft similar to the experiences here. The hemostatic properties are known to our dental colleagues and may be better than the oxidized cellulose we formerly preferred.

H.T. Greenway, M.D.

Keloids and Hypertrophic Scars

Evaluation of Cynthaskin and Topical Steroid in the Treatment of Hypertrophic Scars and Keloids
Yii NW, Frame JD (St Andrew's Hosp, Essex, England)
Eur J Plast Surg 19:162–165, 1996   1–11

Introduction.—Hypertrophic scars and keloids remain difficult to treat, despite advances in the understanding of wound healing and collagen metabolism. A new product under investigation, Cynthaskin TM, is available as lotion that dries to form an adherent and transparent film. In a prospective study, 41 patients were treated with cynthaskin and a topical steroid, triamcinolone acetonide.
Methods.—Cynthaskin TM has been used for more than a decade in Australia for the coverage of donor sites for autografts and partial-thickness burns. The product is a biosynthetic film incorporating GUM ACACIA B.P. and humectants into aqueous emulsions of acrylic polymers. A

TABLE 2.—Response to Cynthaskin-Triamcinolone Treatment in Group A
According to the Etiology of the Scars

Causes	Number of patients	Number of improved patients
Surgical incision	18	16
Burn	9	7
Skin graft donor site	2	2
Other trauma	3	2
Total	32	27

(Courtesy of Yii NW, Frame JD: Evaluation of cynthaskin and topical steroid in the treatment of hypertrophic scars and keloids. *Eur J Plast Surg* 19:162–165, Copyright 1996 by Springer-Verlag.)

topical agent was prepared that combined liquid cynthaskin and 0.1% triamcinolone acetonide. This preparation was applied twice daily in 32 patients with hypertrophic scars and 9 with keloids. Eighteen patients with hypertrophic scars and 4 with keloids had untreated scars and keloids for comparison with the treated areas. Outcome of treated areas was judged on color, elevation, texture, itching, and pain.

Results.—The mean duration of treatment was 4.3 months in the hypertrophic scar group and 3.2 months in the keloid group. Application of cynthaskin-triamcinolone led to improvement in 84.4% of patients with hypertrophic scars. Scars of various causes (Table 2) and at different sites (Table 3) responded to the lotion. Significantly fewer patients (44.4%) in the keloid group showed improvement, but all patients achieved relief of pain and itch.

Conclusions.—Treatment with cynthaskin and a topical steroid was effective in patients with hypertrophic scars but was less successful for those with keloids. No adverse effects, such as dermal atrophy or allergy, were noted. Advantages of cynthaskin include its ability to form a trans-

TABLE 3.—Response to Cynthaskin-Triamcinolone Treatment in Group A
According to the Sites of the Scars

Sites	Number of patients	Number of improved patients
Shoulder	4	1
Sternal area	4	3
Breasts	5	5
Face and neck	5	5
Abdomen	4	4
Back	2	1
Upper extremity	3	3
Lower extremity	5	5
Total	32	27

(Courtesy of Yii NW, Frame JD: Evaluation of cynthaskin and topical steroid in the treatment of hypertrophic scars and keloids. *Eur J Plast Surg* 19:162–165, Copyright 1996 by Springer-Verlag.)

parent film that conforms to the scar and surrounding skin. Makeup can be applied over the film, and it washes off easily for reapplication.

▶ The use of aqueous emulsions of acrylic polymers is progressing from wound dressings to the drug delivery era. The liquid form here with triamcinolone acetonide drying as transparent film signals its use as a carrier for drugs. Obviously, the treatment of hypertrophic scars and keloids is only an initial step for its use in many future disease processes. The Australians continue to offer innovative ideas in our specialty!

H.T. Greenway, M.D.

Adjunct Therapies to Surgical Management of Keloids
Berman B, Bieley HC (Univ of Miami, Fla)
Dermatol Surg 22:126–130, 1996   1–12

Background.—Keloids, an overgrowth of dense, fibrous tissue that occur after healing of a skin injury and extend beyond the border of the original traumatized area, tend to recur after surgical excision. In the present report, the authors' and others' experiences with adjunct therapies to surgical management of keloids, and the effects of these combined interventions on keloid recurrence rates, are reviewed.

Discussion.—Surgical excision of keloids, by itself, results in recurrence rates that reportedly range from 45% to 100%. More encouraging results have been obtained when using excisional surgery in combination with other treatments. For example, when intradermal corticosteroids are used together with surgical intervention, the recurrence rate falls to less than 50%, as reported in the majority of studies. External radiation after excision, often in combination with other treatments, has resulted in a less than 10% recurrence rate. In several studies with small numbers of patients, no recurrences of keloids were noted at 8 months to 4 years, when surgery together with button compression on earlobes (with buttons left in place for 3 weeks to 6 months) was used. Various lasers, including the carbon dioxide laser, the Neodymium-YAG laser, and the argon laser, also have been used in the treatment of keloids, with wide variations in reported recurrence rates. In general, laser treatment results in recurrence rates that are comparable to those noted with conventional surgery. When laser ablation is combined with other treatments, however, improvement in recurrence rates has been observed. Studies investigating cryosurgery as a means of treatment for keloids found that when used alone, 51% to 74% of patients were recurrence-free at mean follow-ups of 30 and 31 months. In a small series of patients treated with a combination of cryotherapy and intralesional corticosteroids, excellent results were reported with follow-up for up to 1.5 years. Injection of interferon (IFN)-α2b into the surgical excision site immediately after surgery represents another adjunct approach to surgical management. In a small series of patients, an 8% recurrence rate was noted after keloid excision with IFN-α2b injections.

Conclusions.—Surgical excision of keloids in combination with other treatment modalities results in lower recurrence rates than those reported for surgical excision alone. Although various therapeutic approaches are available, none have been shown to routinely prevent keloid recurrence. Several potential agents, including procollagen peptides, minoxidil, and pentoxifylline, are currently under investigation. The efficacy of these and other agents in preventing keloid recurrence remains to be determined in future in vitro studies.

▶ Preventing the reformation of a keloid is the key to augmenting its simple surgical removal. The authors review their and others' experiences at achieving this goal. During the years, my practice has embraced many of the "newer" approaches as they arrive on the scene, including lasers, "magical, perhaps they somehow inhibit collagen," and even post-removal interferon injected into the excision site. Postexcisional radiation continues to be the mainstay in our practice, achieving good results with low-dose ranges of 1,500–2,000 rad. Because of its association with acne therapy sequelae, many dermatologic surgeons fail to recognize its benefits in low doses for certain nonmalignant conditions and clearly, its use as adjunctive therapy in keloids appears beneficial.

H.T. Greenway, M.D.

Hemostasis

Surgical Pearl: Hemostasis in the Patient With Uremia
Lawrence N, Kurnik B (Arizona Health Sciences Ctr, Tucson)
J Am Acad Dermatol 33:806–807, 1995   1–13

Introduction.—Patients with uremia have an increased risk of surgical bleeding complications, typically caused by platelet defects. These bleeding complications can precipitate flap or graft failure and primary closure dehiscence. Problems with hemostasis and their management in these patients are discussed.

Causes.—Platelet dysfunction has been linked to elevated plasma concentrations of urea, guanidinosuccinic acid, parathyroid hormone, prostanoid metabolism products, and nitric oxide-endothelium relaxing factor. However, no single cause of platelet dysfunction has been identified. Hemostasis dysfunction can also be induced in uremic patients by drugs such as aspirin, β-lactam drugs, cephalosporins, diazepam, chlordiazepoxide, and diphenhydramine hydrochloride.

Diagnosis.—The Ivy bleeding time is the most reliable indicator of increased surgical bleeding. Three 1-cm incisions are made in the volar forearm. The length of bleeding time with a blood pressure cuff placed above the incisions is monitored.

Management.—Several interventions can normalize bleeding time (Table 1). Either peritoneal dialysis or hemodialysis can improve, but not

TABLE 1.—Approaches to the Treatment of Uremic Platelet Dysfunction

Modality	Dose	Onset	Duration	Mechanism	Comment
RBC transfusion	Transfuse to Hct ≥26%–30%	Immediate	Prolonged if Hct remains elevated	Rheological	Anemia is an overlooked contributory or predisposing factor to bleeding. Consider prophylactic transfusion before high-risk procedures
dDAVP	0.3 μg/kg IV over 15–30 min in 50 ml saline	<1 hr	4–8 hr	Release of stored FVIII–VWF from endothelium	Rapid, reliable effect with few side effects. Useful for acute bleeding or prophylaxis. Short duration and tachyphylaxis after 1–2 doses limits usefulness in prolonged bleeding episodes.
Cryoprecipitate	10 units IV every 12–24 hr	1–4 hr (peak effect 12–24 hr)	8–24 hr	Unknown—? by increasing FVIII–VWF	Delayed onset and longer duration suggest combined use with dDAVP for prolonged bleeding diathesis. Major risk is viral hepatitis.
Conjugated estrogen	Premarin, 0.6 mg/kg IV daily for 5 days	<6 hr with progressive shortening of bleeding time over 5–7 days	≥2 wk	Unknown	May also be effective orally. Could conceivably be used long term. Lesser acute potency decreases usefulness for severe, acute bleeding. Could be used in conjunction with dDAVP or cryoprecipitate.

Abbreviations: FVIII-VWF, Factor VIII-von Willebrand factor; *Hct,* hematocrit; *IV,* intravenous; *RBC,* red blood cells. (Courtesy of Wooley AC: Platelet dysfunction in uremia. *Kidney* 19:415–420, 1987. From Lawrence N, Kurnik B: Surgical pearl: Hemostasis in the patient with uremia. *J Am Acad Dermatol* 33:806–807, 1995.)

correct, platelet dysfunction in uremic patients. Intravenous l-deamino-8-D-arginine vasopressin (dDAVP) has a rapid and short duration of action, whereas conjugated estrogen and cryoprecipitate allow more prolonged normalization of bleeding time.

Conclusions.—Bleeding complications are common among uremic patients and may be related to multiple causal factors. Several management options exist to normalize bleeding times.

▶ Uremic patients can present special problems such as the achievement of hemostasis during removal of cutaneous neoplasms and defect reconstruction. Whereas the authors prefer conjugated estrogen for Mohs procedures, in our practice we have found dDAVP to be an adequate approach, although it requires intravenous administration. We have also found dDAVP to offer adequate coverage for our Mohs cases, including reconstruction, which differs from these authors. The list of drugs that adversely affect bleeding in the uremic patients and cause medicinal hemostatic dysfunction must also be reviewed in these patients.

H.T. Greenway, M.D.

Preparation and Anesthesia

Antibiotic Prophylaxis in Cutaneous Surgery

Rabb DC, Lesher JL Jr (Med College of Georgia, Augusta)

Dermatol Surg 21:550–554, 1995   1–14

Background.—Cutaneous surgery can be complicated by postoperative wound infections, endocarditis, and late contamination of prosthetic implants. The American Heart Association's guidelines on antibiotic prophylaxis were reviewed, and dermatologists were surveyed to determine how practitioners currently address this problem.

Methods.—Of 1,000 questionnaires mailed to members of the American Academy of Dermatology and of the American Society for Dermatologic Surgery, 451 responses were received. A total of 438 from 47 states and 6 foreign countries were evaluable.

Findings.—Practitioners most commonly used prophylaxis for manipulation of infected tissue (in any procedure) and in patients with a prosthetic heart valve. Two percent of the respondents never used antibiotics, and 7.3% always used them. Another 2.8% deferred the decision to the primary phsyician. More than half the respondents chose either a cephalosporin or erythromycin for prophylaxis.

Conclusions.—The risk of bacteremia is known for a wide range of medical and dental procedures (Table 1). Most dermatologists obtain pertinent medical histories and use appropriate prophylaxis when operating on infected tissue in patients with a high-risk cardiac lesion and when operating on patients with prosthetic heart valves. However, dermatologists also appear to use antibiotic prophylaxis when indications for use are unclear.

▶ This article presents a clear pattern of practice for dermatologists and dermatologic surgeons as they approach the problem of when and how to

---

TABLE 1.—Incidence of Bacteremia in Procedures and Daily Activities

Procedure or Activity	Incidence of Bacteremia
Tooth extraction	60–90%
Periodontal surgery	50–88%
Incision of abscess	38%
Tonsillectomy	28–38%
Cystoscopy	17%
Rigid bronchoscopy	15%
Endoscopy	4–8%
Cardiac catheterization	5%
Sigmoidoscopy	2–9%
Normal childbirth	0–5%
Tooth brushing	24–40%
Chewing food	17–24%

Adapted from Everett ED, Hinschmann JV: Transient bacteremia and endocarditis prophylaxis. A review. *Medicine,* 57:61–77, 1977. (Reprinted by permission of the publisher from Rabb DC, Lesher JL Jr: Antibiotic prophylaxis in cutaneous surgery. *Dermatol Surg* 21:550–554, Copyright 1995 by Elsevier Science.)

use prophylaxis. As with other specialists, many of us still tend to practice as we were trained, especially when guidelines are not totally clear. As stated, the American Heart Association guidelines may be of little value to dermatologic surgeons. However, we find it most useful to follow whatever guidelines and protocol the patient has received from their cardiologist. Most of our transplant and immuno-compromised patients also have protocols. In our everyday practice the main questionable area arises in orthopedic prostheses. The chairman of our orthopedic department at Scripps Clinic performs the majority of our hip prostheses, and he is most concerned during the first 2 years, which is when he believes an active inflammatory phase still exists. In reality we almost always provide antibiotic prophylaxis when indicated or when the question arises.

H.T. Greenway, M.D.

Preincisional Single-Dose Ceftriaxone for the Prophylaxis of Surgical Wound Infection
Chalkiadakis GE, Gonnianakis C, Tsatsakis A, et al (Univ of Crete, Greece; Apollonio Hosp, Heraklion, Crete, Greece)
Am J Surg 170:353–355, 1995   1–15

Background.—Preincisional intraparietal antibiotic injections are used to prevent infections after surgery. However, it is unclear whether topically injected antibiotics remain mostly in the surgical wound or are absorbed systemically. The current study determined the actual levels of antibiotic in serum, surgical wound edges, and fluid from the surgical wound during

TABLE 1.—Plasma Concentrations of Ceftriaxone During Operation and Postoperatively (During a 24-hour Period) in 20 Patients Undergoing Abdominal Surgery

Time* (h) After 2-g Preincisional Injection of Ceftriaxone Solution	Plasma Concentration (µg/mL)
0.5	82.50 ± 10.87
1.0	96.13 ± 22.54
1.5	99.47 ± 14.67
2.0	88.60 ± 21.72
3.0	84.93 ± 18.53
4.0	74.79 ± 18.11
5.0	68.27 ± 20.15
6.0	55.07 ± 17.56
12.0	32.15 ± 11.57
24.0	10.42 ± 4.12

Data reported as mean ± standard deviation.
*Sampling time deviation ± 0.05 hour.
(Reprinted by permission of the publisher from Chalkiadakis GE, Gonnianakis C, Tsatsakis A, et al: Preincisional single-dose ceftriaxone for the prophylaxis of surgical wound infection. *Am J Surg* 170:353–355, Copyright 1995 by Excerpta Medica Inc.)

local anesthetic solution. The hypothesis was tested by comparing the subjective experience of pain associated with room temperature and warmed local anesthetic, with each subject acting as his or her control, thus controlling for variability in pain perception.

Methods.—Twenty-six subjects received 1 injection of the room temperature (21°C) local anesthetic and 1 injection of the warmed (40°C) local anesthetic in 2 different sites. The injections had equal volumes and were injected at a standard rate through size-matched syringes. Both the subject and the injector were blinded to the anesthetic temperature. Each subject was asked to verbally rate the pain at each site between 0 and 10 and to evaluate the difference between the 2 injections as none, slight, or significant.

Results.—There was a mean difference of 1.5 in pain score between the 2 injections. Of the 25 subjects, 11 determined that the warmed solution was significantly less painful, 10 determined that the warmed solution was slightly less painful, 2 reported no difference, and 3 reported that the room temperature solution was slightly less painful.

Conclusions.—Warming local anesthetic to 40°C before subcutaneous injection reduces the pain of infiltration. It is an inexpensive, simple, and safe method that can be implemented easily in the office or emergency room setting.

▶ Achieving painless local anesthesia is a technique we strive for daily in our practices. In my practice, which is mainly referral, it continues to amaze me that many, many patients have a fear or dread the scheduled procedure solely based on their previous experiences with local anesthesia. Advances, including the addition of bicarbonate solution, topical EMLA cream, and in the report, warming (we actually do warm our local anesthetic), contribute to a more pleasant and tolerable experience. But we have found it is the actual "technique" that we use (including *time*) that distinguishes our staff and our local anesthesia from our colleagues. Patients do compare, and they do remember!

H.T. Greenway, M.D.

Physical Enhancement of Dermatologic Drug Delivery: Iontophoresis and Phonophoresis

Kassan DG, Lynch AM, Stiller MJ (Harvard Med School, Boston)
J Am Acad Dermatol 34:657–666, 1996   1–17

Introduction.—Passive diffusion alone produces poor absorption through the skin. The percutaneous absorption of drugs has been shown to increase with the use of iontophoresis (electric current) or phonophoresis (ultrasound). These modalities and their enhancement of percutaneous absorption are discussed.

Iontophoresis.—An electromotive force, typically between 0.5 and 20 mA, is applied to enhance absorption of drugs and chemicals across

TABLE 1.—Iontophoresis of Lidocaine

Procedure	Current	Result	Study design
Pulsed dye laser treatment of port–wine stains[25]	20–30 mA/min	10 of 11 patients satisfied	11 patients, double-blind, placebo–controlled
Needle prick[24]	0–4 mA × 7 min	Increased duration of anesthesia	27 patients, double–blind, placebo–controlled
Shave biopsy on nose[21]	3mA	Efficacious	Case report
Various dermatologic procedures[20]	2–4 mA × 5–12 min	80% to 100% efficacy for epidermal procedures	94 procedures in 64 patients
Dialysis needle insertion[23]	3 mA × 10 min	Iontophoresis preferred over injection	13 patients, served as own controls
Cauterization of spider veins[22]	3 mA × 7 min	16 of 16 patients satisfied	16 subjects, unblinded

(Courtesy of Kassan DG, Lynch AM, Stiller MJ: Physical enhancement of dermatologic drug delivery: Iontophoresis and phonophoresis. *J Am Acad Dermatol* 34:657–666, 1996.)

tissues. The mechanisms involved are not clear. However, it has been proposed that the electric potential induces pore formation in the stratum corneum by causing a reorientation of α-helical keratin polypeptide molecules into a parallel arrangement and by forming hair follicles and sweat gland ducts into diffusion shunts. Absorption is most enhanced with ionic compounds and least enhanced with lipophilic substances. Iontophoresis can deliver drugs beyond the cutis and subcutis, to tendon, cartilage, and the systemic circulation. It has been clinically useful in the management of cutaneous anesthesia (Table 1), hyperhidrosis, and herpes simplex and aphthous stomatitis and in the absorption of antibiotics through both injured and uninjured tissue.

Phonophoresis.—The drug to be delivered is used as the coupling agent (instead of gel or water) during the application of ultrasound. The enhanced absorption may be induced by thermal, chemical, and/or mechanical alterations in the ultrasound-treated tissues. This modality has enhanced the penetration of local anesthetics (Table 2), fluocinolone acetonide gel, and amphotericin B and the treatment of suppurative wounds and keloids.

Conclusions.—Iontophoresis and phonophoresis are promising modalities in enhancing the delivery of dermatologic and nondermatologic drugs.

TABLE 2.—Phonophoresis of Topical Anesthetics

Anesthetic	Frequency (kHz)	Energy (W/cm^2)	Duration of treatment (min)	Test method	Effect on drug delivery
4% Lidocaine in oil[67]	Not documented	2	5	Homogenize tissue and optical density measurement	Increased
25% Lignocaine cream[66]	870	2	5	Needle prick	Insignificant
Aqueous lidocaine[68]	48	0.17	5	Reaction to voltage	Increased

(Courtesy of Kassan DG, Lynch AM, Stiller MJ: Physical enhancement of dermatologic drug delivery: Iontophoresis and phonophoresis. *J Am Acad Dermatol* 34:657–666, 1996.)

Determining the optimal techniques and conditions for safe and effective use requires further study.

▶ Both electromotive forces (iontophoresis) and ultrasound (phonopheresis) offer significant potential to dermatologic surgeons especially in the arena of local anesthesia. Although much work needs to be done, the current use of topical anesthesia before local infiltration demonstrates the need for such advances. Although the time required for effect may be increased beyond current infiltration (see Tables 1 and 2), the ease and comfort for the patient warrant further refinements.

H.T. Greenway, M.D.

Efficacy of the Topical Anesthetic Cream, EMLA, in Alleviating Both Needle Insertion and Injection Pain
Raveh T, Weinberg A, Sibirsky O, et al (Hadassah Univ, Jerusalem)
Ann Plast Surg 35:576–579, 1995   1–18

Introduction.—The topical cream known as EMLA is a eutectic mixture of local anesthetics, including lignocaine base and prilocaine base. It can provide effective topical analgesia for many different types of procedures, from superficial skin procedures to harvesting of split-thickness skin grafts. Its use in reducing the pain associated with percutaneous infiltration of local anesthetic before surgical skin biopsy was studied.

Methods.—The randomized, double-blind, placebo-controlled study included 162 excisional biopsies in 54 consecutive patients. Each patient had 3 skin lesions requiring surgery; 1 lesion each was treated with EMLA cream and an occlusive dressing, petroleum jelly (Vaseline) with an occlusive dressing, or just an occlusive dressing. The ointments and dressings were left on for 1 hour. Pain was rated on a verbal scale.

Results.—The application of EMLA cream was associated with significantly reduced pain of needle insertion and of infiltration with lignocaine. However, petroleum jelly also produced significant pain reduction. Little difference in pain relief occurred with 1 versus 4 hours of topical anesthesia, and lesions on the face were no more painful than lesions in other areas.

Conclusions.—Topical application of EMLA cream can help reduce the pain associated with needle insertion and local anesthetic infiltration in patients undergoing surgical skin biopsy. However, a placebo effect is apparent in that Vaseline reduces pain significantly as well.

▶ This brief article studies the effect of EMLA to reduce the pain of injection. The authors found a diminishment in pain with EMLA but also found significant alleviation of pain with placebo. This points out the importance of patient rapport, relaxation, and placebo.

D.C. Whitaker, M.D.

Use of EMLA Cream in the Treatment of Post-Herpetic Neuralgia

Litman SJ, Vitkun SA, Poppers PJ (State Univ of New York, Stony Brook)
J Clin Anesth 8:54–57, 1996   1–19

Introduction.—The eutectic mixture of local anesthetics (EMLA cream), which contains lidocaine and prilocaine, has been shown to produce effective pain relief in patients undergoing venous or arterial cannulation and various dermatologic procedures, including skin grafting. The use of EMLA cream for an extended period in the treatment of postherpetic neuralgia is reported.

Case Report.—Woman, 73, had experienced postherpetic neuralgia affecting the left T_4 to T_6 dermatomes for 14 months. Her pain had been treated with a great variety of medications as well as both noninvasive and surgical treatments. Treatment with a continuous thoracic epidural block was considered, but was contraindicated by the patient's scoliosis, history of chronic obstructive pulmonary disease and myocardial infarction, and poor response to previous treatment with a single-dose epidural anesthetic. Therefore, treatment with topical EMLA cream was chosen. The EMLA cream was applied in a layer that was 1.5–2 mm thick (total dose, 50 g), then covered with a bio-occlusive dressing for 24 hours. After discharge, the patient was instructed to apply the EMLA cream in a dose of 30 g every 24 hours, covered by a bio-occlusive dressing. Pain scores and methemoglobin and lidocaine levels were determined regularly for 36 hours and at 3 days and 2 weeks after discharge. At 3 days, the patient reported that the pain returned 6–8 hours after EMLA application. Therefore, she was instructed to apply 15 g every 12 hours and remove the bio-occlusive dressing after 4 hours. The patient's pain score was reduced from 10 to 3 by 1 week after discharge and was reduced the next week so that there was no pain on palpation. The dosage was decreased to 15 g every 24 hours, which was maintained until 4 weeks. Lidocaine levels were never greater than 1 μg/mL, and the methemoglobin levels were never greater than 0.8 gm%.

Discussion.—High-dose, long-term treatment with EMLA cream is effective in breaking the pain cycle at the level of the cutaneous nerve endings and thereby controlling the pain of postherpetic neuralgia. Repeated applications during the day appear to be more effective than a single daily dose. The treatment did not produce a toxic plasma concentration of the anesthetic drugs. Therefore, EMLA cream is recommended as a simple, safe, noninvasive, cost-effective therapy for postherpetic neuralgia.

▶ As the authors discuss, postherpetic neuralgia may contain several components, with EMLA acting only at the level of the cutaneous nerve endings where it may break the pain cycle. Fifty grams under occlusion provided relief during weeks of therapy. Side effects of both lidocaine and prilocaine (methemoglobinemia) were not observed. Caution was urged in patients taking antiarrhythmic and sulfonamide medications. A number of our patients with postherpetic neuralgia may benefit from this regimen, either under our care or coordinated with anesthesia or pain clinics.

H.T. Greenway, M.D.

Lateral Cutaneous Nerve of the Thigh Blockade as Primary Anaesthesia for Harvesting Skin Grafts

Wardrop PJC, Nishikawa H (St Luke's Hosp, Bradford, England)
Br J Plast Surg 48:597–600, 1995   1–20

Objective.—The thigh is a good site for the harvest of skin grafts, but it can be difficult to provide local anesthesia for such a large area. Orthopedic surgeons commonly perform regional blockade of the lateral cutaneous nerve of the thigh (LCNT) for postoperative analgesia. This block was studied for use in anesthesia in patients who underwent a harvest of split skin grafts from the thigh.

Technique.—The investigators used a standard technique to obtain blockade of the LCNT with 10 mL of 0.5% bupivacaine. The injection was made 1 cm medial to the anterior superior iliac spine, where the LCNT passes beneath the inguinal ligament (Fig 1). Thirty minutes later, the anesthetized area was marked; the distribution tended to be more distal and medial than suggested in anatomic textbooks. Anesthesia of the middle third of the lateral thigh was almost always obtained, however. If a pinprick test revealed inadequate anesthesia, an injection of 10 mL of 1% lignocaine and adrenaline was given, followed if necessary by direct local infiltration of 1% lignocaine and adrenaline 1:200,000.

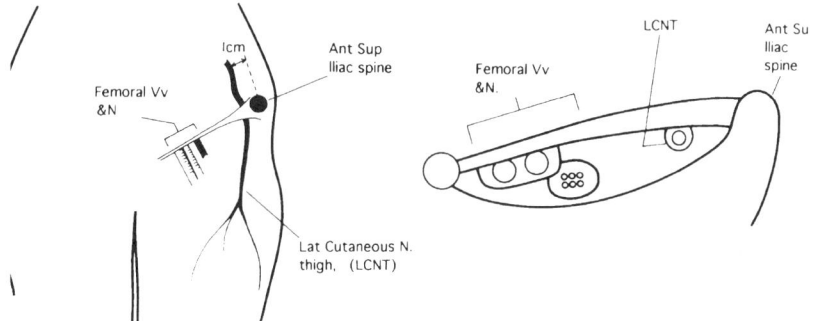

FIGURE 1.—The lateral cutaneous nerve of the thigh is 1 cm medially along the inguinal ligament from the anterior superior iliac spine. (Courtesy of Wardrop PJC, Nishikawa H: Lateral cutaneous nerve of the thigh blockade as primary anaesthesia for harvesting skin grafts. *Br J Plast Surg* 48:597–600, 1995.)

Experience.—The investigators performed LCNT block in 23 patients, mean age 69 years, who underwent a split skin graft. The anesthetic took full effect within 15 to 20 minutes; anesthesia covered a mean area of 569 cm². The block was successful in 17 patients, defined as no pain during graft harvest. The anesthesia failed in 6 patients, mostly early in the experience. The block lasted a mean of 10 hours.

Conclusions.—The LCNT block technique described provides safe and simple anesthesia for harvest of split skin graft from the thigh. Failures can occur, but the technique becomes highly reliable with experience. The LCNT block provides good postoperative analgesia as well as anesthesia, and can even be repeated in the postoperative period, if needed.

▶ Most of our cases are performed under local anesthesia because patients prefer the avoidance of pain. They clearly remember the pleasant and unpleasant aspects of the local anesthetic. This nerve block clearly benefits both patient and physician. As stated, there is a "learning curve," in part related to the understanding of the anatomy. I like topicals such as EMLA (lidocaine 2.5% and prilocaine 2.5%) but nerve blocks are both fun to perform and beneficial to the patient such as in this case with the harvest of split-thickness skin grafts.

H.T. Greenway, M.D.

Sublingual Triazolam Versus Peroral Diazepam as a Premedication for General Anaesthesia

Penttilä HJ, Nuutinen LS, Kiviluoma KT, et al (Oulu Univ, Finland)
Can J Anaesth 42:862–868, 1995   1–21

Background.—Premedication is often given to patients who undergo surgery to reduce anxiety and/or produce sedation. Triazolam is commonly used for night sedation, but its use for day-case surgery is controversial. However, a new form of sublingual triazolam, with a shorter time to peak plasma concentration and elimination half-life than diazepam, has become available. The effects of sublingual triazolam were compared with those of peroral diazepam in patients who underwent surgery with general anesthesia in a double-blind, randomized trial.

Methods.—Eighty-one patients who underwent elective surgery with general anesthesia were randomly assigned to receive either peroral diazepam 10 mg with a sublingual placebo or sublingual triazolam 0.2 mg with a peroral placebo. Blood pressure and heart rate were monitored before and after the operation. Anxiety and sedation were rated objectively and subjectively every 15 minutes before and 30 and 60 minutes after the operation. The patients were also asked to rate their satisfaction with the premedication.

Results.—Both groups demonstrated similar decreases in blood pressure and heart rate after premedication. There were no significant differences between the groups in either objective or subjective ratings of sedation or anxiolysis. Only the triazolam group had statistically significant anxiolysis and sedation before the induction of anesthesia. Fewer patients in the triazolam group required postoperative oxicodon or diclofenac. Patients in the triazolam group were more likely to be satisfied with the effects of the premedication than patients in the diazepam group.

Conclusions.—Sublingual triazolam is as safe and potent as peroral diazepam as a premedicant for general anesthesia and brings greater patient satisfaction. This agent is especially useful for patients who cannot swallow.

▶ Both diazepam and triazolam have been used for anxiety and sedation. These anesthesiologists prefer triazolam 0.20-mg sublingual to diazepam 10-mg oral as a sedative and anxiolytic. Interestingly, the patients were more satisfied. We have used sublingual diazepam and I suspect we will see an increase in this route of therapy and with this new form of triazolam.

H.T. Greenway, M.D.

The Efficacy of a Topical Lidocaine/Prilocaine Anesthetic Gel in 35% Trichloroacetic Acid Peels

Rubin MG (Univ of California, San Diego)
Dermatol Surg 21:223–225, 1995   1–22

Background.—There are several forms of topical anesthesia used in treating superficial skin lesions, but all have various shortcomings. These include ineffectiveness on intact skin and inability to be used on larger areas of skin. EMLA cream is the only anesthetic of this type that gives acceptable anesthesia on large areas of intact skin, but to occlude the entire face is difficult. A similar product is self-occluding because it contains methylcellulose. There are concerns about possible toxicity from absorption of the topical lidocaine and prilocaine. The effectiveness of this topical cream in 35% trichloroacetic acid peels was evaluated.

Methods.—A topical anesthetic gel containing lidocaine 2.5% and prilocaine 3.5% was used in 10 patients who had previously undergone a papillary dermal 35% trichloroacetic acid peel. Patients rated the level of burning compared to their first peel, which had been performed without anesthetic.

Results.—Of the 10 patients, 5 reported 40% less discomfort, and 3 reported 70% less discomfort. Two patients reported no aesthetic effect. In all 10 patients, the anesthetic gel enhanced the depth of the peel. All patients experienced rebound stinging and burning 30 to 60 minutes after the peels.

Conclusions.—This anesthetic gel can increase the depth of trichloroacetic acid peels; this may be caused by the vasoconstrictive effect of the anesthetic. Because there is greater risk of complications with a deeper peel, use of this anesthetic gel should be avoided when using trichloroace-tic in concentrations above 25% for any type of dermal peel.

▶ Mark Rubin is one of the most thoughtful and eloquent presenters of information about medium-depth peeling that I have had the pleasure of knowing. This article is important because it presents information that is readily applicable to our patients and that must be heeded by those per-forming medium-depth chemical peels, whether they are using EMLA or the "green gel." The temporary vasoconstriction described in this article as a possible explanation for the enhanced effect of the peel must be heeded carefully and could, theoretically, make it more difficult to treat vascular lesions with vascular lesion lasers as a result of the use of this topical anesthetic.

D.J. Papadopoulos, M.D.

Lidocaine and Epinephrine Levels in Tumescent Technique Liposuction
Burk RW III, Guzman-Stein G, Vasconez LO (Univ of Alabama, Birmingham)
Plast Reconstr Surg 97:1379–1384, 1996   1–23

Background.—Blood and fluid losses have traditionally limited the use of liposuction. The tumescent technique of liposuction is associated with reduced blood loss, enabling the aspiration of larger volumes of fat. However, concerns have been raised about the safety of the lidocaine doses needed for this technique, particularly in patients undergoing concurrent esthetic procedures requiring additional lidocaine and epinephrine infil-tration. The safety of the technique was explored in both patients under-going tumescent technique alone and those undergoing both tumescent technique and esthetic procedures.

Methods.—Ten patients who underwent tumescent technique liposuc-tion alone and 10 patients who underwent tumescent liposuction with concurrent esthetic surgery (Table 1) were studied. All patients received infiltration of 1,000 mL normal saline with 250 mg lidocaine and 1 mg epinephrine for the tumescent technique liposuction. The concurrent facial and breast surgery required an additional infiltration of 0.5% lidocaine

TABLE 1.—Other Surgical Procedures Performed Concurrent With
Tumescent Liposuction

Blepharoplasty	4
Endoscopic brow lift	4
Rhytidectomy	4
Abdominoplasty	4
Breast reduction	3
Mastopexy	1
Nasoplasty	1

(Courtesy of Burk RW III, Guzman-Stein G, Vasconez LO: Lidocaine and epinephrine levels in tumescent technique liposuction. *Plast Reconstr Surg* 97:1379–1384, 1996.)

TABLE 2.—Volumes of Tumescent Solution Infiltrated, Decanted Fat Aspirated, and Solution Aspirated in Liposuction Population

Average amount of tumescent solution	4796 cc
Range	2000–10,000 cc
Average amount of fat aspirated	3405 cc
Range	650–7500 cc
Average amount of solution aspirated	1393 cc
Range	820–2400 cc

(Courtesy of Burk RW III, Guzman-Stein G, Vasconez LO: Lidocaine and epinephrine levels in tumescent technique liposuction. *Plast Reconstr Surg* 97:1379–1384, 1996.)

with 1:200,000 epinephrine. Serum levels of lidocaine and epinephrine were determined at 3, 12, and 23 hours after infiltration, at which time the patients were questioned about the symptoms of lidocaine and epinephrine toxicity.

Results.—The patients undergoing liposuction alone received a mean dose of 21.6 mg of lidocaine per kilogram (range, 9.8–30.3 mg of lidocaine per kilogram) and of epinephrine of 5.24 mg (range, 4.1–10.0 mg). The patients undergoing concurrent procedures received a mean dose of 22.9 mg of lidocaine per kilogram (range, 11.2–38.3 mg of lidocaine per kilogram) and of epinephrine of 4.96 mg (range, 2.2–7.0 mg). The lidocaine aspirated with the fat varied in volume from 35 to 103 µg/mL (Table 2). The serum lidocaine levels were below 3 µg/mL, the level associated with toxicity, in all patients in both groups and generally peaked at 12 hours in patients undergoing the tumescent technique alone (Fig 1) and at 23 hours in patients undergoing concurrent procedures (Fig 2). The serum epinephrine levels typically peaked at 3 hours at 3–5 times greater than normal levels, normalizing by 12 hours.

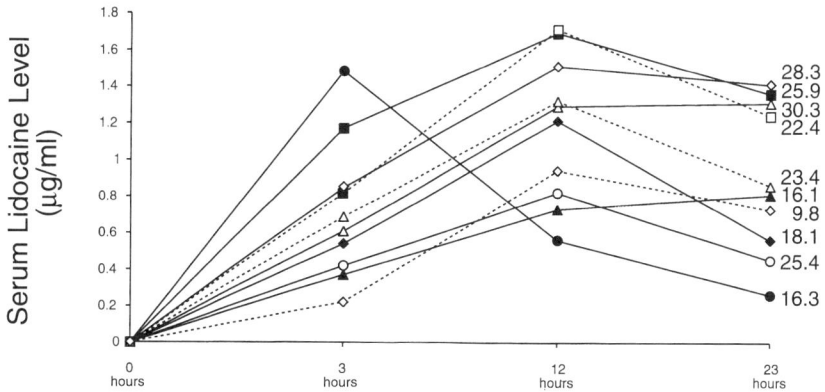

FIGURE 1.—Serum lidocaine levels in patients undergoing tumescent liposuction alone. The total dose of lidocaine (mg/kg) is listed to the right of figures. Patients with the peak lidocaine level at 3 hours receive 50 mg lidocaine IV. (Courtesy of Burk RW III, Guzman-Stein G, Vasconez LO: Lidocaine and epinephrine levels in tumescent technique liposuction. *Plast Reconstr Surg* 97:1379–1384, 1996.)

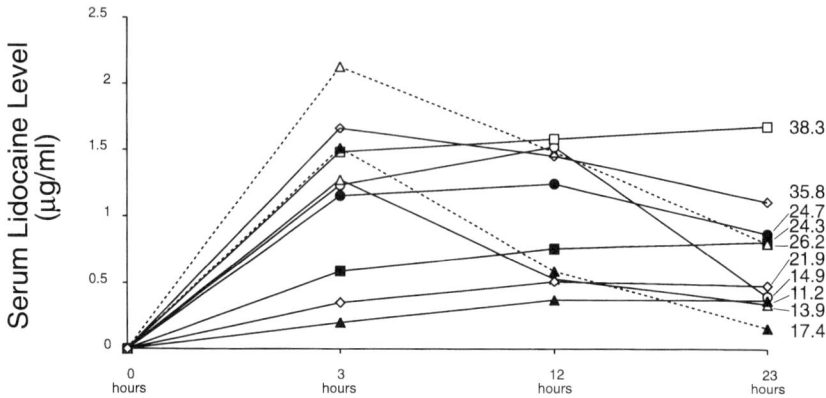

FIGURE 2.—Serum lidocaine levels in patients undergoing tumescent liposuction combined with other esthetic surgery. The total dose of lidocaine (mg/kg) is listed to the right of figures. (Courtesy of Burk RW III, Guzman-Stein G, Vasconez LO: Lidocaine and epinephrine levels in tumescent technique liposuction. *Plast Reconstr Surg* 97:1379–1384, 1996.)

Conclusions.—The tumescent technique for liposuction is safe with a dose of up to 28 mg of lidocaine per kilogram and a dose of up to 10 mg epinephrine. The technique also can be safely combined with esthetic surgery requiring additional infusions of lidocaine and epinephrine.

▶ The authors confirm the previous findings of dermatologic surgeon Jeff Klein, M.D., and others demonstrating the safety of the tumescent technique. By then sharing their findings of concurrent procedures (see Table 1), they encourage us to build on our skills and procedures. Although their mean dose of lidocaine was well below levels used safely in tumescent liposuction, even they feel safe using up to 28 mg of lidocaine per kilogram with up to 10 mg of epinephrine. We appreciate our colleagues' confirmation and support!

H.T. Greenway, M.D.

Lasers

RESURFACING, HAIR TRANSPLANTATION, AND BLEPHAROPLASTY

Laser Skin Resurfacing: Pre- and Posttreatment Guidelines
Lowe NJ, Lask G, Griffin ME (Univ of California, Los Angeles; Skin Research Found of California, Santa Monica)
Dermatol Surg 21:1017–1019, 1995   1–24

Objective.—Experience gained in the management of 30 patients with photodamaged skin changes yielded guidelines for pre- and posttreatment regimens. When the Ultrapulse carbon dioxide laser is used for skin resurfacing, complications can be avoided and optimal results obtained if a course of topical and orally given therapy is followed before and after the procedure.

TABLE 1.—Pretreatment Regimen

–Daily A.M. broad spectrum sunscreen
–Daily A.M. topical hydroquinone (eg, 2% hydroquinone cream,
   10% glycolic acid gel, or 4% hydroquinone liquid or cream)
–Nightly tretinoin 0.025% or 0.05% cream
–Wash with soap-free wash (Aquanil or Cetaphil)
Keflex 250 mg, PO BID, 1 day before treatment
–Zovirax 400 mg, PO BID, 1 day before treatment

Abbbreviations: PO, by mouth; *BID,* twice a day.
(Reprinted by permission of the publisher from Lowe NJ, Lask G, Griffin ME: Laser skin resurfacing: Pre- and posttreatment guidelines. *Dermatol Surg* 21:1017–1019, copyright 1995 by Elsevier Science Inc.)

Methods.—The patients, 28 women and 2 men, had photodamaged skin ranging from Glogau classification II to IV. All underwent a pretreatment regimen for at least 4 weeks before laser resurfacing (Table 1). Initial laser passes of 450–500 mJ/cm^2 were performed with a 2– and 7–W fluence using a 3–mm collimated handpiece. At each pass the ablated tissue was removed by firm wiping with normal saline–soaked gauze. Later passes were based on the severity of photodamage and ranged between 350 and 500 mJ and 2 and 5 W. The posttreatment regimen consisted of orally given and topical therapy and a washing routine starting at week 2 (Table 2).

Results.—In 22 patients treated with the original topical regimen a painful vesicular eruption developed, and the use of Polysporin and Desowen ointment was then discontinued. Posttreatment regimens subsequently included orally given therapy with Keflex and Zovirax, Crisco,

---

TABLE 2.—Posttreatment Regimen

Days 1–3	-Keflex 250 mg, PO BID
	-Zovirax 400 mg, PO BID
	-Crisco applied daily under Vigilon dressing
Days 4–7	-Keflex 250 mg, PO BID
	-Zovirax 400 mg, PO BID
	-Acetic acid soaks BID (5 cc of 5% glacial or distilled white acetic acid in 150 cc water)
	-Crisco applied six times a day
	-Pramasone 1% HC ointment to pruritic areas
Weeks 2–4	-Wash with soap-free wash (Aquanil or Cetaphil)
	-Titanium dioxide containing sunscreen daily (eg, Neutrogena SPF 17)
Week 4	-Broad spectrum sunscreen applied daily
	-Tretinoin cream 0.025% or 0.05% applied nightly
	-Topical hydroquinone applied daily (eg, 2% hydroquinone 10% glycolic acid gel daily if pigmentation occurred)
	-Wash daily with soap-free wash (Aquanil or Cetaphil)

Abbreviations: PO, by mouth; *BID,* twice a day.
(Reprinted by permission of the publisher from Lowe NJ, Lask G, Griffin ME: Laser skin resurfacing: Pre- and posttreatment guidelines. *Dermatol Surg* 21:1017–1019, copyright 1995 by Elsevier Science Inc.)

and dilute acetic acid soaks. Pramasone lotion was applied to pruritic lesions. A diffuse erythema appeared in all patients after the first week. The eruptions occurring in many patients appeared to represent a primary irritant reaction in the laser-treated skin. Hyperpigmentation, a delayed complication, may be treated with alternating tretinoin and hydroquinone preparations.

Discussion.—Improvement of photodamaged skin changes was judged good to excellent in 80% of patients. Supervised pre- and posttreatment regimens help to achieve optimum results from laser skin resurfacing for photodamaged skin. Topical retinoids and skin-lightening agents are recommended during the 4 weeks before therapy. Oral anti–herpes simplex agents and broad-spectrum antibiotics are continued for 7 days after the laser treatment.

▶ Most of our problems with facial laser resurfacing have not been scarring from overzealous treatments but rather events occurring that can, for the most part, be prevented. We owe a debt of gratitude to Dr. Lowe and his colleagues for helping us organize our approach into stepwise thinking during the pre- and posttreatment periods so as to both prevent problems and improve on the normal postoperative period. Preoperatively, proper nutrition and—in some cases—vitamin and antioxidant supplementation also may play a role. Postoperatively, I tend to vacillate between biosynthetic dressings (and between clear and opaque) and topical petrolatum but have not found it necessary to use both over the same given area. I also would tend to classify the postoperative "diffuse erythema" as an expected postoperative sequelae as opposed to a complication, although appropriate preoperative education is necessary. The delayed hyperpigmentation also could be expected and prevented or decreased with this type of protocol.

H.T. Greenway, M.D.

Skin Resurfacing With the Ultrapulse Carbon Dioxide Laser: Observations on 100 Patients
Lowe NJ, Lask G, Griffin ME, et al (Univ of California, Los Angeles; Skin Research Found of California, Santa Monica; Cranley Clinic for Dermatology, London)
Dermatol Surg 21:1025–1029, 1995   1–25

Background.—Patients with photodamaged skin can be effectively treated with the Ultrapulse carbon dioxide (CO_2) laser. Improvement of rhytides, precancerous and benign skin lesions, and superficial benign pigmented lesions has been noted with use of this therapeutic modality. The authors' experience with the Ultrapulse CO_2 laser in treating a group of patients with different severity of photodamaged skin is described.

Patients and Methods.—One hundred patients with skin that was moderately or severely photodamaged were included in a study designed to evaluate the efficacy and toxicity of treatment with the Ultrapulse CO_2

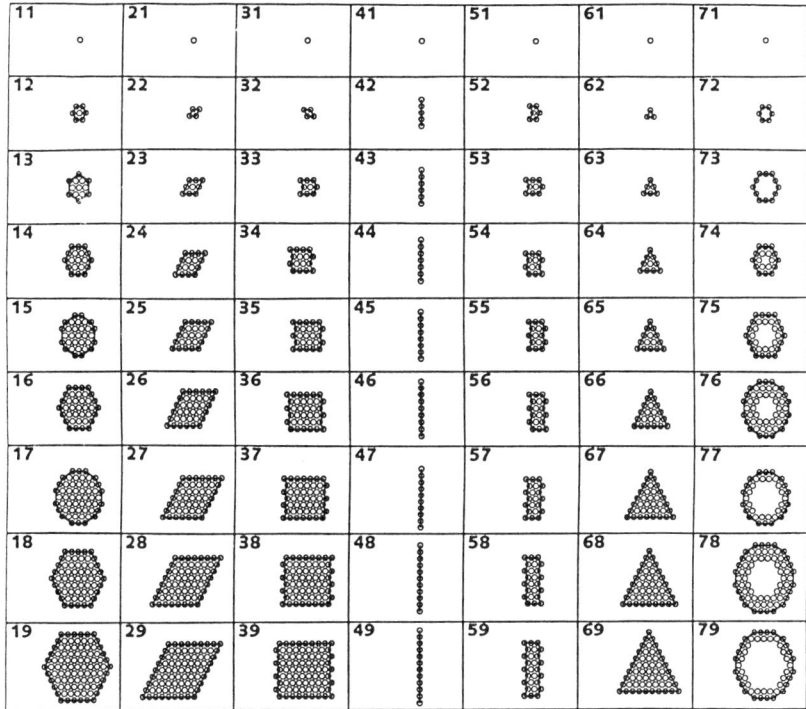

Representative Scan Patterns for the UltraScan Delivery System

FIGURE 1.—Different patterns can be obtained using the computer pattern generator and the Ultrapulse CO_2 laser. (Reprinted by permission of the publisher from Lowe NJ, Lask G, Griffin ME, et al. Skin resurfacing with the Ultrapulse carbon dioxide laser: Observations on 100 patients. *Dermatol Surg* 21:1025–1029, copyright 1995 by Elsevier Science Inc.)

laser. A pretreatment regimen was initiated 2 to 4 weeks before laser treatment was carried out. During treatment with the Ultrapulse CO_2 laser, a 3-mm collimated handpiece was used for most patients. In other patients, a computer pattern generator device that is able to deliver variously sized and shaped treatment patterns was used (Fig 1). Baseline and post-treatment evaluations were conducted to determine the severity of photodamage. In selected patients, skin surface replicas also were obtained and assessed using computer image analysis technology.

Results.—Five patients experienced a dramatic improvement at 1 month after laser treatment. Moderate improvement also was noted in 68 patients, and minimal improvement in 27 patients. At 2 months after treatment, 20 of the 27 patients who had only minimal improvement at 1 month had progressed to moderate or dramatic improvement from baseline. A transient erythema that persisted for up to 6 weeks occurred in all patients, many of whom also experienced a temporary hyperpigmentation that lasted for up to 4 months.

Conclusions.—The Ultrapulse CO_2 laser provides effective treatment for skin resurfacing of photodamaged skin. Although some side effects do occur in association with laser treatment, these effects are manageable and are less of a problem and more consistent and predictable than those resulting from chemical peeling and dermabrasion. Use of the computer pattern generator, together with the Ultrapulse CO_2 laser, can be useful when treating patients with scars or those undergoing whole face resurfacing.

Rapid Laser Scanning for Facial Resurfacing
David LM, Sarne AJ, Unger WP (Inst of Laser Cosmetic Surgery, Hermosa Beach, Calif)
Dermatol Surg 21:1031–1033, 1995   1–26

Background.—Carbon dioxide (CO_2) laser skin resurfacing is being used with increasing frequency in dermatologic practice. The Ultrapulse laser, introduced in 1990, is easily mastered and treatment is relatively simple to perform. Freehand delivery of impacts is, however, fairly time consuming, and accurate and precise placement of impacts can be problematic. Use of the computer pattern generator (CPG), a new computer scanning device, in conjunction with the Ultrapulse laser, may help overcome the difficulties associated with freehand laser resurfacing. Experience with a prototype CPG combined with the Ultrapulse laser is described.

Patients and Methods.—Sixty-one patients aged 19 to 68 years with actinic damage (55 patients) and acne scarring (6 patients) were included in the study. Surgeons experienced in freehand laser resurfacing used the CPG during treatment. Different patterns and sizes were evaluated to identify those most useful for various conditions and locations on the face. Patients were photographed at baseline, during and immediately after treatment, and at 1, 3, 5, and 7 days, and 2 weeks after treatment. Photographs also were obtained at 1 and 3 months whenever possible.

Results.—A square pattern containing "packed" impact proved to be most efficacious for all facial areas. Full-face resurfacing, including eyelids, required about 15 minutes to complete when using the combined CPG and Ultrapulse laser approach, compared with nearly 60 minutes when done freehand. The upper lip required less then 1 minute, and lower eyelids required less than 5 minutes to complete with the combined approach. More uniform, accurate, and precise distribution of impacts also were achieved with use of the CPG. Re-epithelization occurred at 3 to 5 days for lower eyelids and at 7 to 9 days for the upper lip in 60 patients, representing faster healing than that noted for patients not treated with the CPG. In the remaining patient, a postoperative infection involving the upper lip occurred, resulting in delayed healing (2 weeks). No resultant scar was noted in this patient, and an excellent result was ultimately obtained.

Conclusion.—Operative time for full-face resurfacing is markedly reduced when using the new CPG in conjunction with the Ultrapulse laser. Pulses are also delivered with greater uniformity with the CPG, resulting in more uniform and possibly more rapid healing over the treated area. In addition, the added control afforded by the CPG may help reduce overlapping during treatment, thereby minimizing adverse treatment-related effects, including charring and subsequent scar formation.

Laser Skin Resurfacing With the SilkTouch Flashscanner for Facial Rhytides
Lask G, Keller G, Lowe N, et al (Univ of California, Los Angeles; Dela Vina Surgicenter, Santa Barbara, Calif; Skin Research Found of California, Santa Monica)
Dermatol Surg 21:1021–1024, 1995   1–27

Background.—Facial rhytides can be effectively treated using carbon dioxide (CO_2) lasers. The high peak power and short exposure times obtained when using these lasers results in char-free ablation—an effect that can also be achieved when using a SilkTouch Flashscanner attached to a conventional CO_2 laser. The aim of this study was to assess the efficacy of the SilkTouch flashscanner in patients undergoing skin resurfacing.

Patients and Methods.—Forty patients undergoing treatment of fine to deep facial rhytides were included in the study. The SilkTouch Flashscanner was attached to 1 of 2 continuous wave CO_2 lasers (Sharplan 1030 and the Surgipulse XJ150). The depth of penetration achieved when using the scanner on both CO_2 lasers was histopathologically evaluated using preauricular skin from patients scheduled to undergo facelift surgery. Assessments were made just before facelift excision. In 2 patients, silicone surface replicas were obtained both before and 2 months after laser therapy and were subjected to optical micrometric analysis. Clinical evaluation of all patients also was performed before and after treatment.

Results.—No histopathologic differences were noted with use of the SilkTouch scanner on the 2 different CO_2 lasers. Perioral and periorbital areas showed the best response to treatment. Treatment of nasolabial folds on an individual basis were not significantly improved, although when the entire face was resurfaced, improvement of nasolabial folds was noted by an overall tightening effect. Optical micrometry showed a reduction in rhytide volume, indicative of improvement. Healing took place within 7 to 10 days. Persistent erythema was the most frequently noted complication and appeared to be directly associated with depth of ablation. Deeper ablations corresponded to longer lasting erythema. Postinflammatory hyperpigmentation also was noted. This was correlated with patient skin type and was rarely seen in those with skin types I and II. When found in patients with lighter skin types, hyperpigmentation resolved more promptly than in patients with darker skin types.

Conclusions.—Cutaneous resurfacing can be effectively carried out using the Silktouch Flashscanner. The minimal residual thermal damage associated with this approach permits a more controlled, and thus safer, method of ablation.

▶ There have been many debates between physicians using the SilkTouch flashscanner by Sharplan Lasers, Inc. (Allendale, NJ) and those using the coherent UltraPulse CO_2 laser as to which is more effective. I have seen patients treated with both, and have found clinical results to be comparable. We only use the coherent UltraPulse CO_2 laser in our clinic, and I have seen good results with it. I am of the opinion that no matter which of these lasers is used for full-face procedures, that IV sedation or general anesthesia is necessary because of the extreme pain that is felt by the patient, as well as the extreme anxiety that is elicited in the physician and staff as a result of the discomfort to the patient.

D.J. Papadopoulos, M.D.

Skin Resurfacing of Fine to Deep Rhytides Using a Char-Free Carbon Dioxide Laser in 47 Patients
Waldorf HA, Kauvar ANB, Geronemus RG (Laser and Skin Surgery Ctr, New York)
Dermatol Surg 21:940–946, 1995   1–28

Background.—Carbon dioxide (CO_2) lasers that are able to remove thin layers of skin with very little thermal damage to surrounding tissue have been developed. The effects of these lasers, which rely on rapid pulsing or scanning of the laser beam, are both predictable and reproducible. This treatment approach appears to be potentially beneficial for skin resurfacing, and clinical results obtained thus far have been encouraging. No published series is presently available, however. The efficacy and associated side effects of skin resurfacing using a CO_2 laser with a scanning device were therefore evaluated in a group of patients with fine to deep rhytides.

Patients and Methods.—Treatment efficacy, healing time, and side effects were retrospectively reviewed in 47 patients undergoing CO_2 treatment with a flashscanner between November 1994 and April 1995 for perioral, periorbital, or glabellar rhytides. Cosmetic appearance, and the presence of erythema, hyper- or hypopigmentation, and scarring of the treated area was evaluated by 2 independent evaluators using pre- and post-treatment photographs and chart review.

Results.—Good to excellent cosmetic outcomes were noted in all anatomic areas evaluated, with the greatest improvement observed in the periorbital area. Post-treatment erythema was observed in all patients, and this persisted for 1 to 6 months. Other minor complications included contact dermatitis to topical preparations, temporary postinflammatory hyperpigmentation, and milia formation. A primary herpes simplex virus infection was documented in 1 patient during re-epithelization; intravenous therapy was required in this patient. Another patient experienced minor focal atrophy. None of the patients showed evidence of hypertrophic scarring or permanent pigmentation changes after treatment.

Conclusions.—Patients with glabellar, perioral, and periorbital rhytides can be safely treated using a CO_2 laser system with scanning beam and can expect to see improvement, or even complete resolution, of skin wrinkles.

▶ The above 4 articles detail the latest advance in CO_2 laser surgery: skin resurfacing. Although systems may be different, the fact that the treatment of rhytides and facial resurfacing can be achieved successfully with the carbon dioxide laser dramatically increases their potential usage, not only in dermatologic surgery, but also in other specialties. I suspect that as we become more comfortable caring for laser rejuvenated skin, we will use this as a primary modality, whereas others may use this as an adjunct to other procedures. The inclusion of resurfacing in our office during the past year produced dramatic results, as well as changes in our use of modalities such as dermabrasions and chemical peeling. The various authors correctly note the differences in various regions of the face, the need for more than 1 pass with the laser, and the "art" of the physician. Technologic advances, including the computer pattern generator and a scanning device, allow more precise as well as more rapid treatment.

H.T. Greenway, M.D.

Resurfacing of Atrophic Facial Acne Scars With a High-Energy, Pulsed Carbon Dioxide Laser
Alster TS, West TB (Georgetown Univ, Washington, DC; Washington Hosp Ctr, Washington, DC)
Dermatol Surg 22:151–155, 1996   1–29

Background.—Dermabrasion, chemical peels, excisional surgery with closure, punch grafting and elevation, collagen implants, and silicone injections, used alone or in combination, have for many years been the standard therapeutic methods used to treat patients with atrophic acne scars. These methods, however, have resulted in adverse effects, the most noteworthy of which are scarring and pigmentation changes. The recently introduced high-energy carbon dioxide lasers (CO_2) offer yet another treatment alternative. They offer advantages over other available methods, in that thermal injury to uninvolved adjacent tissue structures is reduced during treatment, thereby minimizing the risk of post-treatment complications. The efficacy of a high-energy, pulsed CO_2 laser in the treatment of patients with atrophic facial scars was evaluated.

Patients and Methods.—Fifty patients with skin phototypes I-V and moderate-to-severe atrophic facial acne scars were treated by the same experienced laser surgeon. One high-energy, pulsed CO_2 laser treatment was delivered to each patient using identical laser parameters. Photographs were obtained and clinical evaluations were conduced before treatment, and at 1, 4, 8, 12, and 24 weeks postoperatively. In 10 patients, textural analyses of skin were performed at baseline and post-treatment to verify clinical impressions. Two blinded evaluators independently assessed each patient's clinical response to treatment.

Results.—Considerable improvement in acne scars (average, 81.4%) was observed after high-energy, pulsed CO_2 treatment. No recurrence or worsening of scars was noted during the 6-month follow-up. Skin texture measurements of laser-treated scars were similar to those of normal adjacent skin. Transient hyperpigmentation was common, occurring in 36% of the patients, and persisting for an average of 3 months post-treatment. Persistent erythema, lasting for an average of 2 months, also was commonly observed and was felt to be part of the normal healing process. None of the patients showed evidence of hypertrophic scarring after laser treatment.

Conclusions.—High-energy, pulsed CO_2 lasers, with their associated precision and reduced thermal injury during treatment, offer a safe and effective means for resurfacing atrophic facial scars. Clinicians with experience in selecting the appropriate laser parameters, identifying the number of laser passes that will be needed during treatment, and "sculpting" or "feathering" edges of scars, will be able to manage patients with problem skin types and cosmetic areas with little risk of adverse side effects. Careful monitoring of patients after treatment and prompt clearing of hyperpigmentation using topical hydroquinone preparations should help facilitate patient satisfaction and optimal clinical results.

▶ Advances in CO_2 laser technology, with the development of high energy pulsed systems, have made them highly desirable for the surgical dermatologist's practice. Although certainly applicable in resurfacing of wrinkles, their use in treating atrophic facial acne scars is clearly defined in this article. An average of 81% clinical improvement seems wonderful, especially in light of the user friendliness of these lasers. (However, I did find in my practice that I prefer not to promise anything more than a 50% improvement whether using lasers, dermabrasions, etc.) The prolonged erythema (average, 2 months) continues to be a routine postoperative finding. Postoperative pigmentation (overall in 35% of cases) continues to be a problem in spite of preventive and therapeutic measures (hydroquinones). With such results and the avoidance of blood products associated with dermabrasion, its use for facial acne scarring will continue to develop.

H.T. Greenway, M.D.

Laser Resurfacing in Pigmented Skin
Ho C, Nguyen Q, Lowe NJ, et al (Univ of California, Los Angles; Skin Research Found, Santa Monica, Calif)
Dermatol Surg 21:1035–1037, 1995   1–30

Introduction.—Laser skin resurfacing has been used successfully in treating solar elastosis and acne scars in patients with Caucasian skin phototypes I and II. Results in the patients reported here, Asians and Hispanics with skin types III and IV, show that the laser treatment can be effective in such patients when measures are taken to reduce the risk of dyspigmentation.

Methods.—Twenty-five patients were treated with the Coherent Ultrapulse 5000C CO_2 laser with the Truespot 3-mm collimated handpiece and 5 with the Sharplan SilkTouch flashscanner, 4-mm spot size, attached to the Sharplan 1030 CO_2 laser. All patients had either facial rhytides or acne scars. Before surgery, tretinoin cream 0.05%, hydroquinone 5%, and desonide cream 0.1% were applied nightly for 2-4 weeks and broad sunscreens used each morning. Topical anesthetic cream was applied before the procedure; postoperative care included Vigilon dressing, nonadhesive gauzes, and oral acyclovir and cephalexin. Patients were evaluated at 1 week, 1 month, and 3 months.

Results.—Facial rhytides in perioral and periorbital areas responded well to both laser resurfacing devices. The average response after 1 laser treatment was 50% improvement. Acne scar treatment was less effective, with 25% improvement after 1 treatment. Re-epithelialization of treated areas was noted in 7 to 10 days. The most common side effects were persistent erythema and transient hyperpigmentation. Broad spectrum sunscreen and sun avoidance, together with pre- and postoperative use of tretinoin, hydroquinone, and desonide cream, minimized postinflammatory hyperpigmentation.

Conclusion.—With proper pre- and postoperative management, laser resurfacing can be used to improve facial rhytides and acne scars in patients with skin phototypes III and IV. Hypopigmentation did not occur in any of these cases. The procedure was well tolerated and is less painful than manual dermabrasion treatment.

▶ Skin phototypes III and IV present a challenge for treatment of rhytides and acne scarring by laser resurfacing (or by chemical peeling or dermabrasion in the past). Perhaps more critical than the surgical expertise is the pre- and postoperative regimen after proper patient selection. The lack of significant hypopigmentation even after 3 laser resurfacing passes speaks well for technique. Persistent erythema (6 weeks) with hyperpigmentation persisting 3 to 4 months after the procedure is also seen in other treatment modalities. Of interest was the authors' judgement of improvement: 50% for rhytides and 25% for acne scarring. Appropriate lest we promise our patient too much!

H.T. Greenway, M.D.

▶ Encouraging results in this difficult patient population. Everyone should note that patients were pretreated for 2–4 weeks before the procedure and tests were performed with patients showing prolonged erythema, hyperpigmentation or hypopigmentation excluded. Also, take note that no patients who had used isotretinoin within the past 12 months were treated in this study.

D.J. Papadopoulos, M.D.

Ultrapulse Carbon Dioxide Laser Resurfacing and Facial Cosmetic Surgery

Apfelberg DB (Stanford Univ, Calif; Atherton Plastic Surgery Ctr, Calif)
Can J Plast Surg 3:133–136, 1995   1–31

Background.—The author has used the ultrapulse carbon dioxide laser to perform facial cosmetic surgery since July, 1994. His experience with this technique in more than 100 patients was summarized.

Patients and Treatment.—The laser was used as a scalpel in 41 patients undergoing a facelift, blepharoplasty, and forehead lift and in 74 patients undergoing resurfacing of various facial areas (Table 1). The laser was aided by 4.5 power surgical loops. Skin slices of 100 µm were removed with no blood (Fig 1). The cold beam that was produced carried very little risk of thermal damage and subsequent burn scars. Candidates for complete superficial laserbrasion include patients with fine static rhytides, perioral or periocular wrinkles, full-face photo aging, and acne or chickenpox scars. Patients with a history of keloid, who have taken isotretinoin in the previous 18 months, or who have frequent oral herpes infections must be treated cautiously.

Technique.—Complete superficial laserbrasion is performed at 450 to 500 mJ, 3 to 5 watts, with 10% overlap to remove the epidermis and uncover irregularities. The surgeon wipes the desiccated tissue clean with very moist saline gauze and dries the surface. Two to 4 subsequent passes are made at 350 mJ, 3 to 5 watts, to remove the shoulders or high points of the rhytides, furrows, or scars (Figs 2 and 3). The presence of a reddish-pink color indicates epidermis removal; uniform gray, the depth of the papillary dermis; and chamois yellow, tissue removal to the reticular dermis. The surgeon should stop at this point and redo the area in 2 to 3 months; otherwise there is a risk of scarring. To prevent a sharp line of demarcation, the surgeon feathers the edges of the regular areas by paintbrushing a random pattern with gradually declining laser powers, a random pattern with the same power, or 35% trichloroacetic acid.

TABLE 1.—Resurfacing—Patient and Treatment Data

	Number of patients	Average age	Healing days	Complications
Peri-oral	40	38.9	9–11	2 scars (lip)
Eyelid	20	46.7	9	0
Full face	3	41.3	8–10	0
Scar	7	24.6	6–8	0
Other	4	34.5	5–7	0

Ablation depth can be precisely controlled with pulse energy*

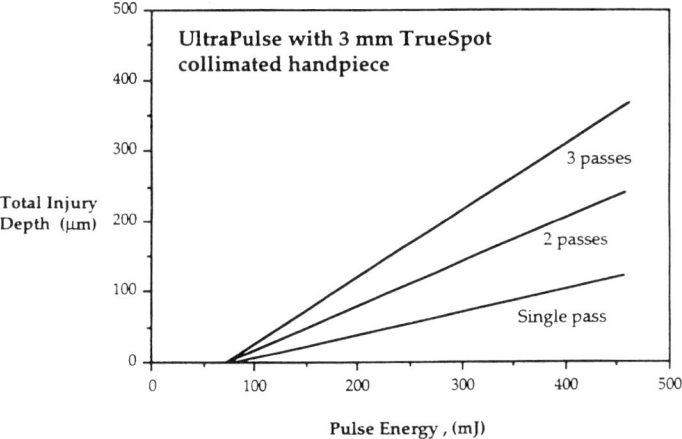

FIGURE 1.—Illustration of depth of tissue destruction at 450 mJ setting. Each pass removes 100 μm of skin. With a collimated handpiece, the fluence to tissue is precisely controlled by adjusting the pulse energy. The depth of ablation with the Ultrapulse can be adjusted by varying the pulse energy from 1 mJ to 500 mJ. (Data from R Fitzpatrick, M.D., Courtesy Coherent Inc.) (Courtesy of Apfelberg DB: Ultrapulse carbon dioxide laser resurfacing and facial cosmetic surgery. Reproduced with permission of *Can J Plast Surg* 3:133–136, 1995.)

Conclusions.—In this author's practice, laser skin resurfacing had replaced chemical peel and dermabrasion. Precise control is possible, and healing occurs with minimal risk of scarring, texture, or pigmentary changes.

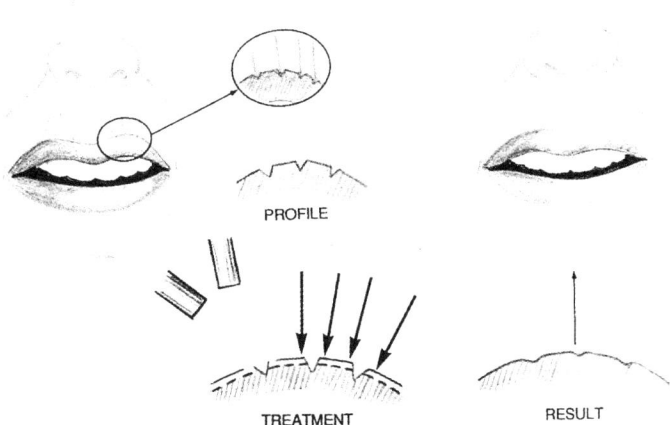

FIGURE 2.—Schematic of upper lip procedure illustrating removal of "shoulders" with resultant smoothing of lip. (Courtesy of Apfelberg DB: Ultrapulse carbon dioxide laser resurfacing and facial cosmetic surgery. Reproduced with permission of *Can J Plast Surg* 3:133–136, 1995.)

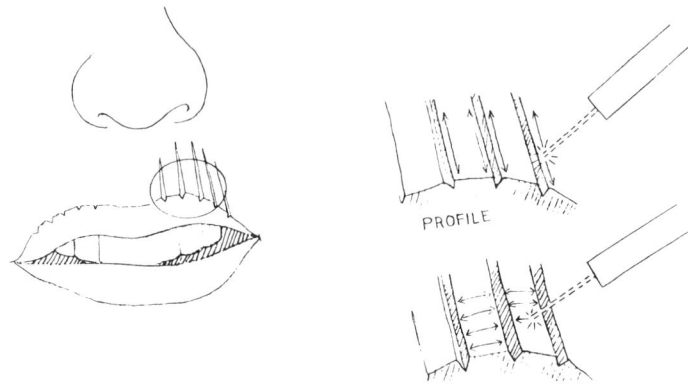

FIGURE 3.—Illustration of either longitudinal or horizontal laserbrasion of high points between depths of rhytides. (Courtesy of Apfelberg DB: Ultrapulse carbon dioxide laser resurfacing and facial cosmetic surgery. Reproduced with permission of *Can J Plast Surg* 3:133–136, 1995.)

▶ The most frequently requested laser resurfacing procedure in my practice is the correction of perioral rhytides, especially those of the upper lip. The approach used by the authors is similar to our approach for the upper lip. One must mark the rhytides to be treated to appreciate how much of the shoulder needs to be corrected. Also, as noted by the authors, after using a wet sponge to wipe the char, the area must be dried thoroughly to avoid laser energy absorption by the residual water on the surface of the skin.

D.J. Papadopoulos, M.D.

Infraorbital Pigmented Skin: Preliminary Observations of Laser Therapy
Lowe NJ, Wieder JM, Shorr N, et al (Skin Research Found of Calif, Santa Monica; Univ of Calif, Los Angeles)
Dermatol Surg 21:767–770, 1995   1–32

Objective.—Although dark circles under the eyes are a common cosmetic concern, there is little information available regarding treatment. A subset of patients with infraorbital dark skin caused by dermal melanin deposition was treated with a Q-switched ruby laser.

Methods.—A Q-switched ruby laser was used to treat 17 patients (2 men), aged 32 to 66, with a 5-mm spot size with fluences of 7.5 J/cm^2. Sites were evaluated every 4 weeks, retreatments were performed at 4-week intervals if necessary, and patients were followed for 6 to 12 months. Responses were graded 1 for 0 to 25% improvement, 2 for 26% to 50% improvement, 3 for 51% to 75% improvement, and 4 for >75% improvement.

Results.—After 1 treatment, 6 of 17 patients had a grade 1 response, 7 had a grade 2 response, and 4 had a grade 3 response. After 2 treatments, 1 of 9 patients had a grade 2 response, 6 had a grade 3 response, and 2 had a grade 4 response. About 30% of patients experienced transient hyperpigmentation that resolved in 4 to 8 weeks. Another 6% experienced hypopigmentation. Dermal melanin deposition in the mid and upper dermis before treatment was markedly reduced after treatment.

Conclusion.—Q-switched ruby laser treatment is an effective treatment for dark circles under the eyes. Maximum improvement is achieved at 3 to 6 months after treatment.

▶ It is important to note that there are many causes for infraorbital pigmented skin and, in my experience, in patients with Fitzpatrick-types I and II skin, this phenomenon is usually the result of a superficial plexus of blood vessels, whereas in patients with type III or darker skin, it is usually the result of pigment. I think performing a biopsy before treating these patients is a very good idea, and I am impressed with the clinical results as presented in this article.

D.J. Papadopoulos, M.D.

Mini-Slit Graft Hair Transplantation Using the Ultrapulse Carbon Dioxide Laser Handpiece

Ho C, Nguyen Q, Lask G, et al (Univ of California, Los Angeles; Skin Cancer Found of California, Santa Monica)
Dermatol Surg 21:1056–1059, 1995   1–33

Background.—Mini-, micro-, and slit grafting techniques have improved the esthetic results of hair transplantation. The Ultrapulse carbon dioxide (CO_2) laser with a slit handpiece can produce ultrashort high-energy pulses that minimize thermal damage to adjacent tissues and may be useful in a mini-slit graft hair transplant.

Methods.—Twenty-five patients underwent laser hair transplantation through the use of the newly developed slit handpiece with the Ultrapulse CO_2 laser. The donor strips were strip harvested from the occipital area with a triple-blade scalpel and divided into 1 × 2-mm minigrafts. The recipient sites were made with the Ultrapulse laser at settings of 300 to 450 mJ, 10 to 15 W, and 0.8-second pulse durations. The sites consistently measured 2 × 0.2 mm. Biopsies from some sites were obtained to assess thermal damage of adjacent tissues. The patients were followed for 4 to 6 months.

Results.—The optimal laser setting was 350 mJ, 12 W, and 0.8-second pulse durations. Approximately 2.5 to 3 hours of operative time was required for 200 to 400 minigrafts. Intraoperative bleeding and charring were minimal. The recipient slits accepted the grafts well with minimal compression. There was no excessive pain or swelling. Crusting lasted up to 2 weeks. More than 98% of the grafts took. There was good long-term hair regrowth from the transplant sites. The biopsies revealed minimal thermal damage to the adjacent tissues.

Conclusions.—The Ultrapulse CO_2 laser with the slit handpiece is effective in the performance of mini-slit graft hair transplantation procedures.

Its advantages over conventional scalpel techniques include minimal bleeding, reduced operative time, consistent recipient slit sizes, easier graft handling, less compression, and minimal adjacent tissue damage. Its disadvantages include its cost, the safety and fire hazard requirements, and the prolonged crusting.

Laser Hair Transplantation: Tissue Effects of Laser Parameters
Fitzpatrick RE (Encinitas, Calif)
Dermatol Surg 21:1042–1046, 1995   1–34

Introduction.—The use of the pulsed carbon dioxide (CO_2) laser for small graft hair transplantation has been proposed as a solution to some of the potential problems, such as intraoperative bleeding, graft compression, elevation, depression, and difficult graft insertion. The results of small graft hair transplantation that used various laser parameters were compared with the results that used standard micro- and minigraft techniques. In addition, residual thermal damage that occurred with the various laser parameters was given a histological evaluation.

Methods.—Eight adult males with male pattern alopecia were treated with transplantation of 100 micro- and minigrafts obtained from the occiput. For each patient, 20 grafts each were performed as follows: micrografts into 18-gauge needle puncture recipient sites, minigrafts into 14-gauge needle puncture recipient sites, micrografts with laser-created recipient sites, minigrafts with laser-created recipient sites, and slit grafts with laser-created recipient sites. Dilators were used in all needle-created recipient sites. The power settings used for all laser sites in 2 patients each were 15, 20, 30, and 50 W. The patients were evaluated monthly for 6 months.

Scalp tissue obtained during scalp reduction surgery performed with laser power settings at 5-W intervals between 5 and 50 W were examined histologically to determine the zone of thermal damage.

Results.—Crusting and healing resolved more slowly at the laser sites, compared with the conventional sites, and the crusting and healing time correlated with laser power. The hair yield was greater and the onset of growth was earlier at conventional sites than at laser sites. At laser sites, hair yield decreased with increased power settings. The operative time was reduced by 50% for the laser recipient sites, but was increased for the laser donor sites because of the need to avoid thermal damage to adjacent hairs.

Thermal necrosis increased as laser power settings increased. Necrosis zones of less than 100 µm could only be achieved with laser powers of 5 and 10 W or repetition rates of less than 20 Hz. The necrosis zone was greater than 200 µm with a laser power setting of 50 W.

Conclusions.—Optimal results of laser hair transplantation can be achieved through the use of a small beam size, continual beam movement, and a power setting of 15 W. These settings minimize lateral thermal necrosis and crusting and healing time and maximize hair growth.

Laser Hair Transplantation III: Computer-Assisted Laser Transplantating
Unger WP (Toronto)
Dermatol Surg 21:1047–1055, 1995   1–35

Introduction.—Laser techniques for hair transplantation result in less bleeding, pain, and postoperative edema. Because lasers can create recipient site slits, rather than round holes, the cosmetic result may be superior. Because a plug of tissue does not need to be removed from the recipient site, preparation of the recipient site is considerably accelerated with lasers. Thermal damage to adjacent tissue is the most important disadvantage of laser use. The types of lasers now used extensively for hair transplantation are described.

Ultrapulse Carbon Dioxide (CO_2) Laser.—Either round hole or slit recipient sites can be prepared with this laser. Hair growth typically occurs 4–6 weeks later than with conventional techniques, but cosmetic results are usually better with laser techniques. Thermal damage is related to watt setting, millijoule setting, spot size, and the speed of spot movement. Computer-driven scanners have been developed to ensure a consistent speed of spot movement with either a sequential or random mode that have improved the predictability of thermal damage.

Silktouch CO_2 Laser.—Whereas the Ultrapulse laser limits tissue exposure through the use of ultrashort pulses, the Silktouch laser limits tissue exposure with a continuous beam that is moved at a computer-regulated high speed. This laser can be used to produce any vaporization pattern. Although the speed of spot movement is controlled, thermal damage can vary in relation to the watt setting and millijoule setting.

Conclusions.—When appropriate settings are used, both lasers produce comparable thermal damage. The following settings appear to be optimal: to produce a coherent 2.5-mm slit with a 60 × .2-mm sequential spot scanner, 300 mJ and 12, 15, or 40 W result in 80 µm of thermal damage; to produce a coherent 2.5-mm slit with a 40 × .2-mm sequential spot scanner, 350 mJ and 12 W result in 50 µm of thermal damage with prototype 2, whereas 3350 mJ and 20 W result in 81 µm of thermal damage with prototype 3; to produce a Sharplan slit, the "+" size setting at 40 W for .05 seconds × 4 results in 54 to 81 µm of damage; and to produce a Sharplan round site, a "+" size setting at 80 W for .05 seconds × 2 results in 54 to 81 µm of thermal damage.

▶ These 3 articles explore the possible advantages of the CO_2 laser in the evolution of hair transplantation. Whereas advantages are promoted and thermal damage recognized, the marketing of this technology certainly plays a pivotal role. Speed and bleeding control are sought-after advantages; the high cost of the technology is a problem. However, lasers can now be rented as a practice is developed prior to outright purchase. At least 2 competing systems may each offer success; I find the computer pattern generator to be extremely user-friendly.

H.T. Greenway, M.D.

Current Trends in Laser Blepharoplasty: Results of a Survey

Glassberg E, Babapour R, Lask G (Univ of California, Los Angeles)
Dermatol Surg 21:1060–1063, 1995   1–36

Background.—The efficacy of blepharoplasty performed by laser has been questioned. The current survey study determined current trends in laser blepharoplasty to further explore the efficacy of blepharoplasty by laser compared with conventional scalpel techniques.

Methods.—A questionnaire was mailed to a select group of surgeons who routinely performed laser blepharoplasty. Sixteen of the 17 surgeons surveyed responded. A total of 4,269 laser blepharoplasties were reported.

Findings.—The most common laser used in blepharoplasty was the carbon dioxide. Seventy percent of the surgeons used a laser as the only cutting tool, and 88% used it as the sole hemostasis tool. The survey respondents reported that intraoperative and postoperative recovery times were decreased significantly with laser blepharoplasty. The incidence of edema, ecchymosis, and postoperative pain were also less severe with the laser than with scalpel techniques. The respondents reported no serious complications associated with laser use.

Conclusions.—Laser blepharoplasty appears to be effective and safe when used by skilled surgeons. Furthermore, this method may have some advantages over conventional blepharoplasty.

▶ Any tool that allows us to be able to perform a surgical task and provides a relatively bloodless field around the eye is valuable. We await continued improvements in delivery systems, as well as the manipulation of powers and pulse widths. As these parameters are adjusted and our laser tools refined, we will be able to perform increasingly more delicate periocular procedures.

D.J. Papadopoulos, M.D.

VASCULAR

Repetitive Pulsed Dye Laser Treatments Improve Persistent Port-Wine Stains

Kauvar ANB, Geronemus RG (Laser and Skin Surgery Ctr of New York)
Dermatol Surg 21:515–521, 1995   1–37

Introduction.—Development of the flashlamp-pumped pulsed dye laser has revolutionized the treatment of port-wine stains, congenital vascular malformations that lead to both medical and psychological complications. Some port-wine stains are resistant to laser therapy, however, and the incidence of 100% clearing is variable. The cases reported here show that repetitive treatments can lead to significant improvement in resistant stains, without an increased risk of adverse effects.

Methods.—Patients included in the study were infants, children, and adults who failed to achieve more than 75% lightening of their stains within 9 treatment sessions using the flashlamp-pumped pulsed dye laser. The 69 patients, 35 adults and 34 children, all had skin phototypes I-III. Higher energy fluences were used for darker lesions and lower energy fluences for eyelid and neck areas and for children with faint macular lesions. Exposure ranged from 5.75 to 8.00 J/cm² at test sites. After these sites were evaluated, the energy fluence was increased to obtain an adequate clinical response. Patients were divided according to number of laser treatments and assessed for degree of lightening and side effects.

Results.—Thirty-six patients underwent 10–15 treatment sessions (group I), 20 had 16–20 sessions (group II), and 13 had 21–25 sessions (group III). Patients in all 3 groups went from a mean midway treatment score of 2.2–2.6, corresponding to 25% to 49% lesional lightening, to a mean last treatment score of 3.2–3.3, corresponding to 51% to 75% lesional lightening. Complete clearance of the port-wine stains occurred in 9% of group I, 15% of group II, and 15% of group III patients. None experienced hypertrophic scarring. Hypopigmentation occurred in 1 patient and hyperpigmentation in 3, but all of these adverse effects resolved in 3 to 6 months.

Conclusion.—Older therapies for treatment of port-wine stains led to unacceptable cosmetic outcomes. The pulsed dye laser, the first laser designed specifically for treatment of cutaneous vascular lesions, can be repeated in many sessions when stains are persistent. Complications were quite low, even with many treatments, and complete clearance of stains was achieved in 12% of cases.

▶ Repetitive treatments for port-wine stains without significant results can be disappointing for patient and physician alike. Dr. Kauvar and Dr. Geronemus clearly demonstrate the importance (and safety) of persistence, i.e., 10–25 repetitive treatments with good results. Certainly the well known saying below (which I keep on my desk) applies here.

PERSISTENCE
NOTHING IN THE WORLD CAN TAKE THE PLACE OF
PERSISTENCE
TALENT WILL NOT: NOTHING IS MORE COMMON
THAN UNSUCCESSFUL MEN WITH TALENT
GENIUS WILL NOT: UNREWARDED GENIUS IS
ALMOST A PROVERB
EDUCATION WILL NOT: THE WORLD IS FULL OF
EDUCATED DERELICTS
PERSISTENCE AND DETERMINATION ALONE
ARE OMNIPOTENT

H.T. Greenway, M.D.

Dynamic Epidermal Cooling During Pulsed Laser Treatment of Port-Wine Stain: A New Methodology With Preliminary Clinical Evaluation

Nelson JS, Milner TE, Anvari B, et al (Univ of California, Irvine; Harvey Mudd College, Claremont, Calif; Israel Inst of Technology, Haifa; et al)
Arch Dermatol 131:695–700, 1995   1–38

Introduction.—The flashlamp-pumped pulse dye laser (FLPPDL) yields reasonably good results in the treatment of port-wine stain (PWS). Absorption of laser energy by melanin in the epidermal pigment layer, however, reduces the light dosage reaching blood vessels and leads to suboptimal blanching of the lesion. Cooling of skin during pulsed laser PWS therapy offers a means of maximizing thermal damage to the lesion while minimizing damage to the overlying epidermis. The dynamic cooling method described here should permit higher incident light dosages to be used.

Methods.—The method uses a test cryogen as a surface cooling agent, delivered in spurts onto the skin surface through an electronically controlled solenoid valve. Skin surface temperature is measured before, during, and after the cryogen spurt and laser pulse by a fast infrared imaging detector. The cryogen is made to cover a nearly circular zone concentric with the laser spot. Fourteen patients took part in an evaluation of the dynamic cooling method. Twelve of 18 test sites had dynamic cooling and 6 underwent FLPPDL without cooling.

Results.—Measurements obtained by the fast infrared imaging detector showed that the dynamic cooling technique was able to reduce surface temperature before laser exposure by as much as 40°C. The PWS test sites cooled with a 20- to 80-msec cryogen spurt after FLPPDL exposure were free of skin surface textural changes at the maximum light dosage possible (10 J/cm²). At similar exposure, uncooled sites exhibited dermal necrosis. Cooling of the epidermis also reduced patient discomfort during the laser therapy. At 6-month follow-up, clinically significant blanching on the cooled sites indicated that laser photothermolysis of PWS blood vessels had occurred.

Conclusion.—Reduction of skin temperature by this dynamic cooling method allows optimal heating of the PWS to occur. This is particularly important in patients with darker skin types who have been unable to undergo higher light dosages because of epidermal damage; and with higher incident light dosages, the number of laser treatments required may be significantly reduced. Further studies are underway to determine optimal duration of cryogen spurts and exposure to the FLPPDL.

▶ A 40°C decrease in surface cooling with dynamic epidermal cooling with a 20–80 msec cryogen spent during pulsed dye laser therapy seems reasonable. This certainly represents a quantum leap from the cube of ice applied before Argon laser treatments in the past. I look forward to the achievement of optimum cooling and laser energy exposures.

H.T. Greenway, M.D.

PIGMENT AND TATTOOS

Allergic Reactions to Tattoo Pigment After Laser Treatment
Ashinoff R, Levine VJ, Soter NA (New York Univ)
Dermatol Surg 21:291–294, 1995   1–39

Background.—Both the Q-switched ruby laser and the Q-switched neodymium:yttrium-aluminum-garnet (YAG) laser have been used as a means to remove decorative tattoos. The present report describes a previously unreported complication of tattoo removal with these 2 Q-switched lasers.

Case Reports.—Two women, 26 and 23, with tattoos on the right lateral lower leg and right upper thigh, respectively, were evaluated for tattoo removal. Neither patient reported having had any problems with their tattoos before treatment.

In the first patient, the tattoo contained blue, black, yellow, green, and purple pigments. One half of the tattoo was treated with the Q-switched ruby laser and the other half with the Q-switched neodymium:YAG laser. About 3 weeks after her initial laser session, the patient noted that the treated area was pruritic and slightly swollen. Several months later, she returned for a second treatment, during which time both Q-switched lasers were again used. Two weeks later, she experienced a generalized and localized pruritic eruption. She was treated with a broad-spectrum oral antibiotic, an oral H1 antihistamine, and a topical medium-potency corticosteroid cream. The patient noted gradual improvement during the next 10 days. Six weeks later, another generalized eruption occurred, and she was treated with the same regimen as before. The lesions resolved during 2 weeks, although the area over the tattoo took longer to clear. A biopsy specimen was taken from an involved area on her upper back. This showed a superficial perivascular infiltrate of lymphocytes and macrophage with spongiosis, consistent with an id reaction.

In the second patient, blue, black, red, and green pigments were noted in the tattooed area. The patient was treated 6 times with both the Q-switched ruby and neodymium:YAG lasers. Seven days after the sixth treatment was completed, the patient experienced a generalized urticarial eruption. She was treated with a medium potency topical corticosteroid and oral antihistamine, and she improved during the next 2 days. Before her next scheduled treatment, she was given a prophylactic course of prednisone and hydroxyzine, beginning 1 day before laser therapy and continuing for 2 days thereafter. No allergic reaction was noted when the patient was treated with these 2 medications. Although the reasons that this patient did not experience a reaction until after her sixth laser session are not clear, 1 possible explanation is that the tattoo fragments produced after laser treatment must be a particular size before an allergic reaction takes place. In this patient, the appropriate particle size may have been produced only after her sixth treatment, resulting in the subsequent allergic reaction.

Conclusions.—Tattoo pigment placed in the skin is mainly intracellular, existing within macrophages and fibroblasts. Tattoo removal with the Q-switched ruby and neodymium:YAG lasers targets the intracellular tattoo pigment by causing a rapid thermal expansion, which fragments the pigment-containing cells. This, in turn, causes the pigment to become extracellular, and as such, is probably recognized by the immune system as a foreign substance. Accordingly, both localized and generalized allergic reactions are likely to take place. Increased awareness of this newly reported side effect, which is associated with Q-switched laser treatment, is needed.

▶ Metal salts in tattoo pigments are well known to cause allergic reactions, with mercury derived red cinnabar being most common. Our initial laser efforts were to destroy the pigment with the CO_2 (and less commonly, the Argon) laser. Newer laser systems, including the Q-switched ruby and neodymium:YAG described here, may involve more risk because of their selective intracellular action. Although excision and primary closure of smaller tattoos remain my therapy of choice, lasers will continue to play a major role in tattoo therapy.

H.T. Greenway, M.D.

Q-switched Alexandrite Laser Treatment (755 nm) of Professional and Amateur Tattoos

Alster TS (Georgetown Univ, Washington, DC)
J Am Acad Dermatol 33:69–73, 1995   1–40

Background.—Q-switched red or near-infrared laser systems have been successful in removing decorative tattoos, because these systems can target pigment selectively with minimal risk of scarring or permanent pigmentary changes. The clinical efficacy and adverse effects of the newest Q-switched system—the alexandrite laser—in removing amateur and professional tattoos were investigated.

Methods.—Twenty-four multicolored professional tattoos and 18 blue-black amateur tattoos were treated with the laser (755 nm, 100 nsec) every 2 months until total clearing was achieved. The 510-nm pulsed dye laser was used on tattoos that contained red pigment.

Outcomes.—A mean of 8.5 treatments with the alexandrite laser were needed to remove professional tattoos completely. To remove amateur tattoos, a mean of 4.6 treatments were needed. An average of 2 sessions with the 510-nm pulsed dye laser successfully removed red pigment. There was no scarring or long-standing pigmentary changes in laser-irradiated skin (Fig 3).

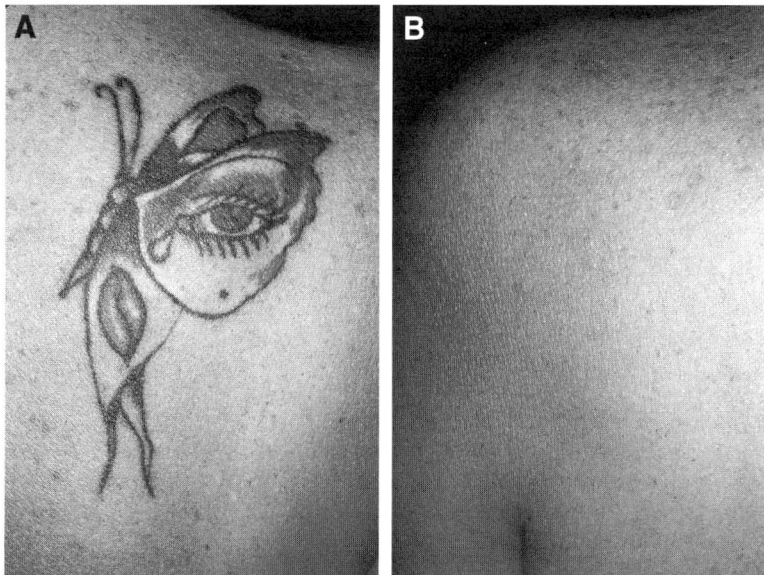

FIGURE 3.—Multicolored professional tattoo before (**A**) and 8 weeks after (**B**) 12 alexandrite treatments (mean fluence, 7 J/cm^2) and 3 pulsed dye laser treatments (mean fluence, 3 J/cm^2). No pigmentary alteration or scarring was noted. (Courtesy of Alster TS: Q-switched alexandrite laser treatment (755 nm) of professional and amateur tattoos. *J Am Acad Dermatol* 33:69–73, 1995.)

Conclusions.—The Q-switched alexandrite laser is effective for removing multicolored professional and amateur tattoos. No adverse effects were associated with such treatment. The 510-nm pulse dye laser effectively removed red tattoo pigment.

▶ As with other complex problems, the combination of lasers (510-nm pulsed dye for the red pigment) appears to offer advantages. I was impressed with the before and after multicolored photographs included in the article. Interestingly, we now see patients who desire tattoo removal via laser sugery so they can have a new tattoo put on in the same site! I would suggest prepayment for this service.

H.T. Greenway, M.D.

MISCELLANEOUS

Lasers in Dermatology
Spicer MS, Goldberg DJ (NJ Med School, Newark)
J Am Acad Dermatol 34:1–25, 1996   1–41

Introduction.—There have been numerous advances in the technology and techniques of laser therapy. With these technical advances, the clinical utility of laser therapy has expanded. Currently, laser therapy can be used to treat various dermatologic conditions with minimal scarring and skin texture changes. Laser physics, laser light-skin interactions, and clinical uses of lasers in dermatologic practice are discussed.

Laser Physics.—Lasers have 2 essential components: a power source and an active medium. The energy from the power source excites the atoms of the medium, which then return to a metastable (intermediately excited) state and eventually a stable state. Heat is produced during the transition from excited to metastable state and light is produced during the transition from metastable to stable state. This light can be delivered to the treatment area as continuous, pulsed, or pseudocontinuous (extremely rapid pulses) beams. Laser light is characterized by irradiance (power density), energy fluence (energy density), and exposure time.

Laser Light-Tissue Interaction.—Most laser light delivered to skin is absorbed by 3 chromophores: melanin in pigmented lesions and oxyhemoglobin and carboxyhemoglobin in vascular lesions. Selective tissue absorption of laser light causes selective destruction of the absorbing tissue. Therefore, optimal treatment involves using the absorption peak wavelength of the appropriate chromophore with pulsed irradiation corresponding to the thermal relaxation time of the target tissue to minimize scarring from thermal diffusion.

Clinical Lasers and Their Uses.—The carbon dioxide laser emits an infrared beam, which much be pulsed to avoid scarring. The beam can be focused (held close to the skin surface) to cut or defocused (held at a distance from the skin) to perform skin ablation. Lasers have been used to ablate warts and condyloma acuminatum, remove keloids and processes of the genital area, and perform surgery in patients who cannot tolerate blood loss. With ultrapulsing, they can be used to treat photodamaged skin and several other superficial skin conditions. The argon laser emits a blue-green beam absorbed nonspecifically by oxyhemoglobin and melanin. The nonspecificity of its absorption increases the risk of skin texture changes or scarring. It is most effectively used to treat benign vascular malformations, telangiectases, and benign pigmented lesions. The argon-pumped dye laser can produce either yellow light, used to treat vascular lesions, or red light, used for photodynamic therapy. The flashlamp-pumped pulsed dye laser (FPDL), with minimal melanin absorption, is currently the treatment of choice for many vascular lesions. The copper laser emits a green beam with shorter and more rapid pulses than the FPDL and is also useful in treating vascular lesions, including nodular grade III and IV port-wine stains. The krypton laser is a new laser that has been used to treat vascular lesions. The pigmented lesion dye laser, using coumarin-containing dye as its active medium, emits 3 wavelengths absorbed optimally by melanin and can treat deep dermal pigmented lesions and benign pigmented lesions. The Q-switched ruby laser emits a red beam, which allows deep dermal penetration, and can remove tattoos and treat benign and deep dermal pigmented lesions. The Nd:YAG laser has no specific chromophore and can be used to treat cavernous hemangiomas and nodular port-wine stains or remove deep, densely pigmented tattoos. The flashlamp Q-switched alexandrite laser emits an infrared beam allowing deep dermal penetration and can remove black, blue-green, red, and yellow tattoo pigment, although hypopigmentation and skin texture changes may occur.

Conclusions.—The uses of laser therapy in dermatologic practice are expanding. Currently, lasers may be used to cut, to perform ablation, or to achieve desiccation. Lasers can also be effective in treating both pigmented and vascular lesions.

▶ Lasers have become an important part of dermatologic surgery. We began in our office in 1984 with an argon laser and subsequently have followed the technology with the addition of other laser systems up to and including the ultrapulsed carbon dioxide laser for severe photo damaged skin and rhytides. Their usage has increased our specialties operating room privileges and we truly have maintained the forefront in cutaneous laser surgery. We owe much to Dr. Leon Goldman, the father of dermatologic surgery who still manages to contribute to laser development and research at his home, now here in San Diego. Thank you, Leon, for your continued inspiration and encouragement.

H.T. Greenway, M.D.

Treatment of Small and Medium Congenital Nevi With the Q-Switched Ruby Laser
Waldorf HA, Kauvar ANB, Geronemus RG (Laser and Skin Surgery Ctr, New York)
Arch Dermatol 132:301–304, 1996   1–42

Background.—Treatment of congenital nevi with excision or dermabrasion can create an unacceptable scar and may require general anesthesia. Treatment with Q-switched ruby laser (QSRL) may be promising. It has been effective in lightening and clearing other benign pigmented lesions. The efficacy of QSRL in the treatment of small-to-medium congenital nevi was investigated.

Methods.—Eighteen patients, aged 1 month to 14 years, with congenital nevi, sized less than 1.5 cm to less than 5 cm in diameter, were treated with contiguous pulses with minimal overlap of the QSRL at regular intervals of 2–4 weeks. Serial photographs were used to monitor treatment effects. A 4-mm punch biopsy specimen was obtained from 1 patient before treatment and after treatment from a clinically clear area.

Results.—All patients experienced clinically apparent lightening by the fourth treatment, at which time there was an average of 57% lightening. By the eighth treatment session, there was an average of 76% lightening of the pigmentation. Five of the patients had more than 90% clearance after an average of 13 treatments. However, 11 patients, including 3 of the 5 patients with more than 90% clearance, had partial repigmentation, which occurred in 2–9 months (average, 4.9 months), resulting in an average final clearance of approximately 50%. The treatment was well tolerated, with mild and transient side effects of erythema or hypopigmentation. There was no scarring or tissue atrophy. The biopsy from a clinically lightened area showed reduced nevus cells in the papillary dermis and upper part of the reticular dermis but not in the lower reticular dermis.

Conclusions.—Pigmentation in congenital nevi can be lightened and sometimes cleared by treatment with QSRL, but not permanently. Treatment effect permanence may be prevented by the persistence of the nevus cells in the deep reticular dermis, which may form a nidus for recurrence. However, the safety and temporary improvement brought by QSRL treatment makes it a viable alternative for making cosmetic improvements in some patients. Further study is needed to assess the long-term results of QSRL treatment.

▶ The authors certainly were able to demonstrate improvement in prepubertal children with congenital nevi of less than 5-cm diameter. Although the QSRL has been effective in other lesions with epidermal pigmentation, the current study clearly acknowledges its weaknesses in these lesions, including the lack of complete elimination of all nevus cells and the possibility of laser irradiation-induced alterations. Finally, the need for long-term follow-up was stressed, and I look forward to follow-up reports on these 18 patients regarding their long-term status.

H.T. Greenway, M.D.

Treatment of Adenoma Sebaceum With the Copper Vapor Laser
Kaufman AJ, Grekin RC, Geisse JK, et al (Univ of California, San Francisco)
J Am Acad Dermatol 33:770–774, 1995   1–43

Objective.—Most patients with tuberous sclerosis, a rare genetic neurocutaneous disease, develop facial adenoma sebaceum after 5 years of age. These angiofibromas have been treated by curettage, cryosurgery, chemical peel, dermabrasion, shave excision, and argon and carbon dioxide laser ablation, all of which carry a risk of scarring or pigmentary change. The copper vapor laser is useful in the treatment of pigmented and vascular lesions. Its utility was examined in 9 patients with multiple facial angiofibromas associated with tuberous sclerosis (Table 1).

Methods.—Under lidocaine occlusion and/or regional block anesthesia, 9 patients with facial angiofibromas, treated previously by various methods, were treated with continuous delivery of yellow light (578 nm) at 0.4 W increasing to 0.6 W with subsequent visits as necessary. Patients healed within 2 weeks and were examined 4–8 weeks after each treatment to determine if additional treatment was necessary. There were at least 6 weeks between treatments.

Results.—All patients had good to excellent results. One patient experienced hypopigmentation that resolved within 4 weeks. Patients received additional treatments as new lesions developed.

Conclusion.—The copper vapor laser is a safe and effective treatment for facial angiofibromas associated with tuberous sclerosis.

TABLE 1.—Clinical and Treatment Characteristics of 9 Patients With Adenoma Sebaceum Treated With the Copper Vapor Laser

Patient	Age (yr)	Sex	Previous treatment	Power (watts)	Light (nm)	No. of treatments	Results
1	12	F	Argon laser	0.38–0.40	Yellow (578)	5	Excellent
2	11	F	None	0.40–0.60	Yellow (578) and green (511)	9	Excellent
3	28	M	Dermabrasion, electrodesiccation	0.50	Yellow	9	Very good
4	22	M	Shave excision	0.40–0.58	Yellow and green	5	Excellent
5	19	F	Dermabrasion; carbon dioxide laser	0.40–0.86	Yellow and green	5	Excellent
6	24	F	None	0.45–0.50	Yellow and green	2	Very good
7	12	M	None	0.60–0.64	Yellow and green	4	Very good
8	13	F	None	0.49–0.55	Yellow	3	Excellent
9	14	M	None	0.46	Yellow	1	(Test area)

(Courtesy of Kaufman AJ, Grekin RC, Geisse JK, et al: Treatment of adenoma sebaceum with the copper vapor laser. *J Am Acad Dermatol* 33:770–774, 1995.)

▶ The authors clearly demonstrate that, whereas my 10-year-old Argon laser and 1996 CO_2 laser are effective treatments for adenoma sebaceum, the copper vapor laser with both selective photothermolysis and nonselective destruction in the experienced physician offers effective treatment with rapid healing. Of interest was their choice of the 2 wavelengths for treatment: the yellow light (578 nm) initially in all patients, followed by the green light (511 nm) in 5 of 9 patients with resistant lesions. Advances continue in laser surgery.

H.T. Greenway, M.D.

Pulsed Dye Laser Treatment of Warts
Kauvar ANB, McDaniel DH, Geronemus RG (New York Univ Med Ctr; Laser Ctr of Virginia, Virginia Beach; Eastern Virginia Med School, Norfolk)
Arch Fam Med 4:1035–1040, 1995   1–44

Background.—Warts, or verrucae, have been managed using a variety of approaches, including application of caustic agents, cryotherapy, electrosurgery, chemotherapeutic agents, surgical excision, and carbon dioxide laser ablation. All these methods are, however, associated with nonselective epidermal damage. Response rates for previously untreated verrucae also have been poor with conventional techniques; data concerning response rates of difficult to manage verrucae are not, to the authors' knowledge, currently available. The treatment of verrucae with pulsed dye lasers has previously been reported in a small number of patients, with encouraging results. Experience with pulsed dye laser treatment of verrucae in a large group of patients is described in the present report.

Patients and Methods.—One hundred forty-two consecutive patients referred to 2 tertiary care laser centers during a 6-month period were included in the study. Photocoagulation of 703 recalcitrant and 23 previously untreated warts was undertaken using the flashlamp-pumped pulsed dye laser. Patients were followed up for 3 to 9 months after treatment, and response to laser therapy was evaluated.

Results.—The overall clearance rate for all wart types was 93%. An average of 2.5 treatments was needed to achieve complete resolution of all treated warts. Seventy-four percent of the warts resolved after delivery of 1 laser treatment. A 99%, 95%, 84%, and 83% overall response rate was noted for body, limb, and anogenital warts, hand warts, plantar warts, and periungual warts, respectively. Side effects related to laser treatment were minimal, and included a nonhypertrophic 2-mm white scar on the proximal phalanx of a finger in 1 patient, and focal transient hyperpigmentation, limited to the treatment sites on the lower extremities, in 1 patient with type IV skin who had undergone photocoagulation of 2 warts. Fifty-five percent of the patients reported experiencing transient pain lasting for several hours after treatment, whereas 16% reported discomfort for up to 24 hours, and 25% reported pain for 2 to 3 days. Only 4% of patients had discomfort for up to 1 week. Very few patients indicated that laser treatment of warts interfered with their daily activities.

Conclusions.—Pulsed dye laser treatment, unlike conventional therapeutic methods, is able to selectively destroy warts without interfering with the surrounding skin. Adverse treatment-related effects are minimal and uncommon. Given its safety and efficacy, pulsed dye laser treatment appears to be a very useful first-line approach for untreated and uncomplicated warts; available data also indicate that this may be the best method for treatment of recalcitrant warts.

▶ Various laser systems have been successful in treating verrucae during the past decade. When our office began treating skin lesions in 1984 with our "new" Argon laser, verrucae were found to be similarly responsive but soon, the CO_2 laser became more expedient for those verrucae requiring laser therapy. Although the pulsed dye laser may be successful, the higher energy required may limit the laser's longevity, and as stated, its use may remain limited to problem warts.

H.T. Greenway, M.D.

Carbon Dioxide Laser Ablation as an Alternative Treatment for Cutaneous Metastases From Malignant Melanoma
Lingam MK, McKay AJ (Gartnavel Gen Hosp, Glasgow, Scotland)
Br J Surg 82:1346–1348, 1995   1–45

Introduction.—Isolated limb perfusion has been shown to be the most effective treatment of local recurrences of metastatic melanoma on the extremities. Not all patients are eligible for isolated limb perfusion or respond to it. The efficacy of carbon dioxide laser treatment in the management of local recurrence was assessed in patients with metastatic melanoma in whom isolated limb perfusion failed or was not suitable.

Methods.—Over a 2-year period, 19 patients underwent carbon dioxide laser ablation for the treatment of cutaneous lesions from malignant melanoma. All patients had too many or too large lesions for local surgical excision. Of the 19 patients, 17 had been treated previously with isolated limb perfusion.

Results.—All lesions could be treated in 1 session that took an average of 10 to 15 minutes. The defects that resulted after treatment were multiple full-thickness punctate burns that healed without grafting. The patients were followed up for a mean of 15 months. Five of the 19 patients died at a mean of 9 months after laser treatment; only 2 had recurrence at the time of death. Of the 14 survivors, 8 had no recurrences and 6 underwent repeated laser ablation.

Conclusions.—Carbon dioxide laser ablation is a safe and effective treatment for local control of cutaneous metastases of malignant melanoma that can be performed without a disruption of the patient's life. Further study with a prospective randomized trial is justified to compare the efficacy of laser ablation with that of isolated limb perfusion in patients without distant metastases.

Use of the Carbon Dioxide Laser to Manage Cutaneous Metastases From Malignant Melanoma
Hill S, Thomas JM (Westminster Hosp, London; Royal Marsden Hosp, London)
Br J Surg 83:509–512, 1996   1–46

Introduction.—Isolated limb perfusion (ILP) is used to treat lesions of malignant melanoma that are confined to the limb of origin. Hyperthermic ILP with melphalan yields poor results, however, in terms of response rates and duration of response. An alternative treatment, carbon dioxide laser ablation, was used in 100 patients with cutaneous metastases from malignant melanoma.

Patients and Methods.—The patients had cutaneous and subcutaneous metastases that were too numerous or recurred too frequently for conventional surgical excision. Forty-one were considered suitable for ILP and 15 had recurrent disease after ILP; in other cases, ILP was contraindicated because of distant spread. Treatment was performed with patients under local or general anesthesia, depending on the number and position of lesions. To prevent thermal damage to adjacent skin, the smoke plume produced by tumor ablation was removed by strong suction.

Results.—The most common sites of primary tumors were the lower leg (61 tumors) and the sole of the foot (10 tumors). Seventy-six of the 100 patients had 1–4 laser treatments; 5 patients required 10 or more treatments. Between 3 and 450 lesions were ablated at a single treatment. Patients had little or no postoperative pain, and most wounds healed completely within 6 weeks. Although less than 2% of lesions recurred after laser treatment, new crops of metastases developed and required further laser treatment. Thirteen patients later underwent ILP when large-volume subcutaneous disease developed. The overall survival at 1 year from the first laser treatment was 68%. Half of the patients with stage IIIa disease had metastases controlled by 3 or fewer laser treatments within the first year of follow-up.

Conclusion.—In patients with stage IIIa disease, ILP using hyperthermia and melphalan does not appear to yield a survival advantage, and the morbidity rate is significant. Carbon dioxide laser treatment offers a simple and effective alternative to ILP, with virtually no morbidity.

▶ These 2 publications (Abstracts 1–46 and 1–47) review experiences either with failed limb perfusion or as an alternative to limb perfusion. We have on occasion treated cutaneous metastasis from melanoma with carbon dioxide laser ablation and found it to be effective with the individual lesions treated (most commonly in cases on the lower extremities in women in our practice). Although it is not curative, it may help decrease tumor load for better results with other therapies, including not only those referred to here but also vaccines and alfa 2-b interferon.

H.T. Greenway, M.D.

Treatment of Hidradenitis Suppurativa With Carbon Dioxide Laser Excision and Second-intention Healing

Finley EM, Ratz JL (Ochsner Clinic, New Orleans, La; Ochsner Med Found, New Orleans, La)
J Am Acad Dermatol 34:465–469, 1996   1–47

Introduction.—Hidradenitis suppurativa (HS) is considered to be an androgen-dependent disorder. Both men and women are affected, and no racial predilection is apparent. The disease may occur in any area with terminal hair in apocrine gland-bearing skin. Medical regimens are successful only in the early stage of HS, and the treatment of choice once the disease progresses is surgery. Seven patients were successfully treated with carbon dioxide laser excision.

Patients and Methods.—The patients, all women, ranged in age from 20 to 46 years. Four had inguinal disease and 3 had axillary disease. During the course of their disease, which ranged in duration from 1 to 10 years, all had received multiple courses of orally given antibiotics and topical antiseptics. Diseased areas were excised with the carbon dioxide laser, achieving margins of 3–4 mm beyond clinically involved tissue. Procedures were performed as same-day or clinic outpatient surgery with the patients under local anesthesia. Treated areas were allowed to heal by second intention.

Results.—Five patients had bilateral procedures, for a total of 12 excisions. Blood loss was negligible and complications have been minimal. To prevent contractures, patients performed full range-of-motion stretch exercises. Treated areas usually healed in 4 to 8 weeks, and cosmetic outcome was judged good in all cases. Procedure-related scars were flat and linear. With 10 to 27 months of follow-up, there has been only a single recurrence, an inflamed nodule on the margin of an excisional scar. Some patients had further HS in untreated areas.

Conclusion.—Carbon dioxide laser excision with second-intention healing is a safe and effective treatment for HS. Wound healing progresses rapidly, recurrence is uncommon, and cosmetic results are good. Prompt surgical intervention is recommended because of the risk of squamous cell carcinoma that arises in HS.

▶ The authors remind us that HS may successfully be managed with the carbon dioxide laser and that these areas may heal nicely by granulation. I also have found that split-thickness skin grafting is acceptable without evidence of too much contraction. It is important that surgical treatment not be delayed when indicated; there were findings of 16 cases of squamous cell carcinoma, with 7 deaths resulting from metastatic disease.

H.T. Greenway, M.D.

Laser Treatment of Erythematous/Hypertrophic and Pigmented Scars in 26 Patients
Dierickx C, Goldman MP, Fitzpatrick RE (Univ of California, San Diego)
Plast Reconstr Surg 95:84–90, 1995   1–48

Background.—Patients with red, pigmented, or hypertrophic scars may seek cosmetic treatment, which should ideally be both effective and free of complications. Treatment with the flashlamp pulsed-dye laser or the pigment lesion dye laser was evaluated retrospectively.

Methods.—Fifteen patients with erythematous or hypertrophic scars were treated with a pulsed-dye laser set at 585 nm with a pulse duration of 450 μs at energies of 6.0–7.5 J/cm² and a beam size of 5 mm. Eleven additional patients with lesions of postinflammatory hyperpigmentation underwent treatment with a pigment lesion dye laser set at 510 nm with a pulse width of 300 ns and a beam size of 5 mm. In all cases, the laser spots were overlapped by 10%, with the entire lesion treated in each session. Polysporin ointment was used until crusting was gone, with avoidance of sun exposure for 1 month. The lesions were examined after 4 to 8 weeks, when treatment was repeated if necessary.

Results.—No patients had adverse sequelae. Overall, an average of 80% improvement was noted after 1.45 treatments, with 100% improvement after 1 or 2 treatments found in 45% of the patients. The effectiveness of the treatment of erythematous or hypertrophic scars did not vary significantly with the varying fluence of the laser, but it was greater in scars less than 1 year old or on the face rather than more than 1 year old or on the extremities or buttocks (Fig 3). The effectiveness of the treatment of postinflammatory hyperpigmentation did not vary significantly with the varying fluence of the laser or with the age of the scar. There was signifi-

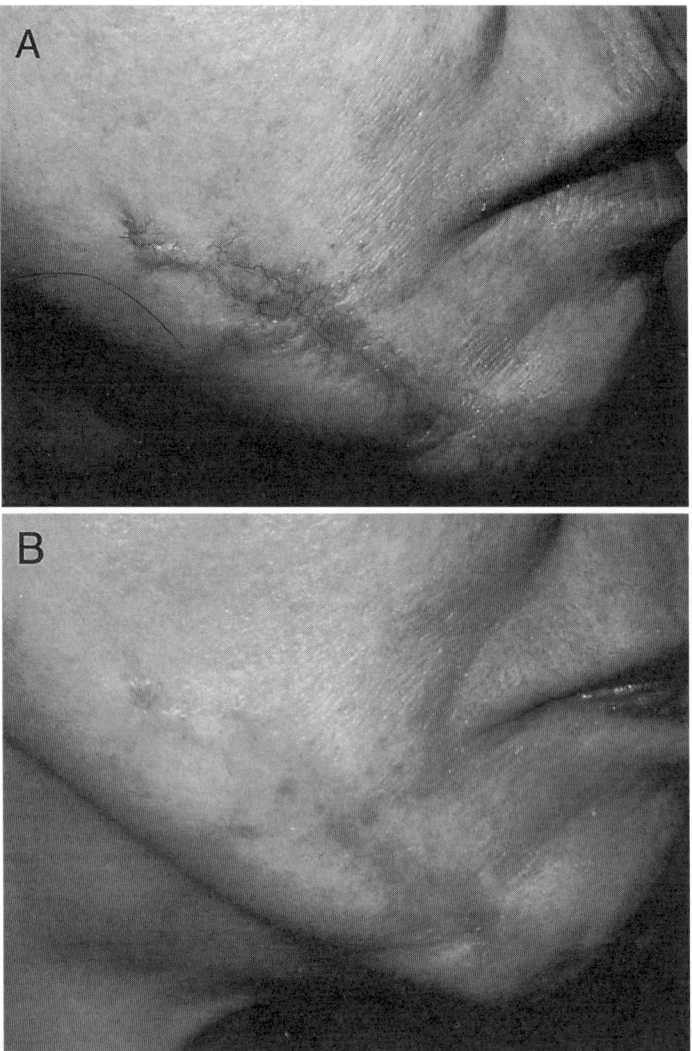

FIGURE 3.—**A,** a woman 63 years of age 9 months after receiving an Obaji chemical peel. The patient had received a series of 6 monthly injections of triamcinolone 10 mg/cc into the scar in an attempt at resolution. **B,** appearance 2 months after the fourth treatment with the Candela flashlamp pulsed-dye laser at 7.0 J/cm². Note 50% resolution of erythema and hypertrophy of the scar. Larger telangiectasias are totally resolved. (Courtesy of Dierickx C, Goldman MP, Fitzpatrick RE: Laser treatment of erythematous/hypertrophic and pigmented scars in 26 patients. *Plast Reconstr Surg* 95:84–90, 1995.)

cant improvement in both pigmentation and scar texture, which was maintained at follow-up examinations 6 to 12 months after treatment.

Conclusions.—Laser treatment is a safe and effective method of managing epidermal pigmentary lesions, such as hyperpigmented or hypertrophic scars.

▶ The "Discussion" on pp. 91–92 of this same journal outlines many of the problems with this article, including the use of 2 laser systems, the age variation of the scars treated, the lack of a controlled study, and so on. Despite all this, the 585-nm flashlamp-pumped pulsed-dye laser may play a role in the treatment of some cases of hypertrophic scarring. I was particularly interested in the case presented in Figure 3 related to scarring after an Obaji chemical peel. As with others, combination treatments yielded the best results.

H.T. Greenway, M.D.

Complications

Postoperative Wound Infection Rates in Dermatologic Surgery

Futoryan T, Grande D (Tufts New England Med Ctr, Boston)
Dermatol Surg 21:509–514, 1995   1–49

Background.—Although most dermatologic procedures are performed in clinical settings rather than in hospital operating rooms, the incidence of postoperative wound infection appears low. The incidence of surgical wound infections after Mohs micrographic surgery and various reconstructive and excisional procedures was evaluated retrospectively. Also evaluated were correlations between surgical wound infection rate and lesion type, anatomical location, postoperative defect size, number of Mohs surgeries required to reach a tumor-free plane, and reconstructive procedure type.

Findings.—Records of 1,047 surgical procedures performed during a 20-month period were examined. Twenty-four infections occurred: 13 after Mohs procedures followed by various reconstructions, and 11 after simple excisions (Table 2) Wound infection rates were within the range expected for "clean" surgical procedures. Six of the 13 infections after Mohs procedures occurred on the ear (Table 4). Large postoperative defects also showed a higher rate of wound infection.

Conclusions.—Dermatologic surgery can be performed in an outpatient setting without significant risk of infection. Infection rates after Mohs micrographic surgery are higher when the procedure is performed on the ear. Wounds that reach the level of the cartilage also appear to be corre-

TABLE 2.—Infections in Dermatologic Surgical Procedures at the New England Medical Center over 20 Months

Procedure	Number of Cases	Number of Infections	Infection Rate
Mohs (excisions followed by various repairs)	530	13	2.45%
Excisions	517	11	2.13%
Total	1,047	24	2.29%

TABLE 4.—Modified Rate for Mohs Procedures on Non-ear Sites

Mohs Procedure	Number of Cases	Number of Infections	Infection Rate
Mohs (excisions followed by various repairs) on all anatomic sites	530	13	2.45%
Mohs (excisions followed by various repairs) on the ear	48	6	12.50%
Modified infection rate for Mohs (excisions followed by various repairs) for all non-ear anatomic sites	482	7	1.45%

(Reprinted by permission of the publisher from Futoryan T, Grande D: Postoperative wound infection rates in dermatologic surgery. *Dermatol Surg* 21:509–514, copyright 1995 by Elsevier Science Inc.)

lated with a higher rate of infection. Antibiotic prophylaxis should be considered for large defects or for surgery on the ear, especially if cartilage is exposed during the procedure.

▶ It is important that we monitor our results, both good and bad, to continue to improve our overall care. Grande and Futoryan's evaluation of more than 1,000 total cases provides much needed data. Their findings of increased numbers of problems in the ear correlates with previous reports and our own experience. The use of prophylactic antibiotics continues to be controversial but is appropriate in selected cases. With newer topical and systemic antibiotics, which may provide better and easier therapy (and maybe prophylaxis) for *Pseudomonas aeruginosa,* the ear may not be as much of a problem in the future. Each of us should monitor our own infection and complication rates on a monthly basis to ensure improved care and quality. At our clinic, I do this by participating in the Department of Surgery monthly morbidity statistic evaluations and have found that to be a most valuable experience.

H.T. Greenway, M.D.

A Prospective, Randomized Surveillance Study of Postoperative Wound Infections After Plastic Surgery: A Study of Incidence and Surveillance Methods

Andenaes K, Amland PF, Lingaas E, et al (Norwegian Natl Hosp, Oslo, Norway; Univ Hosp, Oslo, Norway; Radium Hosp, Oslo, Norway)
Plast Reconstr Surg 96:948–956, 1995   1–50

Background.—Little attention has been paid to wound infection after elective plastic surgery. Such infections may go undetected if the follow-up period is too short. The incidence of wound infection within 30 days after elective plastic surgery was examined.

Methods.—Three hundred fifteen patients who were undergoing elective plastic surgery were randomly allocated to receive either outpatient care on the 30th day after surgery or self-control via questionnaire. Procedures were categorized as to risk of infection (Table 1). The definition of post-operative wound infection has been debated; a new definition scheme was created on the basis of the normal physiologic wound-healing model (Table 2).

Results.—The patients who received outpatient care showed a follow-up rate of 95% and an infection rate of 16.3%. The self-controlled group showed a follow-up rate of 68% and an infection rate of 17.1%. Forty-three patients (16.7%) had wound infections; only 12 infections (28%) were diagnosed during the hospital stay. The monthly wound infection rate decreased as the study progressed. Longer duration of surgery and "dirtier" preoperative contamination class correlated with greater wound infection rate. No significant difference was established in

---

TABLE 1.—Each Operative Procedure Was Either Allocated to 1 of These 2 General Sections or Given a Special Code Number

Code for Operative Procedures—General Sections

Section 1

01	Debridement	Surgical cleaning of a skin defect
02	Excision	Closure after excision included
03	Tangential excision	Tangential excision/shaving/dermabrasion without covering
04	Skin-grafting	All full-thickness—and split-skin—grafting
05	Flap I	All cutaneoous flaps including Z-plasty
06	Flap II	All fascio- and myocutaneous flaps including muscle transfer alone
07	Free flap	All free flaps

Section 2

10	Dermal autograft	All dermal grafting
11	Cartilaginous autograft	All cartilaginous grafting
12	Bone autograft	All bone grafts
13	Mammary prosthesis	All silicone mammary implants, exchange of prosthesis included
14	Silicone prosthesis	All implants made by silicone (except mammary)
15	Gold weight	Gold implant into upper eyelid
16	Chondroplast	All implants of chondroplast
17	Proplast	All implants of Proplast
18	Tissue expansion	All implantation of expanders (removal of expanders should normally be coded as 05 or 06)

Note: Increasing numbers within each section are believed to represent increasing complexity and risk of postoperative wound infection.

(Courtesy of Andenaes K, Amland PF, Lingaas E, et al: A prospective, randomized surveillance study of postoperative wound infections after plastic surgery: A study of incidence and surveillance methods. *Plast Reconstr Surg* 96:948–956, 1995.)

TABLE 2.—Scoring System of Postoperative Wound Condition

Score	Character of the Wound
0	Normal healing
1	One of the following signs or symptoms of infection: erythema, edema, or increased pain
2	Two of the following signs or symptoms of infection: erythema, edema or increased pain, or hemoserous discharge alone
3	All three of the following signs or symptoms of infection: erythema, edema or increased pain, or hemoserous discharge combined with one of the latter
	Infection
4	Pus, or hemoserous discharge combined with two of the following: erythema, edema, or increased pain
5	Pus combined with one of the following: erythema, edema, or increased pain; or hemoserous discharge combined with all of the following: erythema, edema, and increased pain
6	Pus combined with two of the following: erythema, edema, or increased pain
7	Pus combined with erythema, edema, and increased pain

(Courtesy of Andenaes K, Amland PF, Lingaas E, et al: A prospective, randomized surveillance study of postoperative wound infections after plastic surgery: A study of incidence and surveillance methods. *Plast Reconstr Surg* 96:948–956, 1995.)

rate of postoperative wound infection between patients who had normal nasal flora and those who carried potential pathogens. The infection rate did differ according to procedure (Table 9).

Conclusions.—This is the first prospective registration of postoperative wound infections after elective plastic surgery; some general conclusions are enumerated in Table 10. A follow-up questionnaire, because of its

TABLE 9.—Incidence of Postoperative Wound Infection Related to the Different Operative Procedures, Wound Infection Score (*WIS*) of 7 Included

			WIS			
			≥4		7	
Code for Operation	Operative Procedure	Total No.	No.	%	No.	%
2	Excision	50	5	10.0%	1	2.0%
4	Skin grafting	20	6	30.0%	5	25.0%
5	Flap I	22	3	13.6%	2	9.1%
12	Bone autograft	9	1	11.1%	0	0.0%
20	Reduction mammaplasty	20	6	30.0%	2	10.0%
40	Cheiloraphia	19	5	26.3%	2	10.5%
41	Palatoraphia	19	1	5.3%	0	0.0%
43	Secondary cleft lip operations	17	3	17.7%	1	5.9%
45	Secondary celft lip–nose operations	17	2	11.8%	0	0.0%

(Courtesy of Andenaes K, Amland PF, Lingaas E, et al: A prospective, randomized surveillance study of postoperative wound infections after plastic surgery: A study of incidence and surveillance methods. *Plast Reconstr Surg* 96:948–956, 1995.)

TABLE 10.—Conclusions

CONCLUSIONS

1.	Plastic surgery also has got its postoperative wound infection problem, not sufficiently recognized earlier.
2.	A simple questionnaire gives us a useful survey of the rate of postoperative wound infection.
3.	For the purpose of registering postoperative wound infection, we propose a follow-up for at least 30 days after surgery also for patients operated on in plastic surgical units.
4.	Surveillance for postoperative wound infection considerably reduces the incidence.
5.	More postoperative wound infections will be recorded if an extended concept of infection is laid down as a basis and the registration is carried out consecutively, implicating a maximum of variables.
6.	Special precautions should be taken for longer surgical procedures, for certain high-risk operations (e.g., mammaplasty and split-thickness skin grafting), and in the higher contamination classes.

(Courtesy of Andenaes K, Amland PF, Lingaas E, et al: A prospective, randomized surveillance study of postoperative wound infections after plastic surgery: A study of incidence and surveillance methods. *Plast Reconstr Surg* 96:948–956, 1995.)

favorable cost, may be a sufficient means of follow-up for such patients; no significant difference was found in rate of postoperative infection between groups. The method of wound infection scoring used is especially suited to plastic surgery because of the superficial nature of these wounds. Its broader utility also bears examination. Patients who undergo plastic surgery should receive follow-up for a minimum of 30 days; lack of follow-up results in underestimation of wound infection rates.

▶ The authors point out that "the existence of wound infections in plastic surgery is often overlooked," and that "postoperative wound infections following elective plastic surgery have never been prospectively registered." They suggest that the occurrence of infections after discharge from the hospital and lack of follow-up are prime reasons for their underestimation. The tables are most revealing, and dermatologic surgeons would certainly fare well in comparisons for similiar procedures (i.e., see top 3 in Table 9).

H.T. Greenway, M.D.

Intraoperative Fire With Electrocautery

Brechtelsbauer PB, Carroll WR, Baker S (Univ of Michigan, Ann Arbor)
Otolaryngol Head Neck Surg 114:328–331, 1996 1–51

Introduction.—There has been substantial documentation of intraoperative fires caused by endotracheal tube ignition and during tracheotomy.

However, intraoperative fires have also occurred during routine soft-tissue procedures in patients under local anesthesia. Two such cases were reported, and the problem of intraoperative fire is discussed.

> *Case 1.*—Woman, 46, underwent local flap reconstruction to correct a left chin skin defect after Moh's excision of a microcystic adnexal carcinoma. Local anesthetic was used, and pure oxygen was administered through a nasal cannula. When a minor bleeder was electrocauterized approximately 3 inches away from the oxygen tubing, the tubing and a gauze pad on her lips caught fire. The pad and tubing were removed immediately. She sustained partial-thickness burns on her upper lip, columella, and nasal alae, which healed uneventfully with bacitracin treatment.
>
> *Case 2.*—Man, 78, who had previously undergone total laryngectomy, underwent open biopsy of a neck mass under local anesthesia. Oxygen tubing with pure oxygen flow was covered with surgical drapes. Cauterization of a bleeder caused a flash fire in the air, igniting the oxygen tubing. The tubing and drapes were removed immediately, but partial-thickness burns occurred on the patient's anterior neck and upper chest. The flames had occurred over the tracheal stoma, causing erythema and char on the peristomal skin. The patient was treated with intravenous dexamethasone. He had no respiratory distress but had late mild stenosis of his tracheal stoma.

Discussion.—Fire requires 3 elements: a fuel source, a method of ignition, and an oxidizer. In operating rooms, tincture of benzoin, sutures packed in isopropyl alcohol, packaging materials, and skin preparations including alcohol are common fuel sources. Ignition is frequently linked to electrocautery. Oxygen is the most common oxidizer in the operative field. Therefore, it is recommended that oxygen be either completely discontinued during the use of electrocautery whenever possible or used with caution. In particular, oxygen tubing should not be covered by surgical drapes, because a resulting oxygen bubble can cause a flash fire in the air under the drapes. The routine need for supplemental oxygen during operative procedures should be carefully reconsidered.

▶ Electrocautery is used in our offices daily, routinely, without problems. Fortunately, rarely do our patients require supplemental oxygen. When oxygen is required, we normally take the appropriate precautions to limit the required triad of the fuel source, the ignitor, and the oxidizer. The growth in laser dermatologic surgery and its required safety standards has carried over into our other procedures. Although we are familiar with topical flammable materials and solutions, the authors' experience in these cases and their subsequent limitation of oxygen tubing concentration is of value. They recommend, as is the practice in our office, turning off the oxygen and allowing it to dissipate before using electrocautery.

H.T. Greenway, M.D.

Cadaver Skin Allografts and Transmission of Human Cytomegalovirus to Burn Patients

Kealey GP, Aguiar J, Lewis RW II, et al (Univ of Iowa, Iowa City)
J Am Coll Surg 182:201–205, 1996   1–52

Background.—Acute cytomegalovirus (CMV) infections are a frequent complication among burn patients. The mechanisms of CMV transmission are unclear. However, animal studies have shown that acute or latent CMV infections in the donor may cause CMV in the recipient of skin grafts. The potential for cadaver skin allografts to serve as a vehicle for the transmission of CMV to burn patients was examined.

Methods.—A total of 22 burn patients, who were CMV seronegative on admission, required cadaver skin allografts. These patients were all given CMV seronegative cellular blood products. The cadaver allografts were used without regard to the donor's CMV serostatus. The CMV serologic status of the patients was determined weekly during hospitalization and 1, 3, and 6 months after hospital discharge.

Results.—Of the 22 cadaver skin allografts, 20 (90.9%) were CMV seropositive. The 2 patients who received skin allografts from CMV sero-negative donors remained CMV seronegative. Five of the 22 patients (22.7%) experienced CMV seroconversion. Cytomegalovirus infection was manifested as CMV pneumonia in 1 patient, CMV viruria in 2 patients, and persistent fever, abnormal liver enzymes, and diarrhea not attributable to other pathogens in 3 patients.

Conclusions.—Cytomegalovirus infection can be transmitted to CMV-seronegative burn patients through the use of CMV-seropositive cadaver skin allografts. Two strategies should be considered to prevent CMV transmission, particularly in patients requiring extensive skin grafting. The patients could be given prophylactic ganciclovir, although the potential toxicities of this therapy should be carefully weighed against its potential benefits. Alternatively, skin allografts from CMV-seronegative donors should be used exclusively.

▶ The use of cadaver skin allografts and porcine skin grafts as temporary coverage/dressings is common in many dermatologic surgical practices, including our own. In healthy patients, for shorter time periods and with less surface area to treat than burn patients, one would expect less of a problem, but the potential still exists. Our current population of immunosuppressed patients with tumors and subsequent defects may be more at risk, and this must be considered.

H.T. Greenway, M.D.

NSAID as Pre- and Postoperative Medication—A Potential Risk for Bleeding Complications in Reduction Mammaplasty

Blomqvist L, Sellman G, Strömbeck JO (Stockholm Söder Hosp)
Eur J Plast Surg 19:26–28, 1996   1–53

Background.—A large number of intraoperative and postoperative bleeding complications were noted in patients treated for macromastia after reduction mammaplasty, prompting a retrospective study to identify factors associated with an increased risk for bleeding complications.

Methods.—The records of 193 patients undergoing reduction mammaplasty in 1990 and 1991 were reviewed. Operative blood loss and postoperative hematoma formation were noted, and associations between bleeding complications and patient or operative factors were analyzed.

Results.—Of the 193 patients, 10 had profuse intraoperative bleeding, and 20 had postoperative hematoma formation (including 6 who required reoperation). Of the 10 patients with profuse intraoperative bleeding, 9 had been premedicated with diclofenac (Table 2). Hematomas occurred in 3 of the 5 patients treated with ketorolac. There were bilateral hematomas in 50% of the patients treated with nonsteroidal anti-inflammatory drugs (NSAIDs).

Conclusions.—Bleeding complications can occur in previously healthy women after preoperative and postoperative treatment with NSAIDs. These complications can be reversed or prevented with drugs that stimulate coagulation factor release.

▶ Anesthesiologists in this series used a premedication scheme which included non-steroidal anti-inflammatory drugs (NSAID), but dermatologic surgeons routinely avoid NSAID where possible. Interestingly, the drug of choice for therapy for NSAID-induced bleeding was desmopressin (a synthetic vasopressin analogue from Sweden). On occasion in our practice, we

TABLE 2.—Intraoperative Bleeding

	Total number	Intraoperative bleeding (%)	p
Premedication			
Opioids[a]	171	1(0.6)	ns
Sedatives only[b]	76	0	ns
Diclofenac (Voltaren[TM])[c]	34	9(27.3)	<0.001
Ketorolac (Toradol[TM])[c]	6	0	ns
No drug	6	0	ns

[a] morphine 145, ketobemidon 21, pethidin 5
[b] midazolam 75, diazepam 1
[c] Diclofenac and ketorolac were mostly given together with the sedative midazolam but also, in some cases, together with morphine.
Abbreviation: ns, not significant
(Courtesy of Blomqvist L, Sellman G, Strömbeck JO: NSAID as pre- and postoperative medication. A potential risk for bleeding complications in reduction mammaplasty. *Eur J Plast Surg* 19:26–28, copyright 1996 by Springer-Verlag.)

have treated hemophilia and other at risk patients with desmopressin acetate (DDAVP) preoperatively with satisfactory results.

H.T. Greenway, M.D.

Miscellaneous Pearls

Nutrition and the Elderly

Neldner KH (Texas Tech Univ HSC, Lubbock)
J Geriatr Dermatol 4:122–130, 1996   1–54

Introduction.—Aging is determined by both genetic and environmental factors. It involves the progressive deterioration of homeostatic mechanisms, immune function, signal transduction pathways, mean muscle mass, and absorption of various nutrients (Table 1). Although this deterioration is largely genetically determined, recent evidence supports the importance of nutritional factors in modifying this progression.

Aging Skin.—Environmental insults, particularly ultraviolet light damage, primarily affect the epidermis and dermal elastic tissue. The genetic effects of aging are believed to primarily affect the dermal connective tissue and vascular components. However, both of these aging effects are related biochemically to free radical damage. An elaborate system of free radical scavengers has been developed.

Nutrition.—The most important antioxidants are vitamins A, C, and E; beta carotene; and the enzymes glutathione peroxidase (a selenium metalloenzyme), superoxide dismutase (a zinc/copper/manganese metalloenzyme), and catalase. Aging patients may have increased free radical damage associated with nutritional deficiencies caused by systemic disorders; reduced protein intake; reduced cutaneous synthesis of vitamin D; reduced trace element intake; lactose intolerance; and gastrointestinal disorders reducing nutrient absorption, transport, and storage.

Treatment with single nutrient supplements and of particular combinations have had conflicting results, suggesting that each antioxidant has a

---

TABLE 1.—Nutritional and Genetic Risk Factors Confronting the Elderly

- Progressive loss of lean muscle mass
- Gradual reduction in dietary protein
- Immune status decline
- Achlorhydria
- Thiamine and cobalamine deficiency
- Vitamin A, C and E deficiencies
- Impaired cutaneous synthesis of vitamin D
- Decreased calcium absorption
- Zinc intake below the RDA
- Lactose intolerance increased with age
- Selenium status decline
- GI tract disorders with secondary malabsorption

(Courtesy of Neldner KH: Nutrition and the elderly. *Geriatr Dermatol* 4:122–130, 1996.)

specific function in the detoxification of superoxide anions, singlet oxygen, hydrogen peroxide, and hydroxyl radicals. Subclinical or marginal nutritional deficiencies may have significant metabolic effects.

Recommendations.—The best approach to maintaining general health and slowing natural aging is eating a diet with reduced fat plus the proper amounts of protein, carbohydrates, vitamins, and minerals. However, elderly patients with inadequate diets may be prescribed a daily multiple vitamin/mineral supplement with an additional vitamin E supplement.

▶ "You are what you eat" was pointed out to each of us as children at home, at school, and even in our biblical education with the story of Daniel. I am now learning that oxidative damage is a problem, along with my knowledge of the immune system declining with age.

The author's summary of a balanced diet with 5 fruits or vegetables per day, reduced fat, physical and mental exercise, and moderation seem prescribed also for me. I have long been recommending a daily multivitamin for my elderly patients. I am glad to see that the author supports this, although he adds the boost of Vitamin E (400 IU). I must continue to upgrade my training in nutrition to both better the care for my patients, and also to be able to talk with them!

H.T. Greenway, M.D.

Angiogenesis and the Skin: A Primer
Arbiser JL (Harvard Med School, Boston)
J Am Acad Dermatol 34:486–497, 1996   1–55

Background.—Angiogenesis is a multistep process, relying on the secretion of growth factors, which bind to specific receptors, stimulating endothelial cells and creating a pathway of migration and finally tube formation (Fig 1). It is a normal, necessary process during embryonic development and wound healing, but it may also occur as part of a pathologic process in dermatologic disease. Factors mediating angiogenesis were studied.

Angiogenic Stimulators.—Several angiogenesis-stimulating factors have been isolated (Table 1). They include basic fibroblast growth factor, acidic fibroblast growth factor, vascular endothelial growth factor, platelet-derived endothelial cell growth factor, angiogenin, heparin-binding endothelial growth factor-like growth factor, oncostatin M, and interleukin-8. These factors have varying specific targets, including keratinocytes, fibroblasts, endothelial cells, melanoma cells, smooth muscle cells, and tumor cells. Malignant transformation appears to be associated with secretion of these factors.

Angiogenic Inhibition.—In vitro and animal studies have showed the inhibition of angiogenesis associated with the following factors: thrombospondin, thalidomide, angiostatic steroids, fumagillin analogues platelet factor 4, angiostatin, and interleukin-12.

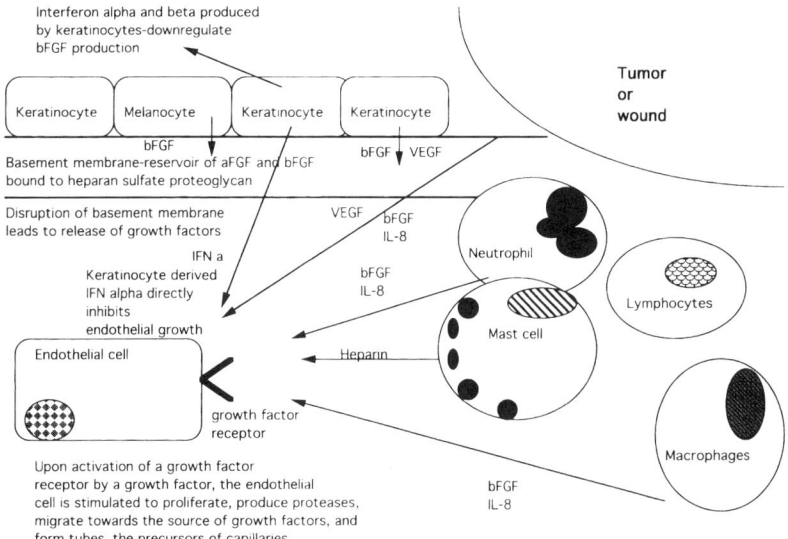

FIGURE 1.—Steps of cutaneous angiogenesis in response to wound or tumor. *Abbreviations: IFN,* interferon; *aFGF,* acidic fibroblast growth factor; *bFGF,* basic fibroblast growth factor; *IL-8,* interleukin 8; *VEGF,* Vascular endothelial growth factor. (Courtesy of Arbiser JL: Angiogenesis and the skin: A primer. *J Am Acad Dermatol* 34:486–497, 1996.)

TABLE 1.—Stimulators of Angiogenesis

Factor	Target of action	Molecular weight (kd)	Clinical relevance
Acidic fibroblast growth factor (aFGF, FGF-1)	Keratinocytes, fibroblasts, endothelial cells, chondrocytes	16	Experimentally, accelerates dermal wound healing, granulation tissue formation, and reepithelialization
Basic fibroblast growth factor (bFGF, FGF-2)	Endothelial cells, melanoma cells, neuronal differentiation, other tumor cells	18	Experimentally, accelerates wound closure, reepithelialization, found in proliferating hemangiomas but not in vascular malformations
Vascular endothelial growth factor/vascular permeability factor (VEGF/VPF)	Endothelial cells	45	Produced in hypoxic tumors (i.e., gliomas) and in psoriasis
Platelet-derived endothelial cell growth factor (PD–ECGF)	Endothelial cells	45	Stimulates endothelial cell migration, produced by fibroblasts, squamous cell carcinoma
Angiogenin	Endothelial cells	14	Unknown
Heparin–binding EGF-like growth factor (HB–EGF)	Smooth muscle cells, fibroblasts	22	HB–EGF precursor binds diphtheria toxin, found in wound fluid
Oncostatin M	Kaposi's sarcoma endothelial cells, inhibits melanoma growth	28	Potent mitogen for Kaposi's sarcoma cells from patients with AIDS
Interleukin–8	Produced by melanoma, stimulates endothelial cell growth, recruits macrophages to tumors	8	May be important for melanoma invasion and metastasis, also possible benefit in other skin cancer

Abbreviations: aFGF, acidic fibroblast growth factor; *bFGF,* basic fibroblast growth factor; *PD-ECGF,* platelet-derived endothelial cell growth factor; *VEGF,* vascular endothelial growth factor; *HB-EGF,* heparin-binding EGF-like growth factor.

(Courtesy of Arbiser JL: Angiogenesis and the skin: A primer. *J Am Acad Dermatol* 34:486–497, 1996.)

Angiogenic Modulators.—The binding of growth factors is dependent on the availability of heparan sulfate receptors anchored to the cell surface by syndecans, a family of proteins. In addition, endothelial integrins are cell surface molecules that mediate alterations in cell shape and attachment to substrates. Integrin inhibitors cause apoptosis of tumor endothelial cells.

Clinical Significance.—Treatments targeting the growth factors important in angiogenesis have great potential in managing various dermatologic disease, including psoriasis, verrucas, and cutaneous malignancies. In particular, corticosteroids or interferon alfa-2a may be useful in treating hemangiomas, and interferons α and β both may be effective against basal cell and squamous cell carcinomas. Further research is needed to examine the contribution of angiogenesis in disease processes and the potential of anti-angiogenic therapy.

▶ The importance of angiogenesis in all types of skin cancer cannot be underestimated. Perhaps through control of angiogenesis we can produce and maintain dormancy in malignant lesions, including melanoma. Although this may require a different thought process for those who achieve "cure" via surgical modalities, it is within the realm of the dermatologic surgical oncologist. Each of us who has large skin cancer practices has a group of patients in whom "control" better explains our treatment regimens. Anti-angiogenic therapy along with other novel treatments may not be far away.

H.T. Greenway, M.D.

Gene Transfer
Slama J, Andree C, Winkler T, et al (Brigham and Womens Hosp, Boston; Harvard Med School, Boston; Agracetus Inc, Middleton, Wis)
Ann Plast Surg 35:429–439, 1995   1–56

Introduction.—Clinical trials of gene transfer methods have expanded to a broad range of disease targets. The principles and techniques of gene therapy technology were reviewed, with particular emphasis on gene transfer to skin and wounds.

Definitions.—The process of gene transfer involves the introduction of DNA or RNA molecules into cells. Current research protocols are limited to germ transfer directed toward somatic cells. Transfer of a gene into a cell can result in the addition of a function or the inhibition of a pre-existing function. Transferred DNA may be stably incorporated into the chromosome of the host cell or may exist as a separate molecule. One strategy (ex vivo gene transfer) involves isolation of cells from the patient, gene transfer to these cells once they are established in tissue culture, and their subsequent re-engraftment into the patient. The in vivo approach does not involve tissue culture or engraftment but requires transfer only to target cells.

Gene Transfer Techniques.—The techniques summarized are viral vectors, chemically mediated gene transfer, electroporation, injection of DNA, and particle-mediated gene transfer. With each of these techniques, it is important for outcome studies that input DNA or cells be accounted for.

Gene Transfer Applications.—The applications discussed include inherited diseases; neoplasia, infectious diseases, and other acquired diseases; systemic diseases; and gene transfer to skin and wounds. Skin is a feasible target for gene therapy because it is easily accessible and has an excellent blood supply. Keratinocyte transplantation back to the host after in vitro culture offers promise in the treatment of dermatologic diseases and in modifying deficiencies or toxicities present in the systemic circulation. For healing wounds, useful proteins could be delivered locally in consistently high concentrations over the treatment period.

Discussion.—Gene transfer in the treatment of diseases is an evolving technique that raises a number of ethical, religious, political, regulatory, legal, and proprietary issues. Current proposals for human gene therapy in the United States require approval by both the Food and Drug Administration and the NIH Recombinant DNA Advisory Committee. Although more than 100 protocols have been approved, the issues raised will take many years to resolve.

▶ New frontiers continue to explode and we cannot expect to practice as we were originally trained in our residencies. The addition of a function or inhibition of a previous function via gene therapy offers excitement in the treatment not only of wound healing but of a variety of other dermatologic indications. "Antisense" and other terms will enter the vocabulary of dermatologic surgeons as we function as cutaneous surgical and medical oncologists.

H.T. Greenway, M.D.

"Pull-through": A New Technique for Breast Reduction in Gynecomastia

Morselli PG (St Orsola-Malpighi Hosp, Bologna, Italy)
Plast Reconstr Surg 97:450–454, 1996   1–57

Introduction.—A new technique for breast reduction in gynecomastia involves pulling the glandular parenchyma through 2 incisions previously made for liposuction. This technique, which has been used successfully in 11 patients, eliminates the incision in the areolar area and its related complications.

Surgical Technique.—The procedure is performed with the patient under general anesthesia. While the patient is still conscious and in an upright position, the area to be treated is marked. After 2 10- to 12-mm incisions are made for the cannula, liposuction is performed with dissection of the parenchyma from a deeper layer. The glandular tissue is mobilized and the pectoral fascia and a thin layer of breast tissue and fat are preserved. With the thumb and index finger, the parenchyma to be excised is pinched and clamped. The instrument is pulled through the incision, the glandular tissue exposed, and the parenchyma excised. Upper and central parts of the parenchyma are pulled through the axillary incision and inferior and central parts through the inframammary incision. A small amount of parenchyma is removed each time to ensure uniform dissection and a smoothly contoured mammary area.

Discussion.—Plastic surgeons attempt to minimize the number and dimensions of surgical scars in breast surgery. With the pull-through technique, only 2 small incisions are required to remove breast parenchyma in patients with fatty glandular gynecomastia. The central esthetic unit of the breast remains intact and complications associated with areolar incisions are avoided. The 11 patients whose experience is the basis of this report have had no complications during 11 months of follow-up.

▶ Tumescent liposuction offers improvement in some cases of gynecomastia, notably the fatty type. The 2 remaining types, glandular and fatty glandular, offer more of a challenge to those dermatologic surgeons performing liposuction. Although it is not mentioned in the article, care must be taken to avoid changes (i.e., dimpling) of the nipple, which can be achieved by remaining 1–2 cm away at depth.

H.T. Greenway, M.D.

Treatment of Nevus Ota by Liquid Nitrogen Cryotherapy
Hosaka Y, Onizuka T, Ichinose M, et al (Showa Univ, Tokyo; Chiba Univ, Tokyo)
Plast Reconstr Surg 95:703–710, 1995   1–58

Background.—Nevus Ota, a dermal pigmentation disorder common in Asians, is caused by an abnormal occurrence of melanocytes within the connective tissue. This disfiguring condition has been treated by carbon dioxide snow cryotherapy, a method that often leaves scarring. Liquid nitrogen is now preferred in Japan because of its ease of handling and its lower temperature during surgery. The techniques of liquid nitrogen cryotherapy and cases of patients who had a deeply situated type of nevus Ota were reviewed.

Patients and Methods.—From 1977 to 1991, 600 patients were treated with liquid nitrogen cryotherapy at 1 Japanese university hospital. The apparatus used was the CRYO-MINI, a portable gun-type device with a variety of tips for different treatment purposes. Application times varied from 2–3 seconds to 9–10 seconds based on severity of the lesion and skin

TABLE 1.—Treatment Response of Facial Pigmented Lesions to Liquid
Nitrogen Cryotherapy Using CRYO-MINI

Type of Lesion	No. of Patients	Results
Nevus Ota	164	Excellent–good
Nevus Ota–like melanosis	15	Good*
Nevus spilus	34	Good–fair†
Blue nevus	12	Good
Senile lentigines	237	Excellent–good
Nevus pigmentosus	138	Good–fair
	600	

*Postoperative pigmentation is more likely to occur than nevus Ota.
†Recurrence of the lesion is frequently observed, and postoperative pigmentation often follows.
(Courtesy of Hosaka Y, Onizuka T, Ichinose M, et al: Treatment of nevus Ota by liquid nitrogen cryotherapy. *Plast Reconstr Surg* 95:703–710, 1995.)

thickness. Shorter times were used for children whose skin was thinner and on sites such as the eyelid; forehead/nose sites and adult skin had longer application times. Local anesthetics helped reduce postoperative pain. Children and apprehensive adults had the procedure under general anesthesia.

Four previously untreated patients had deeply situated type II (moderate) or type III (intensive) nevus Ota. In such cases, repeated applications of liquid nitrogen in combination with dermabrasion often are required. It is important to avoid excessive treatment in the eyelid area. A new technique was developed to desiccate eyelid lesions by electrocoagulation, using a specially designed hair-removing needle.

Results.—Treatment response to liquid nitrogen cryotherapy was excellent to good in the most common lesions, nevus Ota and senile lentigines (Table 1). Patients with deeply situated nevus Ota were a man 26 years of age (Fig 6), a boy 6 years of age, and 2 women, both 21 years of age (Fig 5). Pigmentation was greatly reduced in these patients after a series of cryosurgery sessions.

Conclusion.—Liquid nitrogen cryotherapy minimizes the damage to surrounding skin and reduces scarring. Treatment suppresses the melanin synthesis in epidermal melanocytes and selectively destroys dermal melanocytes. Because results are not apparent at once, treatment sessions are scheduled 4 to 5 months apart so that results of the earlier session can be evaluated. The CRYO-MINI instrument simplifies treatment, but care must be taken to determine optimal application times for each patient.

▶ Cryotherapy was used both to suppress melanin synthesis in epidermal melanocytes and to destroy dermal melanocytes. Although nevus Ota is rare in this country, in Japan and other areas this may be a frequent problem. The use of a disk-shaped copper tip was believed by the authors to be significant and was used in both superficial and deep lesions. I was fortunate during my residency to be exposed to cryosurgery with a variety of solid probes and disks. Like all devices, they have their special place and seem to have been most effective, as judged by the results and photos in this report.

H.T. Greenway, M.D.

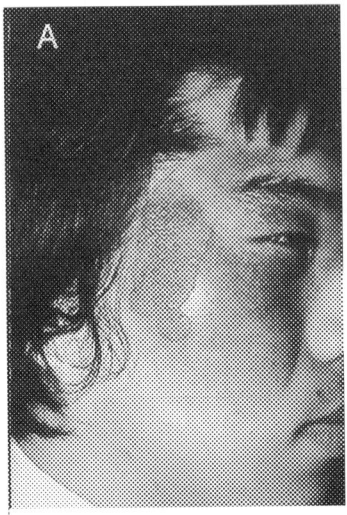
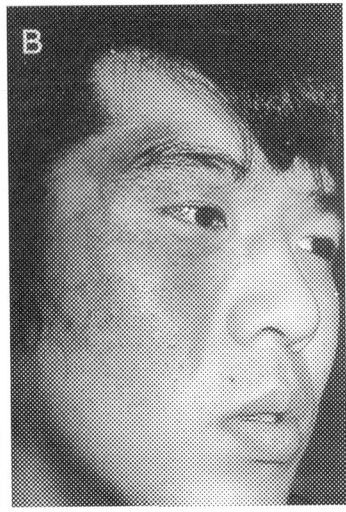
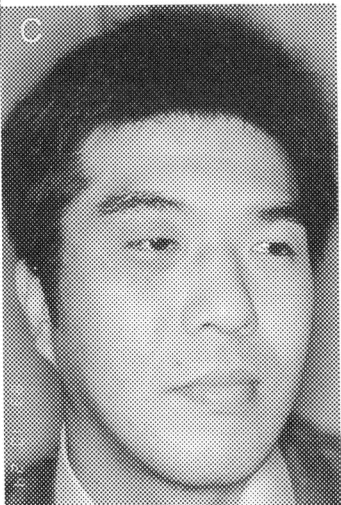

FIGURE 6.—A man 26 years of age with nevus Ota. The distribution of pigmentation was the same as in the patient in Figure 5. **Left,** lateral view showing the bulla formed after trial applications of the cryoprobe. **Center,** lateral view, 3 months after the trial applications. **Right,** lateral view, 2 years and 5 months after the second cryotherapy. (Courtesy of Hosaka Y, Onizuka T, Ichinose M, et al: Treatment of nevus Ota by liquid nitrogen cryotherapy. *Plast Reconstr Surg* 95:703–710, 1995.)

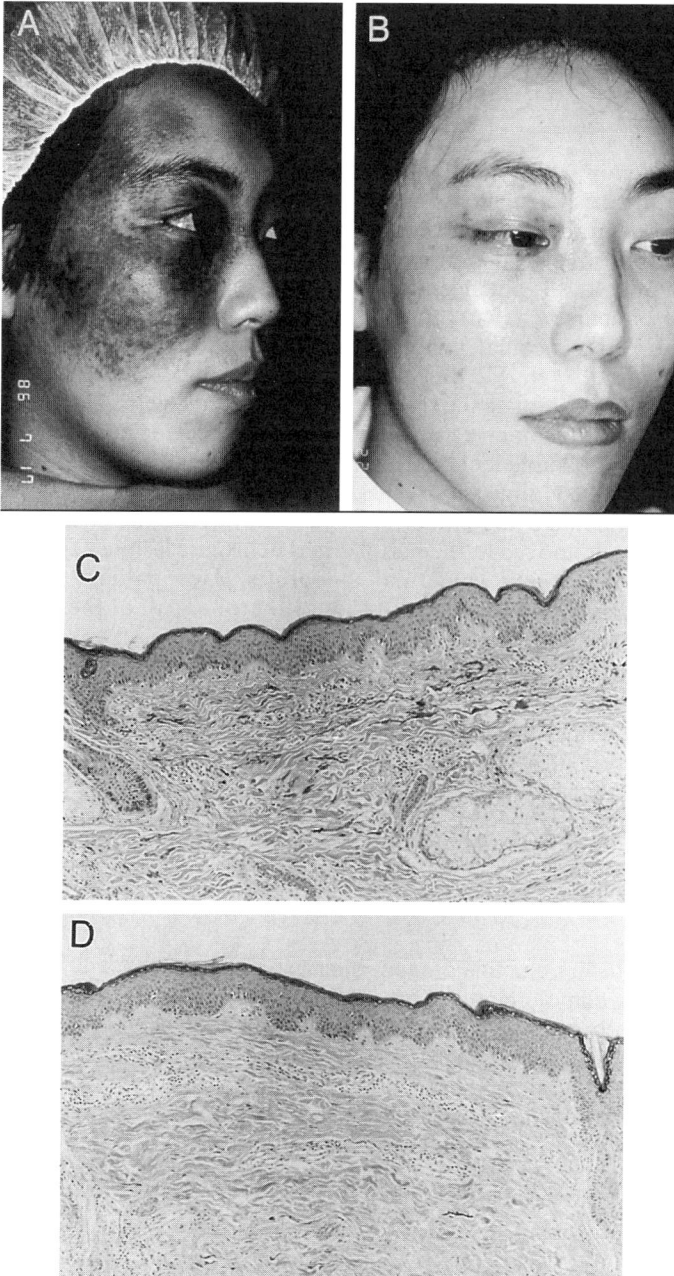

FIGURE 5.—A woman 21 years of age with nevus Ota. The pigmentation spread over the eyelid, forehead, and cheek regions. **Above, left,** lateral view, preoperative. **Above, right,** lateral view, 2 years and 5 months after the fifth therapy. **Below,** biopsies from the periocular region with stain at 100×: **left,** preoperative and **right,** after the fourth treatment. (Courtesy of Hosaka Y, Onizuka T, Ichinose M, et al: Treatment of nevus Ota by liquid nitrogen cryotherapy. *Plast Reconstr Surg* 95:703–710, 1995.)

Surgical Combination Therapy for Vitiligo and Piebaldism

Falabella R, Barona MI, Escobar C, et al (Universidad del Valle, Cali, Colombia; Fundación Valle del Lili, Cali, Colombia)
Dermatol Surg 21:852–857, 1995   1–59

Introduction.—Vitiligo is a dermatosis of unknown etiology characterized by destruction of melanocytes and subsequent depigmentation. Piebaldism is characterized by a white forelock and symmetrical depigmented macules that involve the anterior thorax or abdomen, and the lateral or dorsal trunk, and is a congenital stable autosomal dominant leukoderma. In some patients with vitiligo or piebaldism, melanocyte transplantation may restore the normal pigmentation. The efficacy of additional mini-grafting with 1.0 to 1.2 mm punch grafts during surgical correction of leukoderma to complete the restoration of achromic defects was evaluated.

Methods.—Melanocyte transplantation was performed on 8 patients with refractory stable leukoderma. Five patients had segmental vitiligo, 2 had generalized vitiligo, and 1 had piebaldism. Three patients with segmental vitiligo had an epidermal shave in which the hyperpigmented macules were removed at the periphery of achromic lesions. Three patients had in vitro cultured epidermal autografts. Two patients had suction epidermal grafts. In the areas of residual achromia, all of the patients had additional mini-grafts.

Results.—In 7 patients, the depigmented defects were 100% restored. One patient had 80% improvement. All patients had variable degrees of repigmentation when treated with epidermal grafting, mini-grafting, or in vitro culture autografts. All patients said they were satisfied with the results.

Conclusion.—To restore depigmented defects, surgical methods, followed by additional mini-grafting may be helpful. For routine daily practice, the design of simplified procedures is necessary to restore extensive and refractory leukoderma.

▶ My friends in Columbia present their experiences with a difficult problem that is more common in their practice. The concept of dealing not only with the leukodermic areas but also with the hyperpigmented areas at the periphery of the vitiligo suggests continued refinements in this challenging problem seen daily in practices in certain areas of the world. Repigmentation with cultured melanocytes and the use of cell stimulant growth factors for pigment cells may offer future improvements.

H.T. Greenway, M.D.

Ethical, Medical/Legal Issues

Influence of Specialist Title on Perceived Surgical Ability

Kreidstein ML, Thomson HG, Neligan PC (Univ of Toronto)
Can J Plast Surg 2:149–154, 1994   1–60

Background.—Patients seeking facial surgery may consult a surgeon from a traditional specialty with rigorous criteria for certification, such as a plastic surgeon or otolaryngologist, or a "subspecialist," such as a cosmetic surgeon, aesthetic plastic surgeon, or facial plastic surgeon. Patients may believe that subspecialists are more skilled and may view subspecialists' surgical results more favorably.

Methods.—One hundred thirty patients were selected randomly from a population at a medical walk-in clinic. These participants were given a set of before-and-after photographs showing 6 unrelated facial operations. Each set of pictures was randomly attributed to a plastic surgeon, plastic surgery resident, aesthetic plastic surgeon, facial plastic surgeon, otolaryngologist, or cosmetic surgeon. The study participants completed a questionnaire assessing the quality of the result of each operation. They then indicated which type of surgeon was most likely to achieve the best results for each operation.

Findings.—Most often, study participants felt that cosmetic surgeons were more likely to achieve the best results in rhytidectomy or rhinoplasty. Plastic surgeons were most often selected as best for facial laceration repairs or facial skin tumor removal. Ratings were intermediate for plastic surgeons and otolaryngologists. Aesthetic plastic surgeons and plastic surgery residents received low ratings.

Conclusions.—As expected, subspecialists were perceived by patients as having superior surgical ability. Cosmetic surgeons were believed to provide the best cosmetic procedures, and facial plastic surgeons the best reconstructive procedures. However, study participants' assessments of operative outcomes were not influenced by the type of surgeon credited with doing the procedure.

▶ Mohs surgeons and dermatologic surgeons should look at the information presented in this paper very closely as it certainly applies to our subspecialty. I am still amazed at how many of my patients think it is in their best interest to have a difficult facial skin cancer removed by a plastic surgeon. I think the time has come that we must convey in the much wider range of capacity to the American Board of Medical Specialties, and that our residents probably deal effectively with more facial skin cancers during their period of specialization than do physicians in any other specialty. Furthermore, I believe that Mohs surgeons are the most qualified to deal with facial skin cancers and have made invaluable contributions to reconstruction of facial defects, placing these surgeons in the position of being the most experienced in this area. This by no means implies that we do not seek the assistance of our plastic, surgical, and ear, nose, and throat colleagues in our approach to these patients. We have always and will always accept with open arms their participation. The reverse is not always necessarily true. In my experience, the person who loses most if there is nonincorporation of a Mohs surgeon in the extirpation of a facial skin cancer and in the subsequent reconstruction is the patient. Therefore we have to work very hard to get the word out that we can help. Toward that end, I feel changing the name of our parent board from The American Academy of Dermatology to The American Academy of Dermatology and Cutaneous Surgery is a good first step.

D.J. Papadopoulos, M.D.

Capitation Begins to Transform the Face of American Medicine
Korcok M (Lauderdale, Fla)
Can Med Assoc J 154:688–691, 1996   1–61

Introduction.—Fee capitation can control physicians' fees, the way resources are used, and how physicians and patients relate to each other. In the United States, capitation rewards physicians for doing less and penalizes them for doing too much. Capitation requires physicians to accept a flat, monthly fee per patient. If a patient requires frequent or expensive care, physicians must choose between losing money and denying medical services. Capitation transfers the financial risk of providing health care to the physician.

Capitated Contracts.—Despite the disadvantages of capitation contracts, many physicians are signing them because that is where the patients are. Because of pressure from insurers, employers, and the government, many patients are choosing capitation programs over traditional insurance programs. About 25% of physicians in the United States have some patients covered by capitation contracts.

Discussion.—A recent lawsuit by anesthetists at 3 hospitals in New York against Aetna Life and Casualty Company was 1 of the first legal actions taken by physicians against an insurer on the grounds that it was threatening quality of care. Legal experts say there may be more lawsuits as capitation contracts try to change the way physicians practice and view their patients.

▶ An interesting article concerning how physicians north of the border view the transformation of American medicine from a patient-focus to a cost-focus system. Understanding how managed systems and specific capitation agreements work is mandatory now for both private practice and university physicians. We must be aggressive in trying to take back control of the health care system because we are the ones providing patient care. Furthermore, although there may be negative economic repercussions for our profession in the short run with concomitant "middle men" in the insurance industry making obscene profits, we must never forget that the real loser in the tragedy continues to be the patient. The vast majority of physicians in this country practice ethical, necessary, insurance-dependent medicine. We must continue to be patient advocates, informing them appropriately about what it is that they are paying for in this new climate.

D.J. Papadopoulos, M.D.

The Emotional Impact of Mistakes on Family Physicians
Newman MC (Med Coll of Pennsylvania and Hahnemann Univ, Philadelphia)
Arch Fam Med 5:71–75, 1996   1–62

Introduction.—Literature on the emotional effect of mistakes on physicians is sparse. Randomly selected family physicians were interviewed about the emotional impact of the most memorable mistake of their career.

Methods.—Thirty of 40 physicians contacted agreed to undergo audiotaped hour-long interviews. Physicians were interviewed about the most memorable mistake of their career, the support they needed and received, and how they would respond to a hypothetical scenario (a missed fatal myocardial infarction) involving a colleague's decision that was associated with a fatal outcome. A content analysis of the taped interviews was completed by a physician and 2 sociologists.

Results.—Twenty-three physicians (77%) admitted that they had made a mistake. Five (17%) were unsure of whether they made a mistake, and 2 (7%) said they did not make a mistake. Most physicians admitted that their most memorable mistake took place during private practice and not during residency. They reported that their mistake occurred with about equal frequency in their office as in the hospital. The most commonly identifiable responses to a mistake were as follows: 27 (96%), self-doubt; 26 (93%), disappointment; 24 (86%), self-blame; 15 (54%), shame; and 14 (50%), fear. All except 1 physician stated a need for support: 17 (63%) needed someone to talk to, 13 (48%) needed validation of their decision-making process, 16 (59%) needed reaffirmation of their professional competence, and 8 (30%) needed reassurance of their personal self-worth. Physicians most valued having someone to talk to about their mistakes. Eighteen (67%) reported receiving support from persons other than their colleagues. For 15 physicians (55%), the greatest support came from a spouse. In response to the hypothetical scenario, in which a colleague's judgment was associated with a fatal mistake, all physicians acknowledged the colleague's devastation and all except 1 recognized the need for support. However, only 9 (32%) said they would have been unconditionally willing to offer support to the colleague. Nineteen (68%) physicians said that they would have conditionally offered support only if the colleague were a close friend or partner and only if the colleague solicited support.

Conclusion.—Making career mistakes unfavorably affects the practicing physician and creates a strong need for support. Making mistakes is an inevitable part of practicing medicine. Physicians need to create a community of compassion in which they can share stories and support one another. Further investigation is needed to address how physicians can be encouraged toward therapeutic self-disclosure and peer support.

▶ The information presented in this study could be extrapolated and applied to our own subspecialty. It is inconceivable that mistakes will not happen during the course of our professional career. What is disturbing in this study is that colleagues tended not to support a colleague who had a mistake. This is wrong! All of us know the dictum that "good results come from experience and that, unfortunately, experience comes from bad results." We are human, we consider, we make judgments, and we act. We must accept the fact that mistakes will be made and that if we want to learn from our mistakes and gain valuable experience, we must lend each other support. Unfortunately, the legal climate and competition between us has transformed our honorable professional world into a dog-eat-dog existence. We must find a way to get back what we once were proud of—the collegial sharing of ideas and methods, right or wrong, that move our profession forward.

D.J. Papadopoulos, M.D.

Medical Educators Confront the Future
Marwick C
JAMA 274:1747–1748, 1995   1–63

Introduction.—Medical educators met at the annual meeting of the Association of American Medical Colleges (AAMC) to discuss the response of academic medicine to the contemporary realities of constrained resources and increased accountability that have evolved with managed health care.

Areas of Concern.—Three areas of concern require immediate attention. The first area is information, which will be addressed by the new Center for the Assessment and Management of Change in Academic Medicine. Second, the federal advocacy efforts of the AAMC will be intensified by more involvement of constituents, increased interaction with selected professional organizations and private-stake shareholders, and strengthened public relations. Third, the AAMC will advocate realignment of the size and composition of the physician workforce to meet the needs of society better.

Problems.—The service aspect of medical education is vulnerable as cost becomes the top priority in health care. Nonteaching facilities can outbid medical schools as providers of specific services. Reductions are proposed in Medicare funds, on which medical schools have become increasingly dependent.

Responses.—Agreements between medical schools and for-profit health care chains, such as that recently reached between the Tulane University School of Medicine and Columbia/HCA, offer potential for the teaching facility to gain access to capital and to enlarge its primary care base and research participant base. Such agreements must be considered carefully, however, because the first responsibility of a for-profit entity is satisfaction of its shareholders, not "goodwill" toward the needs of academic medicine. Another option, such as that taken by the University of Pennsylvania School of Medicine, is for the medical school to create its own health care system. The merging of medical schools may also prove financially beneficial, as appears to be the case with the 2 medical schools, 4 university hospitals, 2 community hospitals, the research administration institute, and the community-based physician network owned by the wealthy, not-for-profit Allegheny Health, Education, and Research Foundation of Pittsburgh.

▶ Cost has become the top priority in many, if not all, areas of health care. This perspective reminds us that although "we think research and education are important, most people don't." Dermatology training positions are being reduced, and alliances are being formed. Despite self-developed studies and quality of care assurances, in managed care only cost and geographic availability of services seem to be utmost in importance. San Diego is a center of managed care and was recently referred to as the "Bosnia of US healthcare." Health planners see an excess of more than 2,000 physicians in San Diego alone. Rethinking and retooling may be necessary for each of us.

H.T. Greenway, M.D.

2 Oncology

Introduction

Cutaneous oncology is one of the most exciting and constantly changing fields in all of medicine. The reviews in this section are among the very best peer review publications on this topic in the past year. Oncology is all encompassing because it includes diagnosis, treatment, and rehabilitation. This field of dermatologic surgery is especially gratifying for physicians because the cure rate for most tumors is quite high, and the functional and aesthetic outcome is often excellent. It is critically important to improve techniques that contribute to early diagnosis and better clinical evaluation. Patient care requires the most advanced surgical techniques and therapeutic modalities. We believe the authors included in this section meet those high standards and have contributed significantly to our knowledge and care of our patients.

Duane C. Whitaker, M.D.

Malignant Melanoma

The Incidence of Malignant Melanoma in the United States: Issues as We Approach the 21st Century

Rigel DS, Friedman RJ, Kopf AW (New York Univ; NYU Med Ctr; NYU Melanoma Cooperative Group)
J Am Acad Dermatol 34:839–847, 1996   2–1

Introduction.—The twentieth century has seen a dramatic increase in the incidence rate of melanoma in the United States. The current lifetime risk of invasive melanoma is 1 in 87—an increase of more than 1,800% since the 1930s—and is expected to reach 1 in 75 by the year 2000. Some reasons to regard the increasing incidence of melanoma as real, rather than artifactual, were cited and future trends were predicted.

Discussion.—Although public awareness and surveillance of melanoma have increased, these do not appear to be responsible for the rising U.S. incidence of melanoma. Melanoma rates continue to rise even after removal of earlier-detected cases from the population pool. Also, the incidence of melanoma has been rising in countries other than the United States, including many countries with no organized educational programs. No evidence suggests the apparent increase is the result of better cancer-counting methods, in general—and it may be that the incidence of melanoma is being increasingly underestimated. There has been no change in the histologic diagnostic criteria for melanoma, and the mortality rate has continued to increase despite an increase in overall survival.

Past trends suggest that the incidence of melanoma will probably continue to increase for the next 10–20 years, because the effects of educational programs will not become apparent until then. The demographic characteristics associated with melanoma may change, especially among the young women to whom educational programs have been targeted. Nondermatologists will need educational interventions to enhance their ability to diagnose melanoma at an early stage. Public education programs must be established and appropriately focused. Better diagnostic techniques are needed and, once developed, must be integrated into clinical practice. Finally, better screening programs and more accurate methods of assessing the incidence must be developed and implemented.

Summary.—The increasing incidence of melanoma is real and is expected to continue into the early twenty-first century. Public awareness and early diagnosis are currently the only available means to reduce morbidity and mortality caused by this cancer. Dermatologists should expect to have an increased role in public education about and treatment of melanoma.

▶ This article makes the important point that melanoma incidence is increasing and will probably continue to increase during the next 10–20 years, even if behavior is modified and better sun protection measures are taken. It will be important for dermatologists to play key roles in educating the public, as well as other physicians, and in improving efficacy of screening and diagnostic techniques for melanoma.

D.C. Whitaker, M.D.

Resection Margins of 2 Versus 5 cm for Cutaneous Malignant Melanoma With a Tumor Thickness of 0.8 to 2.0 mm: A Randomized Study by the Swedish Melanoma Study Group
Ringborg U, Andersson R, Eldh J, et al (Karolinska Hosp, Stockholm; Umeå Regional Hosp, Sweden; Sabbatsberg Hosp, Stockholm; et al)
Cancer 77:1809–1814, 1996   2–2

Background.—Traditional surgical treatment for cutaneous malignant melanoma has included wide excision with a 4- to 5-cm margin. However, margins of 1–2 cm have been found to be adequate with thin tumors, suggesting that prospective trials should evaluate the safety and efficacy of smaller margins for the surgical resection of thicker tumors. Therefore, the treatment results of surgical resection of primary malignant melanomas with tumor thicknesses of 0.8 to 2 mm with resection margins of either 2 or 5 cm were compared in a multicenter, prospective, randomized trial.

Methods.—Between 1982 and 1990, 769 patients with cutaneous malignant melanoma and tumors with a thickness exceeding 0.8 mm but less

TABLE 1.—Distribution of Patient Characteristics

	Narrow excision	Wide excision
Age (mean:yrs)	52.3	51.4
Sex		
Male	184 (49.3)	187 (47.2)
Female	189 (50.7)	209 (52.8)
Margin of excision (mean:cm)	2	4.5
Site of melanoma		
Head-neck	6 (1.6)	2 (0.5)
Trunk	204 (54.7)	210 (53)
Arm	47 (12.6)	58 (14.6)
Leg	1.10 (29.5)	118 (29.8)
Data unavailable	6 (1.6)	8 (2)
Total number of patients	373	396

Note: Figures in parentheses are percentages.

(Courtesy of Ringborg U, Andersson R, Eldh J, et al: Resection margins of 2 versus 5 cm for cutaneous malignant melanoma with a tumor thickness of 0.8 to 2.0 mm: A randomized study by the Swedish Melanoma Study Group. *Cancer* 77: 1809–1814, 1996. Reprinted by permission of Wiley-Liss, Inc., a division of John Wiley & Sons, Inc.)

than 2 mm were randomly assigned to resection margins of either 2 cm or 5 cm (Table 1). No patients had metastases or had tumors in the hands, feet, head, neck, or genital areas (Table 2). Follow-up was performed every 3 months for 3 years, then every 6 months for 2 years.

Results.—There was a median tumor thickness of 1.2 mm in both treatment groups. Local recurrences were found in 3 patients in the narrow-excision group and 4 patients in the wide-excision group. The 2

TABLE 2.—Distribution of Tumor Characteristics

	Narrow excision	Wide excision
Histogenetic type of melanoma		
Superficial spreading melanoma	271 (72.7)	289 (73)
Nodular melanoma	40 (10.7)	52 (13.1)
Lentigo maligna melanoma	0 (0)	2 (0.5)
Arcal lentiginous melanoma	5 (1.3)	5 (1.3)
Melanoma in situ	0 (0)	2 (0.5)
Malignant melanoma unclassified	16 (4.3)	12 (3)
Data unavailable	41 (11)	34 (8.6)
Level of invasion		
I	0 (0)	2 (0.5)
II	44 (11.8)	67 (16.9)
III	235 (63)	234 (59)
IV	82 (22)	81 (20.5)
V	1 (0.3)	0 (0)
Data unavailable	11 (2.9)	12 (3)
Ulceration	73 (25)	85 (25.9)
Data unavailable	81 (21.7)	68 (17.2)
Tumor thickness (median:mm)	1.2	1.2
Total number of patients	373	396

Note: Figures in parentheses are percentages.

(Courtesy of Ringborg U, Andersson R, Eldh J, et al: Resection margins of 2 versus 5 cm for cutaneous malignant melanoma with a tumor thickness of 0.8 to 2.0 mm: A randomized study by the Swedish Melanoma Study Group. *Cancer* 77:1809–1814, 1996. Reprinted by permission of Wiley-Liss, Inc., a division of John Wiley & Sons, Inc.)

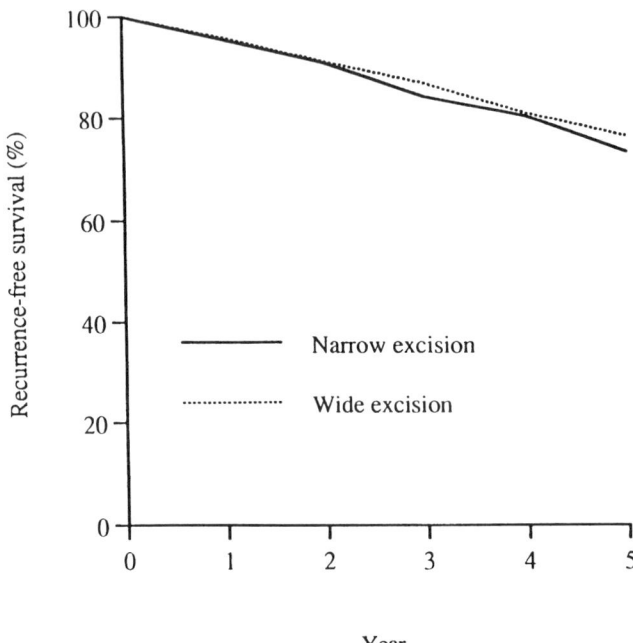

Year

FIGURE 3.—Recurrence-free survival for patients treated with narrow (373 patients) or wide (396 patients) excision. (Courtesy of Ringborg U, Andersson R, Eldh J, et al: Resection margins of 2 versus 5 cm for cutaneous malignant melanoma with a tumor thickness of 0.8 to 2.0 mm: A randomized study by the Swedish Melanoma Study Group. *Cancer* 77:1809–1814, 1996. Reprinted by permission of Wiley-Liss, Inc., a division of John Wiley & Sons, Inc.)

groups were similar for the frequency of regional cutaneous metastases, distant metastases, and deaths. There was a nonsignificantly greater rate of regional lymph node metastasis in the narrow-excision group. There were very similar 5-year rates of observed survival, corrected survival, and recurrence-free survival in the 2 treatment groups (Fig 3).

Conclusion.—A resection margin of 2 cm may be adequate for the treatment of cutaneous malignant melanoma when the tumor thickness is 0.8–2 mm. Longer follow-up is needed to validate these treatment findings.

▶ This is a randomized study with a large number of patients and, therefore, should represent generalizable data for physicians in the United States and worldwide. This publication supports the finding that tumors up to 2.0-mm thickness excised with a 2-cm margin will have similar outcomes to those excised more widely. These data indicate that such melanomas are optimally treated with a 2-cm margin and that there is no justification for wider resection.

D.C. Whitaker, M.D.

Management of Cutaneous Malignant Melanoma by Dermatologists of the American Academy of Dermatology. I: Survey of Biopsy Practices of Pigmented Lesions Suspected as Melanoma
Salopek TG, Slade J, Marghoob AA, et al (New York Univ; State Univ of New York, Stony Brook)
J Am Acad Dermatol 33:441–450, 1995   2–3

Background.—Although the incidence of malignant melanoma (MM) has risen rapidly in the past 50 years, little is known about the role of dermatologists in its surgical management. A survey of the members of the American Academy of Dermatology (AAD) was conducted to determine who performed biopsies of pigmented lesions suspected of being MM, which biopsy technique was used most often, and what factors affected who performed the biopsies and the technique used. Recent changes in biopsy practices and geographic differences were also determined.

Methods and Findings.—All 7,412 members of the AAD practicing in the United States were mailed the questionnaire. The response rate was 40%. Ninety percent of the respondents said they performed the biopsies of pigmented lesions suspected of being MMs. Findings of a 1982 survey were similar. Sixty-eight percent of the current sample and 58% of the 1982 respondents reported using excisional biopsy. Type of biopsy and who performed the initial biopsy of a suspected MM were associated with number of years in practice, type of practice, and whether the dermatologist subsequently performed the definitive surgery for the MM. There were regional variations in biopsy practices.

Conclusions.—Most dermatologists responding to this survey performed biopsies of lesions highly suspected of being MM. A greater percentage of dermatologists are currently performing excisional biopsies than did so 10 years ago.

▶ This study gathered its data via questionnaire to AAD members and, therefore, it is recognized that there may be a response bias in the findings. A clear trend during the last decade indicates that a greater proportion of dermatologists are performing excisional biopsies. Clearly, one factor is the increased training and skills of dermatologists in dermatologic surgery.

D.C. Whitaker, M.D.

Management of Cutaneous Malignant Melanoma by Dermatologists of the American Academy of Dermatology. II: Definitive Surgery for Malignant Melanoma
Salopek TG, Slade JM, Marghoob AA, et al (New York Univ; State Univ of New York, Stony Brook)
J Am Acad Dermatol 33:451–461, 1995   2–4

Background.—Interest and training in dermatologic surgery has been increasing in the past few decades. Data obtained from a survey of American Academy of Dermatology (AAD) members were analyzed to determine who performs definitive surgery for in situ and invasive malignant melanomas (MM), what margins are used or recommended for MMs of different thicknesses, and which factors are associated with definitive surgery and these margins. Changes in the management of MM in the past decade and the possible existence of geographic differences were also investigated.

Methods and Findings.—Of 7,412 questionnaires mailed to AAD members, 40% were evaluable. Sixty-four percent of respondents said they performed definitive surgery for in situ melanoma. This is a substantial increase from a 1982 survey, in which 14% of respondents said they performed definitive surgery in such cases. Although significantly more dermatologists performed the definitive surgery for invasive melanoma in 1992 than in 1982—28% and 14%, respectively—most continued to refer patients to surgeons for definitive treatment. The surgical margins used or recommended for melanomas of all thicknesses have been narrowing in recent years. Regional differences were identified in dermatologists' involvement in the surgical management of patients with MM.

Conclusions.—A growing percentage of dermatologists are involved in the surgical treatment of patients with MMs. Most dermatologists apparently concur with the currently recommended guidelines for surgical margins.

▶ This survey is strong evidence that practicing dermatologists are current and well informed on the surgical treatment of melanoma. It also indicates that members of the AAD have incorporated current knowledge into their practice and their care of patients. This is important information to gather since the AAD has also been a leader in melanoma education and in increasing the awareness of the public that melanoma is a curable disease if diagnosed and treated early.

D.C. Whitaker, M.D.

Melanoma
Rivers JK (Univ of British Columbia, Canada; British Columbia Cancer Agency, Canada)
Lancet 347:803–807, 1996   2–5

Objective.—Among whites, melanoma is the tumor whose incidence is increasing most rapidly. Melanoma is now a major public health problem; mortality may be decreasing, perhaps as a result of earlier detection. Current knowledge about melanoma is reviewed.

Causes and Clinical Features.—Melanoma has been linked to sun exposure, especially exposure sufficient to cause sunburn. However, 20% of cases occur in Africans and Asians and are clearly unrelated to sunlight. Multiple acquired melanocytic nevi are a major risk factor, and risk grows as the number of such nevi increases. Evidence exists for an autosomal dominant melanoma gene. Melanomas can be diagnosed very early, often as a pigmented lesion that grows or changes rapidly. The 3 major features in the melanoma screening checklist are a change in size, color, or shape; the 4 minor ones are inflammation, bleeding or crusting, sensory change, and a lesion diameter of 7 mm or greater. A number of different diagnostic aids are available for early detection of melanoma.

Diagnosis and Staging.—Tumor thickness is the major prognostic factor in patients with localized primary cutaneous melanoma, hence the biopsy should involve complete excision to be certain a complete specimen is available for pathologic review. Tumors representing primary localized disease are designated stage I or II, those with regional lymph node and/or in-transit involvement are stage III, and those with distant metastases are stage IV. The whole of the skin and the regional lymph nodes must be assessed carefully in patients with newly diagnosed melanoma. Abnormal lymph nodes should undergo fine-needle or open biopsy; imaging studies may be indicated for patients with stage III or IV disease.

Treatment.—Early detection and prompt excision of melanomas is potentially curative. Excision margins for localized melanomas have been established, but the need for regional lymph node dissection in patients without clinical evidence of nodal disease is controversial. Adjuvant therapy may be performed to reduce the tumor burden. Dacarbazine has a 20% response rate in patients with stage-IV melanoma, and biologic response modifiers show some activity. Promising developments in gene therapy have been reported as well. Efforts at primary prevention of melanoma focus on reducing sun exposure. Early detection programs involving physician and patient education have also given promising results.

Summary.—The causes, diagnosis, and treatment of melanoma are reviewed. Public health efforts can promote early diagnosis, especially in high-risk patients, thus increasing the chance of cure. Physicians play an important role in informing the public about the dangers of sun exposure.

▶ This article opens with the statement "Melanoma is now the most rapidly increasing cancer in white populations." This article summarizes information known by dermatologists and does not present new information. However, it is succinct and serves an important role in highlighting the dramatic increasing incidence of melanoma in the past 25 years. The article is well referenced. It also reviews primary prevention and early detection strategies that are used in Australia, the United Kingdom and the United States. This is very important reading for nondermatologists.

D.C. Whitaker, M.D.

Carbon-11-Methionine PET Imaging of Malignant Melanoma

Lindholm P, Leskinen S, Nårgen K, et al (Univ of Turku, Finland)
J Nucl Med 36:1806–1810, 1995   2–6

Introduction.—Of all the nuclear medicine techniques studied for this purpose, whole-body [^{18}F]fluorodeoxyglucose positron emission tomography (PET) seems best for assessing the extent of metastatic melanoma. Amino acids and their analogues may be useful for specific imaging of melanoma, and PET imaging with L-[methyl-^{11}C]methionine (^{11}C-methionine) has been successfully used in imaging several types of cancer. A preliminary study of ^{11}C-methionine PET imaging of malignant melanoma is reported.

Methods.—The study included 10 patients with melanoma but no liver metastases. Eight had metastatic melanoma of the skin and 2 had primary melanoma. Carbon-11-methionine PET scanning was performed in all patients before they started treatment for their melanoma. Seven patients underwent dynamic scanning for 40 minutes and the other 3 for 10 to 20 minutes. Scanning was performed 25 to 45 minutes after ^{11}C-methionine injection. The PET findings were compared with those of clinical and imaging follow-up and autopsy.

Results.—The ^{11}C-methionine PET technique detected 22 of 22 melanoma lesions measuring greater than 1.5 cm in diameter. However, it missed 5 smaller areas of pulmonary involvement. The untreated melanoma lesions had average standardized uptake values of 6.3, with an uptake rate (influx constant) of 0.085 min^{-1}. The quality of PET scans was good. They effectively imaged metastatic melanoma of the inguinal and iliac nodes and had no problem in demonstrating tumors close to the bladder.

Conclusions.—The use of ^{11}C-methionine PET scanning for metabolic imaging of malignant melanoma is reported. This technique demonstrates all melanoma metastases measuring larger than 1.5 cm in diameter and may also be of value in measuring in vivo tumor metabolic activity. Predicting the response to treatment on the basis of early changes in ^{11}C-methionine uptake may also be possible.

▶ Positron emission tomography imaging is being used in many centers in the evaluation and follow-up of patients with melanoma. The sensitivity and overall value of imaging is yet to be determined. This study concludes that tumor masses of at least 1.5 cm in diameter will routinely be detected. Though this is helpful, higher resolution, greater specificity, and the ability to detect smaller tumor masses will be necessary to increase the utility of PET imaging.

D.C. Whitaker, M.D.

Prognostic Factors in 1,521 Melanoma Patients With Distant Metastases

Barth A, Wanek LA, Morton DL (Saint John's Hosp, Santa Monica, Calif)
J Am Coll Surg 181:193–201, 1995   2–7

Purpose.—The incidence of malignant melanoma of the skin is increasing rapidly, with 7,200 deaths from metastatic melanoma expected in 1995. However, little prognostic information for patients with metastatic melanoma is available. Variables predicting outcome in patients with melanoma with distant metastases were assessed retrospectively.

Methods.—The analysis included 1,521 patients with American Joint Committee on Cancer (AJCC) stage IV melanoma who were treated at 1 cancer center from 1971 and 1993. The median age was 51 years, and 61% of the patients were male. The patients received a wide range of treatments. Ten clinical and pathologic variables were evaluated as potential predictors of outcome by Cox proportional hazard regression analysis. The review also sought to determine if survival for this patient group had changed over the years.

Results.—Just 2% of the patients had stage IV disease when first seen. The patients had a median survival time of 7½ months and an estimated 5-year survival rate of 6%. Independent predictors of survival were initial site of metastases, disease-free interval before distant metastases occurred, and disease stage before distant metastases occurred. The site of the initial metastases could be used to divide the patients into 3 prognostic groups. Those with cutaneous metastases had a median survival time of 12½ months and an estimated 5-year survival rate of 14%; those with nodal metastases had a survival time of 8 months and a 5-year survival rate of 4%; those with liver, brain or bone metastases had a survival time of 4 months and a 5-year survival rate of 3%. Survival was significantly longer for patients with a disease-free interval before distant metastases of 72 months or longer. Across the 22-year experience, survival rate did not improve significantly.

Conclusions.—Initial site of metastases, disease-free interval before distant metastases, and stage of disease before distant metastases are independent prognostic factors for survival in patients with malignant melanoma. These variables should be taken into account in planning future treatment trials. The last 2 decades have seen no significant improvement in survival for patients with AJCC stage IV melanoma, despite advances in diagnostic imaging and the development of new treatment techniques.

▶ This group reviewed all melanomas seen at their cancer institute during a 20-year period. They then reviewed survival of patients with stage IV melanomas. The authors conclude that median survival for widespread melanoma ranges from 5 to 11 months. Therefore, unfortunately, survival has not significantly improved for patients with advanced melanoma in the past several decades.

D.C. Whitaker, M.D.

Relation Between Size of Skin Excision, Wound, and Specimen

Hudson-Peacock MJ, Matthews JNS, Lawrence CM (Royal Victoria Infirmary, Newcastle-Upon-Tyne, England)
J Am Acad Dermatol 32:1010–1015, 1995   2–8

Background.—Skin wounds generally differ in size and shape from the planned excision, and skin shrinks after excision and fixation. These phenomena suggest possible difficulties in planning closure technique and assessing excision margins, yet they have never been quantified. The size and shape of planned excisions, wounds, and specimens were prospectively compared in patients undergoing cutaneous surgical procedures.

Methods.—The study included 86 patients undergoing excision of 93 benign or malignant skin lesions. All were full-thickness excisions. The length and width of the lesions were measured before excision, and the same measurements were made of the planned excision, the postexcision wound, and the excision specimen before and after fixation. The data were analyzed to determine how the dimensions were affected by patient age and sex and by lesion type and site.

Results.—In 90% of cases, the final wound size was greater than the planned excision size. This was so in all patients, though the effect was greater in young patients and in patients with lesions on the trunk or limbs. The lesions shrunk after fixation—the area of the lesion after fixation averaged 48% of the planned area. Shrinkage was greater for benign tumors than malignant tumors.

Conclusions.—Various factors influence the differences in size between the planned excision size of skin wounds, the postexcision wound, and the specimen size, including patient age and the size and type of the lesion. Wound size does not appear to be equivalent to tumor size, as is often assumed in Mohs' surgery. In addition, measuring tumor clearance margins in fixed tissues does not indicate the true distance between the lesion and normal tissue in vivo. The differences between planned and actual wound dimensions must be considered in planning for wound closure.

▶ Experienced surgeons know that excised tissue shrinks. They also know that freshly excised wounds gape or stretch in size. These authors have attempted to quantify the relation between the size of a wound and the specimen excised. From the standpoint of the reconstructive surgeon, the resultant defect measurement is most relevant. When a specimen is submitted for pathologic examination normally the gross specimen is measured and documented on the pathologic report. In fact, the authors concluded that postfixation specimens shrinks 80%. In cases where the measured surgical margin is required documentation in the medical records, it is important that pathologists and clinicians recognize this discrepancy.

D.C. Whitaker, M.D.

Recommended Width of Excision for Primary Malignant Melanoma

O'Rourke MGE, Bourke C (Adult Public Hosp, Brisbane, Australia)
World J Surg 19:343–345, 1995   2–9

Background.—For many years, wide local excision—with surgical margins of 5 cm or even greater—was recommended for patients with melanoma. However, this recommendation was based on all melanomas as a group, rather than primary early stage melanomas. More recently, narrower excision margins have been recommended for primary malignant melanomas. The authors review the literature and report their experience with limited excision margins for patients with primary malignant melanoma.

Experience.—The authors have been using a limited excision margin—generally 1 cm—for all melanomas since 1975. They have followed this practice regardless of melanoma thickness. Two recent studies have suggested that such narrow margins do not increase either the locoregional recurrence rate or the death rate, compared with wide surgical margins. Recurrence rate is no higher in previously biopsied lesions. Most of the morbidity involves dehiscence of the central part of the suture line, usually associated with hematoma in patients with back wounds. Based on the finding that melanoma invades vertically, the excision is actually more extensive in depth than in width. A wide margin of excision is recommended for satellite lesions, dermoplastic melanoma, and recurrent melanoma.

Discussion.—A surgical margin of 1 cm is recommended for patients with primary malignant melanoma, regardless of tumor thickness. This practice does not increase the recurrence or cure rates compared with the earlier practice of wide excision margins. The authors stress the need for meticulous excision in the operating room, preferably with light general anesthesia.

▶ These authors advocate that all melanomas be excised with a 1-cm margin irrespective of tumor thickness. They state that no difference in local recurrence and no change in death rate occur when these margins are applied. This recommendation, of course, differs from the present guidelines of wider margins for deeper tumors. The recommendations of these authors may prove to be true; however, further long-term studies would be necessary before these recommendations are adopted on a universal basis.

D.C. Whitaker, M.D.

An Estimate of the Incidence of Malignant Melanoma in the United States: Based on a Survey of Members of the American Academy of Dermatology

Salopek TG, Marghoob AA, Slade JM, et al (New York Univ; State Univ of New York, Stony Brook; Univ of Alberta, Edmonton, Canada)
Dermatol Surg 21:301–305, 1995   2–10

Introduction.—The incidence of malignant melanoma (MM) in the United States is increasing by about 4% per year, with a reported incidence rate of about 11 per 100,000. Accurate information on the incidence of MM is needed for several reasons, including evaluation of its costs to the health care system and to society and of the effectiveness of prevention programs. Most patients with MMs are probably seen by dermatologists. Dermatologists were surveyed to estimate the incidence of MM in the United States.

Methods.—All 7,412 members of the American Academy of Dermatology who were practicing in the United States were sent a questionnaire. The dermatologists were asked to estimate the number of new MM cases they had seen in 1982 and 1992, and this information was used to calculate the estimated incidence. There were 2,628 usable responses, a rate of 35.5%.

Results.—The mean number of MM cases seen per dermatologist increased from 6.2 in 1982 to 10.7 in 1992. The number of in situ and invasive MMs increased from 32,000 in 1982 to 80,000 in 1992, calculations suggested. The estimated U.S. incidence rate of MM in 1992 was 32 per 100,000 persons.

Conclusions.—The true incidence of MM in the United States may be higher than previously suggested. Thus the impact of MM on the health care system and on society may be greater than generally thought. The authors suggest some strategies to address the problem of underreporting of MM.

▶ The authors make a strong case that the currently reported incidence of melanoma in the United States is much lower than the actual incidence. The projected incidence rate is 32 malignant melanomas per 100,000 persons. This extrapolates into an actual incidence of perhaps 70,000 to 80,000 MMs per year. This means that a much greater percentage of resources is devoted to detection and treatment of melanoma than is currently known. Future cost for the care of melanoma will probably be substantially greater than other published statistics would indicate.

D.C. Whitaker, M.D.

Management of Stage I Malignant Melanoma
Greenstein DS, Rogers GS (Boston Univ)
Dermatol Surg 21:927–937, 1995   2–11

Purpose.—As the incidence of melanoma rises, dermatologists take on increased responsibility for making complex decisions about its management. Because of the new emphasis on early detection of melanoma, most patients have only stage I disease when their melanomas are diagnosed. The diagnosis, staging, and surgical and other treatments of stage-I melanoma are reviewed.

Diagnosis.—Excisional biopsy should be performed when a cutaneous lesion is suspected of being melanoma. Complete excision permits thorough evaluation of the melanoma, including tumor thickness. Partial biopsy—with punch or incisional biopsy—is sometimes performed to minimize morbidity and does not increase the risk of recurrence or metastasis.

Staging must be accurate to determine the patient's prognosis and plan treatment. Stage-I melanomas are those in which only the primary skin lesion is involved, stage-II melanomas are those involving spread to the regional lymph nodes, and stage-III melanomas are those that have spread to distant sites. The Breslow thickness, as measured from the top of the epidermal granular layer to the maximum depth of the tumor, is the major prognostic factor. The history and physical examination are a critical part of the staging process, focusing on signs and symptoms of metastases. Debate exists over how much additional testing is needed in patients with stage-I melanoma; radiographs and liver function studies may be helpful. More aggressive screening is justified in patients with deeply invasive melanomas, and patients found to have a single metastasis need a complete metastatic workup.

Treatment.—Surgical excision is indicated for most patients with stage-I melanomas and can often be performed as an office procedure. Traditionally, wide excision margins have been used to ensure the removal of microscopic satellites, but the recent trend has been toward narrower margins for lower morbidity. Guidelines for surgical margins based on tumor thickness have recently been reported. Most tumors can be removed with a standard elliptical excision, but the first step is always to measure and draw the proper resection margin. Tumor location determines depth of excision. With narrower margins and adequate undermining, most excisions can now be closed primarily. A multicenter, randomized trial is underway to compare the controversial Mohs micrographic surgical approach with conventional surgery for patients with melanoma.

New treatments for melanoma are always sought, especially for patients with unresectable or high-risk stage-I melanomas. Debate is ongoing as to whether patients with stage-I melanoma should undergo elective lymph node dissection, specifically those with lesions between 0.76 and 4.0 mm in thickness. Many other alternative and adjuvant therapies have been investigated, including hyperthermic isolation limb perfusion, radiotherapy, cryotherapy, chemotherapy, immunotherapy, interferon treatment, and antitumor therapeutic vaccines.

Summary.—The principles of management for stage I melanoma include early detection, accurate diagnosis and staging, and prompt surgical excision. Though various alternative therapies have been proposed, none can yet be recommended for routine use. Treatment must consider the unique characteristics of each patient and tumor.

▶ This is part of a series of continuing education articles regarding the management of melanoma. It presents a very good review with nearly 100 references. It provides a good summary of treatment useful for dermatologists. It also should be of interest to primary care physicians. It does address the controversies regarding elective lymph node dissection that remain unresolved. It highlights some of the latest conclusions on immunotherapy and therapeutic vaccines.

D.C. Whitaker, M.D.

Tumor Vascularity Is Not a Prognostic Factor for Malignant Melanoma of the Skin
Busam KJ, Berwick M, Blessing K, et al (Harvard Med School, Boston; Mem-Sloan Kettering Cancer Ctr, New York; Univ of Aberdeen, Scotland; et al)
Am J Pathol 147:1049–1056, 1995   2–12

Introduction.—Prognostic factors in addition to tumor thickness are sought for patients with cutaneous melanoma. One proposed prognostic variable is tumor vascularity, but studies of this issue so far have been inconclusive. Tumor vascularity was compared in metastasizing and nonmetastasizing cutaneous melanomas.

Methods.—Sixty patients with documented metastases from primary cutaneous melanoma were matched to the same number of patients with primary melanomas that had not metastasized through a mean follow-up of 9 years. The 2 groups were matched for tumor thickness, tumor site, age, and sex. Tumor vascularity was assessed using various vascular markers without knowledge of which group the patient was from.

Results.—Because of its sensitivity and relative freedom from background staining, Ulex europaeus agglutinin I was the best vascular marker. The 2 groups were similar in tumor vascularity, as assessed by either the mean number of microvessels or the highest microvessel count; neither was the tumor vascular pattern predictive of metastases. No significant correlation was evident between tumor thickness and tumor vascularity.

Conclusions.—Tumor vascularity may not be a helpful prognostic factor in attempting to predict the occurrence of metastases in patients with cutaneous melanoma. A larger number of cases must be studied to settle the question, however.

▶ This retrospective study re-evaluates the role of tumor vascularity as a prognostic factor. The study is useful because it examines 60 cases of melanoma that have already metastasized and matches them with nonmetastasizing cases. On this basis the authors felt that vascularity offered no prognostic value. This is a useful finding because clinicians and pathologists continue to search for other features besides tumor thickness that aid in prognostication.

D.C. Whitaker, M.D.

Subungual Melanoma of the Hand

Quinn MJ, Thompson JE, Crotty K, et al (Royal Prince Alfred Hosp, Sydney, NSW, Australia)
J Hand Surg [Am] 21A:506–511, 1996   2–13

Objective.—Although subungual melanoma of the hand has long been recognized, its management and prognostic factors have not been well described. An experience with these rare tumors was described.

Methods.—Thirty-eight patients (24 men and 14 women; median age; 59 years) with subungual melanoma of the hand who were treated at 1 referral center during a 44-year period were included for study. The clinical and histologic features of the tumors were reviewed, along with the patients' treatments and outcomes.

Results.—Most cases involved the thumb. Symptoms had been present for a median of 12 months before diagnosis, and most patients had undergone a previous surgical procedure, most frequently nail avulsion preceding antifungal therapy. Twenty-one patients linked their tumor to a traumatic episode. Twenty-nine patients had ulceration, and 14 of the tumors were amelanotic. The median Breslow thickness was 3 mm; tumor stage was I in 7 patients, II in 22, III in 9, and IV in none.

Definitive treatment consisted of amputation and prophylactic or therapeutic lymph node dissection. On univariate analysis, ulceration and lack of pigmentation were the only significant prognostic factors. The level of amputation—proximal or distal to the interphalangeal joint in the thumb, or the middle of the middle phalanx in the other fingers—made no difference in the local recurrence rate. The median survival was 9 years, with an overall survival of 55% at 5 years and 44% at 10 years.

Conclusions.—Misdiagnosis and delayed diagnosis of subungual melanoma of the hand is common. In their most recent patients, the authors have used selective lymphadenectomy to manage the regional lymph node field.

▶ This article correctly points out both the rarity and difficulty in diagnosis of subungual melanoma of the hand. Such lesions will commonly be seen by primary care physicians, but will ultimately be biopsied and diagnosed by dermatologists or hand surgeons. Because subungual melanomas are rare and present as apparently benign conditions, early diagnosis is difficult. Early diagnosis is further confounded by the fact that nailbed or matrix biopsy may result in a permanent dystrophy.

D.C. Whitaker, M.D.

Cutaneous Melanoma in Women: II. Phenotypic Characteristics and Other Host-Related Factors
Holly EA, Aston DA, Cress RD, et al (Univ of California, San Francisco; Stanford Univ, Calif)
Am J Epidemiol 141:934–942, 1995   2–14

Background.—Melanoma screening of high-risk individuals with certain phenotypic features has been advocated. Although previous studies have identified fair hair and skin and many nevi as high-risk characteristics, the interrelationship of these features and their modification by sun exposure is unclear.

Methods.—A population-based, case-control study was done between 1981 and 1986 in the San Francisco Bay area to identify phenotypic and other host factors associated with cutaneous melanoma in women, after adjustment for sun exposure. Four hundred fifty-two women with cutaneous malignant melanoma and 930 control subjects, aged 25 to 59 years, were included. Interviews were conducted to elicit data on various phenotypic characteristics and medical history. Histologically, 79% of the women had superficial spreading melanoma; 13%, nodular melanoma; and 3%, lentigo maligna melanoma. Five percent of the patients had unclassified melanomas.

Findings.—When all patients with cutaneous melanoma were combined, univariate analysis demonstrated that increased risk was associated with the presence of nevi larger than 5 mm in diameter; light eyes, hair, and complexion; freckles; a history of skin cancer other than melanoma; a history of skin cancer in relatives; and maternal and paternal Northern or Central European ancestry. After adjustment for each other and for sun exposure factors, several phenotypic and host factors were associated with all types of cutaneous malignant melanoma and superficial spreading melanoma. These were large nevi, light hair color, light complexion, and maternal Northern or Central European ancestry. After adjustment for other factors, host factors related to nodular melanoma were the presence of large nevi, light hair color, having ever been overweight by 20 lbs or more, and freckles.

Conclusions.—Melanoma risk is associated with the presence of large nevi, fair coloring, and an ethnic background typical of historically lighter pigmented populations. A history of previous nonmelanoma skin cancer also contributed to a slightly greater risk of cutaneous melanoma. These relationships persisted after adjustment for one another and for sun exposure. The most useful factors for identifying persons who would most benefit from screening and education are number of large nevi, light hair, and light complexion.

▶ This study had a variety of interesting findings and reconfirmed that large numbers of nevi is one of the most consistently correlated phenotypic host factors. The authors found that a host factor of being overweight by 20 lbs or more was associated with nodular melanoma. No theory is offered regarding this association, but this and the other findings suggest interesting avenues for study.

D.C. Whitaker, M.D.

Primary Cutaneous Melanoma: Prognostic Classification of Anatomic Location
Garbe C, Büttner P, Bertz J, et al (Steglitz Med Ctr, Berlin; Fachklinik Hornheide, Münster, Germany)
Cancer 75:2492–2498, 1995   2–15

Background.—Although anatomic location has been identified as a significant prognostic factor in patients with primary cutaneous melanoma (CM), the specific sites associated with high and lower risk have not been established. The prognostic impact of anatomic CM sites was evaluated with multivariate analyses.

Methods.—A total of 5,093 patients with invasive primary CM were examined every 3–6 months for up to 10 years. The anatomic location was classified into 13 sites. Survival probabilities were calculated. Cox proportional hazard analysis was used to determine the prognostic significance of various factors for predicting the increased risk of death from CM.

Results.—Mean tumor thickness varied by anatomic site from 1.83 mm at the lower arm and lower age to greater than 2.50 mm at the scalp, foot, buttocks, and hand. The 10-year survival rates were related to tumor thickness, but not consistently. The univariate 10-year survival rates varied from 63.4% with tumors of the scalp to 87.7% with tumors of the lower arm. In women, the most favorable site-specific survival rates occurred with tumors in the lower arm, followed by the thigh, the buttocks, and the lower leg. In men, the most favorable site-specific survival rates occurred with tumors in the abdomen, followed by the lower leg, the face, and the hand. Using the survival outcome associated to tumors of the lower leg as the baseline, the risk associated with the other anatomic sites was analyzed, controlling for tumor thickness, level of invasion, and sex. The back and breast, upper arm, neck, and scalp (TANS regions) were identified as high-risk sites, whereas the lower trunk, thigh, lower leg, foot, lower arms, hands, abdomen, buttocks, and face were identified as low-risk sites.

Conclusions.—The prognostic significance of anatomic location of primary CM was confirmed, with tumors in the TANS regions identified as the areas of greatest risk. The locations of the low- and high-risk sites suggest that lymphatic drainage may be important factors in determining survival.

▶ These authors analyzed more than 5,000 patients in an attempt to determine if anatomic location of melanomas serves as an independent risk factor. Readers will recall the previous BANS concept as identification of high risk locations. These authors arrive at a different high risk location referred to as the TANS as an independent risk factor. Cutaneous oncologists should be aware of this conclusion, but it will be important to see if the findings can be duplicated.

D.C. Whitaker, M.D.

Intraoperative Radiolymphoscintigraphy Improves Sentinel Lymph Node Identification for Patients With Melanoma
Albertini JJ, Cruse CW, Rapaport D, et al (Univ of South Florida, Tampa; Univ of Texas, Houston)
Ann Surg 223:217–224, 1996   2–16

Background.—There is considerable controversy regarding the surgical management of regional lymph nodes in patients with clinical stage I or II melanoma, particularly those with melanomas thicker than 0.75 mm. However, the ability to identify the first lymph node draining the primary tumor, called the sentinel lymph node (SLN), has led to the use of more limited surgical management of the regional lymphatic basins. Nevertheless, there have been technical difficulties with intraoperative lymphatic mapping procedures that have compromised the reliability of this strategy. The ability to identify all SLNs with a combination of the vital blue dye and radiolymphoscintigraphy with the gamma probe was studied.

Methods.—A total of 106 patients with clinical stage I or II cutaneous melanomas with thickness greater than 0.75 mm were evaluated preoperatively with lymphoscintigraphy to identify 129 lymphatic basins at risk for metastatic disease. All 129 lymphatic basins were biopsied and evaluated intraoperatively with vital blue dye and radiolymphoscintigraphy and with a gamma probe.

Results.—The dual intraoperative lymphatic mapping technique resulted in the identification of at least 1 SLN in 124 of the 129 basins in 102 of the 106 patients. Biopsies revealed metastatic melanoma in the SLNs in 16 patients, of whom 14 underwent elective lymph node dissection of the affected basin. The metastatic involvement was found in 18 of the 25 sampled SLNs and only 1 of the 228 non-SLNs in these patients. The success rate for identification of SLNs was 96% with the use of the combination technique, compared with 80% with the vital blue dye mapping technique alone.

Discussion.—Use of the combined techniques of vital blue dye and radiolymphoscintigraphy and of gamma probe increases the ability to identify SLNs in lymphatic basins at risk for metastatic disease in patients with early-stage melanoma. It is recommended that SLN localization be based on the identification of any node with blue-staining afferent lymphatics draining into a blue-stained node and/or an in vivo gamma probe hot spot-to-background activity ratio of at least 3:1 or an ex vivo SLN-to-non-SLN ratio of at least 10:1.

▶ The authors show that perioperative lymphoscintigraphy, combined with intraoperative use of a gamma probe, and vital blue dye injection identified SLN in 96% of cases. This percent is higher than vital blue dye mapping alone for determination of SLN. The mean follow-up for the study group, however, was 144 days and, therefore, could not demonstrate survival benefits for patients and for the technique as a whole. All melanomas in the study were simply classified as more than 0.5 cm thick with no clinical adenopathy present. Micrometastases were identified in 15% of SLNs. It would be useful for readers if the melanomas were further stratified by thickness.

D.C. Whitaker, M.D.

▶ The findings from these 2 cancer centers (Moffit and M.D. Anderson) add to our continuing to improve our technique for sentinel lymph node identification. My friend and co-author Dr. Merrick Ross (of M.D. Anderson) who completed a research fellowship at Scripps has continued to impress me in this area. We currently believe the need for sentinel node evaluation in melanomas over 1.5 mm thick, no need in less than 1.0 mm thick, and questionable (due to low yield) in 1.0–1.5 mm thickness primary tumors. Of course, the question of improvement of long-term survival is unanswered.

H.T. Greenway, M.D.

Interferon Alfa-2b Adjuvant Therapy of High-Risk Resected Cutaneous Melanoma: The Eastern Cooperative Oncology Group Trial EST 1684
Kirkwood JM, Strawderman MH, Ernstoff MS, et al (Univ of Pittsburgh, Pa; Dana-Farber Cancer Inst, Boston; Morristown Mem Hosp, NJ; et al)
J Clin Oncol 14:7–17, 1996   2–17

Background.—Deep primary melanoma or melanoma that has metastasized to regional lymph nodes is associated with a high relapse rate and poor survival. No adjuvant therapy has been found that can significantly alter this course. However, metastatic melanoma has been shown to respond to treatment with recombinant interferon alpha-2 (IFNα-2). It was hypothesized that treatment with IFNα-2 could have even greater impact if administered as an adjuvant therapy. The efficacy of high-dose IFNα-2 as an adjuvant therapy for the prevention of relapse and death was evaluated in a randomized controlled study.

Methods.—Patients who underwent curative surgery for primary cutaneous melanoma were stratified by disease stage and randomly assigned to either receive intravenous IFNα-2 at a dose of 20 MU/m²/d 5 days per week for 4 weeks and then subcutaneous IFNα-2 at a dose of 10 MU/m²/d 3 times per week for 48 weeks or close observation. The patients were monitored for a median of 6.9 years (range 0.6–9.6 years). The dates of relapses and death were recorded.

Results.—The trial arms were similar for all known prognostic factors. The median duration of relapse-free survival was 1.72 years in the IFN group and 0.98 years in the control group. Median overall survival was 3.82 years in the IFN group and 2.78 years in the control group. The estimated 5-year relapse-free survival rate was 37% in the IFN group and 26% in the control group, and the estimated 5-year overall survival rate was 46% in the IFN group and 37% in the control group. These differences were statistically significant. The impact of therapy was different in the groups defined by disease stage, with the greatest reduction in the risk of relapse occurring in patients with early-stage disease. With multivariate adjustment for other factors affecting outcome, IFN treatment was associated with a 50% improvement in relapse-free and overall survival. Half of the patients required dosing delays or reductions due to toxicity, which was significant, but tolerable, in the majority of the patients. However, 59% of the patients received at least 80% of the target dose of IFN. Most of the treatment withdrawals occurred within 4 months of treatment initiation.

Conclusions.—Maximum-tolerated doses of IFNα-2b administered for 1 year can significantly reduce the recurrence of melanoma and prolong survival by approximately 1 year after curative surgery.

▶ This is the first time an article has clearly documented an effective adjunctive therapy for high-risk melanoma patients. Certainly because of the dosages and side effects, the therapy will actually be administered by our oncology collagues. However, as cutaneous oncologists, we must be aware of those patients to refer for consideration for this treatment. With time I expect the parameters may broaden and even certain node negative medium-thickness primary lesions (not just the current 4.0 mm thickness or greater) may be candidates for adjunctive interferon alfa 2-b.

H.T. Greenway, M.D.

Malignant Melanoma and Pregnancy: Ten Questions
Dillman RO, Vandermolen LA, Barth NM, et al (Hoag Mem Hosp Presbyterian, Newport Beach, Calif)
West J Med 164:156–161, 1996   2–18

Background.—The relationship of melanoma to pregnancy has been of concern for many years. Numerous reports describing the appearance or progression of melanoma during pregnancy have been published. Eight additional patients were described and the literature was reviewed to further explore this apparent association.

Methods and Findings.—The patients, 19 to 40 years, had been previously diagnosed with melanoma while nulligravida. Metastatic disease was then discovered during or shortly after the first pregnancy. The medical literature was analyzed to answer 10 questions on the risk and prognosis of malignant melanoma in pregnancy. This analysis demonstrated no evidence that pregnancy influences risk of melanoma. Also, no evidence suggests that abortion is therapeutic for women with melanoma or necessary to prevent melanoma in the fetus. Though the prognosis of pregnant women with melanoma may be somewhat worse than that of nonpregnant women, the difference becomes nonsignificant when patients are matched for age, location and depth of the primary tumor, and disease stage. Malignant melanoma in pregnant women may be more invasive or advanced because of hormonal or growth factor effects or delays in diagnosis.

Conclusions.—In some women, pregnancy may adversely affect the biologic behavior of melanoma. However, pregnancy termination is not indicated. Melanoma treatment and prognosis are based on disease stage at diagnosis. Because pregnant women with melanoma are more likely to have deeper lesions at diagnosis, physicians must be especially alert to the potential of melanoma and not simply dismiss nevi changes as the result of pregnancy. Women wishing to become pregnant who have been diagnosed as having deeper melanomas and are thus at high risk of recurrence may be advised to defer conception until after 2 to 3 years of disease-free survival.

▶ The authors review 52 references to provide some answers for 10 common questions related to melanoma and pregnancy. Physicians recognize that these answers change over time and different investigators might draw alternative conclusions. This article is meant to be practical and provide some useful information and literature review. It does accomplish those things to a reasonable extent.

D.C. Whitaker, M.D.

▶ Melanoma therapy, management and education, requires a multidisciplinary approach. The head author in this review is Bob Dillman M.D., who formerly was an oncologist in our group at Scripps Clinic before becoming medical director of the Hoag Cancer Center in Newport Beach, California. Dr. Dillman is a most intelligent and caring physician. This is an excellent review and will help us as we confront this problem.

H.T. Greenway, M.D.

Fate of Melanoma Cells Entering the Microcirculation: Over 80% Survive and Extravasate

Koop S, MacDonald IC, Luzzi K, et al (Univ of Western Ontario, London, Canada; London Regional Cancer Centre, Ontario, Canada; John P Robarts Research Inst, London, Ontario, Canada)
Cancer Res 55:2520–2523, 1995   2–19

Background.—Most cancer cells shed from a tumor are thought to be destroyed before they escape the microcirculation; only a few go on to form metastatic tumors. However, recent studies have suggested that most injected cancer cells entering the microcirculation extravasate before undergoing positive or negative growth regulation. A new in vivo videomicroscopy procedure was used to find out what happens to tumor cells after they are injected into the circulation.

Methods.—The study used the chick embryo chorioallantoic membrane (CAM) model, in which fluorescent-labeled B16F10 melanoma cells—either parent or transfectants that overexpressed tissue inhibitor of metalloproteinases 1—were injected into the CAM of chick embryos. Intravital videomicroscopy was then performed to determine how many of the injected cancer cells that reached the CAM microcirculation were still viable in tissue 1 day later, and how many successfully extravasated. Two techniques were used to assess cell survival: injection of 15-μm microspheres with the cancer cells, with comparison of the proportion of viable cells to microspheres before and after injection; and continuous monitoring of individual cancer cells at intervals over the first 24 hours.

Results.—Both the fluorescent labeling studies and the individual cell monitoring studies showed little or no cell loss or destruction in the first 24 to 31 hours after injection. About 80% of cells, either parental or transfected, that originally reached the CAM extravasated within the first 24 hr after injection. The percentage of cells lost in this time was only 11% for the parental cells and 4% for the transfected cells.

Conclusions.—At least in this chick embryo model, most cancer cells that reach the microcirculation successfully extravasate. Thus the inability of individual cells to survive and grow in the target tissue may be an important reason why metastasis is such an inefficient process. Strategies to control the metastatic process may be aimed at regulating tumor cell growth after extravasation.

▶ This study investigated metastatic processes, particularly the fate of melanoma cells after entering the microcirculation. Their findings indicate that a large majority of cells survive the microcirculation. Metastatic processes probably involve a variety of factors; however, regulation of postextravasation growth may be an important component.

D.C. Whitaker, M.D.

▶ Although one cannot completely correlate with the chick embryo model, this is a most interesting study. In my fellowship with Dr. Frederic Mohs, he was (and still is) a proponent of topically applying his zinc chloride fixative to the tumor site before his definitive Mohs excision. He thought the fixative would "fix" any melanoma cells dangling within the microcirculation. Secondly, this article provides insight that control and regulation (and not necessarily 100% cure and elimination) may be important in metastatic disease.

H.T. Greenway, M.D.

Utility of Follow-Up Tests for Detecting Recurrent Disease in Patients With Malignant Melanomas
Weiss M, Loprinzi CL, Creagan ET, et al (Mayo Clinic and Mayo Found, Rochester, Minn)
JAMA 274:1703–1705, 1995   2–20

Introduction.—The follow-up of patients treated for malignancies historically includes frequent evaluation with interval histories, physical examinations, laboratory tests, and imaging studies. However, the value of laboratory or radiologic evaluation has not been conclusively proven. The value of follow-up laboratory and radiologic tests in improving the duration or quality of life for patients with resected melanomas was investigated with the retrospective analysis of prospectively collected data.

Methods.—The records of 261 patients with surgically resected intermediate- and high-risk malignant melanomas were reviewed. The patients had participated in a randomized trial with a follow-up protocol including a history, physical examination, complete blood cell count, blood chemistry panel, and chest x-ray film. Follow-up evaluations were performed monthly for 2 months, then every 2 months for the first year, every 4 months for the second year, every 6 months for the next 3 years, and then annually. The procedures signaling recurrent disease were analyzed.

Results.—Recurrences developed in 161 of the 261 patients. Of the 145 evaluable patients with recurrences, 68% were symptomatic at the time of recurrence. The recurrent melanomas were identified by history in 68% of the patients and by physical examination in 26%. Abnormal chest x-rays signaled the recurrences in the remaining 6% of the patients. Although 11% of the patients had abnormal laboratory studies, these were not the sole indicators of recurrence in any patients.

Conclusions.—Although follow-up laboratory studies and chest x-ray films were performed frequently, recurrent melanoma was detected by physical examination and history alone in 94% of the patients. The local skin and/or locoregional recurrences detected by physical examination are also those most likely to be cured with surgical excision.

► Using follow-up time of 4 years or more, the authors found minimal value in blood analysis and chest x-rays in follow-up of medium-and high-risk melanomas. This is a useful study and probably is not surprising to physicians who treat and follow-up patients with melanoma. This type of study, when replicated, can modify guidelines and the standard of care for patients with melanoma. Such modifications can ultimately decrease cost and prevent the patient from being exposed to unnecessary tests.

D.C. Whitaker, M.D.

▶ Within the last year as part of my initial metastatic workup of my new melanoma patients, I have diagnosed a primary lung carcinoma in two patients via their chest x-ray examination. Surgery for each was curative with no evidence of metastasis in either case. So while I can agree regarding follow-up, at least my initial metastatic evaluation includes a chest x-ray examination even in patients with thin primary melanomas.

H.T. Greenway, M.D.

The Prognosis and Treatment of True Local Cutaneous Recurrent Malignant Melanoma
Brown CD, Zitelli JA (Dallas)
Dermatol Surg 21:285–290, 1995   2–21

Background.—The prognosis of and optimal therapy for true local cutaneous recurrent malignant melanoma have not been established, partly because of ambiguity in definitions of local recurrence. The current authors defined this entity as melanoma with an in situ component recurring contiguous with the scar of the primary excision. The authors then hypothesized that the prognosis of true local cutaneous recurrent melanoma may differ from that of local recurrence from satellite or in-transit metastases.

Methods and Findings.—Fifty patients with true local recurrent melanoma were studied. The surgical margin needed to reach a tumor-free plane using Mohs surgery was calculated, and patient survival was determined. Complete excision of 76% of the tumors was possible with a margin of less than 1 cm. However, to treat all patients successfully, a margin of up to 2 cm was needed. Significantly larger margins were needed to treat thicker tumors. In a Kaplan-Meier analysis, the 5-year overall survival rate was 89%, and the 5-year melanoma survival rate was 98%. Disease-free survival at 5 years was 66%.

Conclusions.—The prognosis of true local recurrent melanoma depends on the thickness of the tumor. A full-thickness excision of the entire previous scar is recommended, including a 2-cm margin or Mohs surgery if a narrower resection margin is desired.

▶ This is a well thought-out retrospective study of 50 patients with melanoma. This investigation distinguishes true local recurrent melanoma from local metastases and lymphatic spread. Distinguishing between the two is clearly important. The recommendations given are based on good data.

D.C. Whitaker, M.D.

▶ As Whitaker states, good data and recommendations can be found in this article. However, is a tumor at a few months "recurrent" or "residual"? Fifty patients in 9½ years with local recurrence seems an awful high number. Then again, my friend and colleague, Dr. John Zitelli, is well known for his great work and has a referral practice.

H.T. Greenway, M.D.

Multiple Primary Melanomas: Data and Significance
Ariyan S, Poo W-J, Bolognia J, et al (Yale Univ, New Haven, Conn)
Plast Reconstr Surg 96:1384–1389, 1995   2–22

Background.—A second primary melanoma will develop in about 5% of patients with primary cutaneous melanoma. Patients with multiple primary melanomas were studied to determine the thickness of these subsequent cutaneous malignancies, their location, and the prognosis.

Methods and Findings.—Twenty-seven patients with a total of 59 individual primary melanomas were studied. A second primary tumor developed in 22 patients, and a third developed in 5. Second malignancies were diagnosed within 1 month of the first malignancy in 8 patients and were considered synchronous. Of the remaining 24 second melanomas, 4 were discovered in the first year, 7 in the second year, and 13 thereafter. The thickness of the first melanoma ranged from 0.2 to 6 mm, whereas all subsequent melanomas were in situ or less than 1-mm thick. The presence of multiple melanomas did not affect prognosis.

Conclusions.—In this series, all patients with subsequent melanomas had thin second lesions. The prognosis of patients with multiple primary melanomas did not differ from their original prognosis.

▶ This study is interesting because it interprets data from patients with 2 or more primary melanomas. The authors conclude that the patients' prognoses are reflected in the thickest melanoma. They suggest that the prognosis is not worsened purely by the existence of multiple primaries.

D.C. Whitaker, M.D.

Treatment of Patients With Melanoma of the Extremity Using Hyperthermic Isolated Limb Perfusion With Melphalan, Tumor Necrosis Factor, and Interferon Gamma: Results of a Tumor Necrosis Factor Dose-Escalation Study
Fraker DL, Alexander HR, Andrich M, et al (Natl Cancer Inst, Bethesda, Md; NIH, Bethesda, Md)
J Clin Oncol 14:479–489, 1996   2–23

Background.—In patients with extremity melanoma undergoing isolated limb perfusion (ILP), the addition of high-dose tumor necrosis factor (TNF) and low-dose interferon gamma (IFN) to melphalan reportedly improves response rates. Response rates and toxicity of hyperthermic ILP using escalating-dose TNF, melphalan, and IFN in patients with in-transit metastases of extremity melanoma were reported.

Methods.—Thirty-eight patients participated in 2 trials. All received IFN, 0.2 mg² for 2 days, followed by a 90-minute ILP with TNF and IFN given at time 0 and melphalan at 30 minutes. Twenty-six patients received 4 mg of TNF, and 12, 6 mg of TNF. All but 2 patients were evaluated 1 month after therapy.

Findings.—The patients receiving 4 mg of TNF had a mean peak perfusate TNF level of 4.8 µg/mL. Those receiving 6 mg had a mean level of 7.4 µg/mL. Seventy-six percent of the patients given 4 mg TNF had a complete response, compared with 36% given 6 mg. The overall objective response rates in the 2 groups were 92% and 100%, respectively. Differences in disease burden or previous regional treatment did not account for the lower complete response rates in the group given 6 mg. Systemic drug toxicity, related more to perfusate leak than to TNF perfusate dose, was short-lived and managed easily. Patients receiving the 6 mg dose had greater regional toxicity, especially myopathy and neuropathy, which was considered dose-limiting.

Conclusions.—In most patients with extremity melanoma, ILP with 4 mg of TNF, INF, and melphalan results in complete local response. Increasing the TNF dose to 6 mg resulted in increased regional toxicity and did not improve the complete response rate.

▶ This National Cancer Institute study found complete local response combining TNF and melphalan in ILP therapy for melanoma. Their findings may be applicable to certain patients with clinical stage III or IV disease.

D.C. Whitaker, M.D.

Screening for Cutaneous Melanoma by Skin Self-Examination
Berwick M, Begg CB, Fine JA, et al (Yale Univ, New Haven, Conn; Mem Sloan-Kettering Cancer Ctr, New York; Cancer Prevention Research Inst, New York)
J Natl Cancer Inst 88:17–23, 1996   2–24

Background.—Some evidence suggests that early detection of cutaneous melanoma helps prevent the development of lethal disease. The value of skin self-examination in reducing the risk of lethal melanoma was investigated in a population-based, case-control study.

Methods.—A structured questionnaire was administered and personal interviews conducted to elicit data on participants' performance of careful, deliberate, purposeful examinations of the skin. A total of 1,199 white Connecticut residents were included. Six-hundred fifty had recently been diagnosed as having cutaneous melanoma. The healthy subjects were frequency-matched by age and sex. Nevi on the arms and backs of the participants were counted during the interviews. One-hundred ten lethal cases of melanoma occurred during 5 years of follow-up.

Findings.—Only 15% of all subjects performed skin self-examinations. However, self-examination was associated with a decreased risk of melanoma incidence. Self-examination also appeared to reduce the risk of advanced disease among patients with melanoma. However, longer follow-up is needed to confirm this latter finding. If these estimates are correct, skin self-examination may reduce by 63% the rate of death caused by melanoma.

Conclusions.—Skin self-examination may be a beneficial screening method for decreasing the incidence of melanoma and the development of advanced disease. Further research is needed to replicate these findings.

▶ Skin self-examination is recommended by many dermatologists and is usually an integral part of the management of patients with dysplastic nevi. This study provides some data supporting the efficacy of self-examination. However, the authors appropriately recommend that further study be done before strategies to increase the practice of self-examination are promoted further.

D.C. Whitaker, M.D.

Favorable Prognostic Factors in Recurrent and Metastatic Melanoma

Buzzell RA, Zitelli JA (Southern Illinois Univ, Springfield; Shadyside Med Ctr, Pittsburgh, Pa)

J Am Acad Dermatol 34:798–803, 1996   2–25

Background.—The prognosis of recurrent and metastatic melanoma varies greatly. Improved survival is correlated with several clinical and pathologic factors. A knowledge of these factors is useful for patient counseling and identifying candidates for more aggressive treatments.

Prognostic Factors.—Patients with true local recurrences from insufficient excision of the primary tumor have an excellent chance for long-term survival after re-excision. Prognosis in these patients is related to features of the primary tumor, such as thickness and level of invasion. Local

TABLE 3.—5 Year Survival Rates of Patients With Melanoma and Regional Lymph Node Metastases Based on Thickness of the Primary Tumor

| | Primary tumor thickness | |
Authors	<3 mm	>3 mm
Callery et al.[25]	49%	18%
Day et al.[34]	59%*	22%*
Roses et al.[36]	56%	24%

*Day et al. used ≤ 3.5 mm.
(Courtesy of Buzzell RA, Zitelli JA: Favorable prognostic factors in recurrent and metastatic melanoma. *J Am Acad Dermatol* 34:798–803, 1996.)

TABLE 4.—Survival of Melanoma Patients With Systemic Metastases
After Complete Metastasectomy

| | Median survival (mo) | |
Authors	Nonvisceral*	Visceral
Ryan, Kramar, Borden[54]	7.2	2.8†
Amer, Al-Sarraf, Vaitkevicius[55]	14‡	1.8‡
Karakousis et al.[58]	16§	2
Balch et al.[60]	8	3
Sirott et al.[69]	8	4.7†

*Skin, subcutaneous tissue, or nonregional lymph nodes.
†Mean survival.
‡Skin metastases.
§Liver metastases.
(Courtesy of Buzzell RA, Zitelli JA: Favorable prognostic factors in recurrent and metastatic melanoma. *J Am Acad Dermatol* 34:798–803, 1996.)

recurrences from tumor metastasis are usually correlated with systemic disease and 5-year survival rates of only about 33%, similar to those in patients with lymph node involvement. Patients with regional lymph node metastases have a survival advantage when only 1 lymph node is involved and the primary tumor is thin (and especially if located on an extremity). Overall, the 10-year survival among patients with regional lymph node metastases is 33%. Although long-term survival in patients with systemic melanoma is less common, a better prognosis is seen in patients with solitary and nonvisceral metastases. Also, several studies have shown that survival may be prolonged in 25% of patients with disease amenable to aggressive surgical metastasectomy (Tables 3 and 4).

Conclusions.—Although the ability to predict survival among patients with recurrent and metastatic malignant melanoma is limited, several useful prognostic factors have been identified. The outlook for such patients is improving.

▶ This useful article differentiates prognoses among patients with metastatic melanoma. Although the prognosis is usually grave, the length of survival is variable. The authors also point out that survival of patients with true local recurrence corresponds to the characteristics of thickness of primary tumor. The information included in this paper may help patients and their families better gauge the length of survival.

D.C. Whitaker, M.D.

Cutaneous Malignant Melanoma and Sun Exposure: Recent Developments in Epidemiology
Katsambas A, Nicolaidou E (Univ of Athens, Greece)
Arch Dermatol 132:444–450, 1996   2–26

Purpose.—Around the world, the incidence of malignant melanoma among white populations is increasing rapidly. There is an urgent need to identify the most important risk factors for this disease. Sun exposure is one major risk factor, but the link between sun exposure and malignant melanoma is a complex one. The epidemiologic evidence regarding the association between sun exposure and malignant melanoma was reviewed.

Latitude of Residence.—Melanoma becomes more frequent with increasing proximity to the equator in countries with homogeneous and fair-skinned populations, such as Scandinavia. Because of pigmentation differences, however, the mortality from melanoma is much higher in Scandinavia than in the Mediterranean countries. Thus, the influence of latitude on melanoma incidence can only be assessed in homogeneous populations. The anatomical distribution of melanomas does not always correspond to the level of sun exposure of different skin areas.

Sun Sensitivity.—Skin and hair color are recognized risk factors for melanoma. Still, not all studies have confirmed the association between these pigmentation traits and disease. Melanoma risk is increased for people who get sunburned easily and do not tan. These factors are closely correlated with pigmentation, and it is difficult to separate their effects. The number of sunburns sustained is not always found to be related to melanoma, however.

Patterns of Sun Exposure.—Attempts to assess lifetime sun exposure have given inconsistent results, and some aspects of the epidemiology of melanoma cannot be explained by total lifetime sun exposure. Such findings have led to the hypothesis that melanoma risk is affected by intermittent episodes of intense sun exposure to previously unexposed skin, such as that occurring during vacations. Both intermittent and cumulative exposure appear to play a pathogenetic role in melanoma. Intermittent exposure may be associated with superficial spreading melanomas occurring on areas not usually exposed to the sun, whereas lentigo maligna melanomas occurring on the face and other sun-exposed areas may be related more to constant exposure.

Childhood Sun Exposure.—Melanoma risk may be greatly affected by sun exposure during childhood and adolescence. It has been suggested, although not proven, that a history of sunburn in childhood increases the risk of melanoma. The link between increased sun exposure in childhood and melanoma may be related to the greater numbers of common melanocytic nevi observed in children with high levels of sun exposure. Freckling is an independent risk factor, whether as a marker of skin sensitivity or sun exposure.

Conclusions.—Epidemiologic evidence on the complex associations between sun exposure and risk of malignant melanoma was reviewed; and, on balance, it suggests that children, individuals who are sensitive to the sun, and those individuals with a history of intermittent, intense sun exposure are at increased risk. These groups have a special need to protect themselves against sun exposure.

▶ This thoughtful paper tries to make sense of etiologic factors in melanoma such as underlying skin type, density of nevi, timing of sun exposure, and others. Even though the causal relationships are far from being fully understood, these authors suggest that intermittent exposure may be the most dangerous to sun-sensitive individuals. This is one more area of protection about which we can counsel our patients.

D.C. Whitaker, M.D.

Does Palpability of Primary Cutaneous Melanoma Predict Dermal Invasion?

O'Donnell BF, Marsden JR, O'Donnell CA, et al (Gen Hosp, Birmingham, England; Univ College, Dublin)

J Am Acad Dermatol 34:632–637, 1996   2–27

Background.—Few researchers have investigated whether histologic melanoma thickness can be predicted accurately by clinical estimations of thickness by palpation. If palpability could reliably predict dermal invasion, it would be useful for determining surgical margins.

Methods.—One hundred sixty-five patients with melanoma were studied. One clinician classified the melanomas as flat, just palpable, palpable, or nodular. These classifications were then compared with histologic measures of tumor thickness.

Findings.—Overall, the degree of palpability was well correlated with the presence or absence of dermal invasion, Breslow thickness, and Clark level. However, there was a weaker correlation between palpability and Breslow thickness for invasive melanomas less than 1-mm thick. Also, elevation and Clark level were not significantly associated with invasive melanomas of less than 4-mm thick (Table 3)

Conclusion.—Melanoma palpability is not an adequate predictor of the presence or absence of dermal invasion or degree of dermal invasion. Thus, this criterion cannot be used to determine surgical margins.

TABLE 3.—Mean and Median Breslow Thicknesses, Median Clark Levels, and Their Ranges for All Melanomas and for Invasive Melanomas

	Breslow thickness (mm)			Clark level	
	Mean	Median	Range	Median	Range
All melanomas					
Flat	0.2	0	0–1	I	I–IV
Just palpable	0.39	0.3	0–1.3	II	I–IV
Palpable	1.03	0.85	0–3.8	IV	I–V
Nodular	4.25	3.2	1.5–12	IV	II–V
Invasive melanomas					
Flat	0.49	0.45	0.2–1	II	II–IV
Just palpable	0.58	0.57	0.15–1.3	III	II–IV
Palpable	1.18	0.9	02.–3.8	IV	II–V
Nodular	4.25	3.2	1.5–12	IV	II–V

(Courtesy of O'Donnell BF, Marsden JR, O'Donnell CA, et al: Does palpability of primary cutaneous melanoma predict dermal invasion? *J Am Acad Dermatol* 34:632–637, 1996.)

▶ This article reminds us that we cannot be certain of diagnosis or depth by clinical examination. Therefore, trying to perform definitive surgery at the time of diagnosis is very risky. Pigmented lesions should be biopsied to establish diagnosis. Definitive surgery with appropriate margins should be performed after melanoma thickness is determined.

D.C. Whitaker, M.D.

Interobserver Variability on the Histopathologic Diagnosis of Cutaneous Melanoma and Other Pigmented Skin Lesions

Corona R, Mele A, Amini M, et al (Istituto di Ricovero E Cura A Carattere Scientifico, Rome; Ospedale S Giovanni, Rome; Ospedale di Viterbo, Italy; et al)

J Clin Oncol 14:1218–1223, 1996   2–28

Background.—Histopathologic microstaging is critical in patients with primary melanoma, as some histologic features are strong predictors of prognosis and essential for guiding treatment. Thus assessing interobserver agreement on the diagnosis and classification of cutaneous melanoma is important.

Methods and Findings.—Four experienced histopathologists assessed 140 slides of cutaneous melanoma, including a small number of benign pigmented skin lesions. For the diagnosis of cutaneous melanoma vs. benign lesions, the kappa value was 0.61. Some discordance in the diagnosis occurred in 26% of the cases. The greatest kappa values for the histologic classification of cutaneous melanoma were obtained for Breslow thickness and presence of ulceration. For other histologic features, such as

TABLE 4.—Interobserver Agreement on the Histopathologic Classification of Cutaneous Melanoma

Histologic Feature	No. of Cases	Proportion in Agreement	Kappa	SE	95% CI of Kappa
Ulceration	75	0.95	0.87	0.047	0.78–0.97
Breslow thickness (mm)	75	0.82	0.76	0.025	0.71–0.81
Histologic type	78	0.75	0.55	0.035	0.48–0.62
Cross–sectional profile	78	0.67	0.54	0.028	0.49–0.59
Nevus association	77	0.88	0.50	0.041	0.42–0.58
No. of mitoses/mm^2*	31	0.66	0.44	0.096	0.25–0.63
Mitotic activity	76	0.72	0.41	0.047	0.32–0.50
Level of invasion (Clark)	80	0.55	0.38	0.027	0.33–0.43
Vascular invasion	80	0.71	0.29	0.036	0.22–0.36
Lymphocytic infiltration	80	0.54	0.27	0.033	0.21–0.33
Regression	76	0.79	0.22	0.043	0.14–0.30
Cell type	81	0.33	0.19	0.022	0.15–0.23
Neural infiltration	77	0.90	0.06	0.037	−0.01–0.13

*Data based on only 3 observers.

(Courtesy of Corona R, Mele A, Amino M, et al: Interobserver variability on the histopathologic diagnosis of cutaneous melanoma and other pigmented skin lesions. *J Clin Oncol* 14:1218–1223, 1996.)

level of dermal invasion, presence of regression, and lymphocytic infiltration, agreement was generally poor (Table 4).

Conclusions.—The reliability of histologic diagnosis and classification of cutaneous melanoma needs to be improved. The inconsistencies among pathologists' assessments are probably the result of the lack of universally accepted criteria and the diagnostic difficulties associated with the initial, thin melanoma.

▶ The investigators recommend that 2 pathologists independently examine pigmented lesions with a third adjudicating when there is a discrepancy. The table indicates that approximately 20% of the time, there is disagreement regarding Breslow thickness. As dermatologic surgeons, we may need to request secondary pathologic review in cases of melanoma or suspected melanoma.

D.C. Whitaker, M.D.

Intraobserver Agreement in Interpretation of Digital Epiluminescence Microscopy

Stanganelli I, Burroni M, Rafanelli S, et al (Santa Maria delle Croci Hosp, Ravenna, Italy; Romagna Cancer Registry, Forlì, Italy)
J Am Acad Dermatol 33:584–589, 1995   2–29

Introduction.—It has been suggested that epiluminescence microscopy (ELM) can aid in the diagnosis of pigmented skin lesions and reduce the need for biopsy in some cases. However, few studies have correlated ELM and histologic findings. Additionally, standard classification criteria for ELM have not been established. An attempt was made to establish defined ELM variables and descriptors and assess the ability to report consistent findings in melanocytic lesions using these criteria.

Methods.—The published literature on ELM of pigmented skin lesions was reviewed and a list of all ELM variables and descriptors was compiled. A series of digital (D)-ELM images were selected based on 3 essential ELM criteria. These images were classified by 1 investigator using 44 selected descriptors and, 2 months later, evaluated again by a second investigator. A third investigator assessed both investigators' findings for intraobserver agreement. For each descriptor assessed, the percentage of agreement and the value for agreement were calculated.

Results.—For all descriptors, a median value of 0.66 was calculated. For the 4 classification systems used, no significant difference in the distribution of the values for individual descriptors was found. Median values for the 4 classification systems used were 0.67, 0.66, 0.61, and 0.66 for the B classification (using 15 descriptors), S classification (10 descriptors), K classification (22 descriptors), and the PS classification (22 descriptors), respectively. Descriptors of present/absent were found to have the highest reproducibility (median = 0.77). Descriptors of distribution, pigmentation, or of width, thickness, and size were found to have lower values (0.77, 0.21, 0.39, respectively).

Conclusion.—With the exception of present/absent descriptors, most of the ELM descriptors had moderate-to-poor agreement. These descriptors associated with moderate-to-poor agreement are likely to be descriptors that are more poorly defined.

▶ These investigators looked at the question of whether one ELM observer would agree with his interpretation of a lesion when viewing the same image 2 months later. High levels of intraobserver variance were found, i.e., an observer may rate the same image differently when viewed at a different time. The highest variability occurred when more complex judgments, i.e., more than the simple presence or absence of a characteristic was required. These findings are a reminder that ELM is a clinical technique that may prove to be useful but is subject to the variability of other clinical observations.

D.C. Whitaker, M.D.

Cutaneous Melanoma and Atypical Spitz Tumors in Childhood
Barnhill RL, Flotte TJ, Fleischli M, et al (Harvard Med School, Boston)
Cancer 76:1833–1845, 1995   2–30

Introduction.—The rarity of malignant melanoma in childhood compounds the difficulty of discovering its biology and natural history. Most reports on this disease have not been population-based and are characterized by significant referral bias. The tumors in many series have not been subjected to careful histopathologic analysis and microstaging. There is a lack of objective criteria for the distinction between Spitz nevi and melanoma. Because of this, some reports have included only melanomas associated with metastasizing melanomas. Reported are the histopathologic descriptions of 23 childhood melanomas and atypical Spitz tumors.

Methods.—Records from 1959 to 1995 of patients with cutaneous malignant melanoma up to age 15 at time of diagnosis were reviewed retrospectively for: demographics, anatomical site of primary melanoma or tumor, presence and location of recurrences or metastases, follow-up, interval to metastases and death, and histopathological parameters. Complete records and microscopic slides were available for 23 patients who met criteria for inclusion.

Results.—Mean patient age of 11 males and 12 females was 9.4 years. The tumors were categorized histopathologically into 4 subgroups: 1) 5 small cell melanoma; 2) 6 adult-like melanoma; 3) 3 Spitz-like melanoma; and 4) 9 atypical Spitz tumor.

The small-cell variant was localized exclusively to the scalp and was associated with a highly aggressive course. These tumors contained a significant component of relatively small cells with oval or round nuclei. Cytoplasm was scant and was usually disposed in sheets. One melanoma developed in association with a congenital nevus, with diffuse infiltration of the entire reticular dermis by nevus cells in an interstitial pattern. It principally involved the reticular dermis with deep extension into subcutaneous fat.

The adult variants were similar to typical tumors occurring in adults. Generally, the cell type was a spindled pleomorphic cell with scant cytoplasm. Hyperchromatism was commonly exhibited by the nuclei.

The Spitz-like variant was defined by an epithelioid cell type resembling the cells in Spitz nevi and a clinical course of metastases. The one death in this subset was from a melanoma that developed on the neck of a boy, age 15 years. The 2 other patients developed lymph node metastases, but were alive at 3 and 9 year follow-up, respectively.

The 9 atypical Spitz tumors were initially diagnosed as malignant melanoma, but were judged to have features insufficient for unequivocal melanoma upon review. These tumors were characterized by significant thickness and abnormal features, including prominent cellularity and mitotic activity. Generally, most tumors were enlarged with abundant ground-glass cytoplasm and angular contours.

Conclusion.—The small cell variant is a potentially unique subtype of childhood melanoma. It appears that the Spitz-like melanomas are vanishingly rare. The anatomical site, cell type, and tumor thickness may be crucial prognostic factors for childhood melanoma. These preliminary findings need to be buttressed by further investigation.

▶ Spitz nevi in children often present challenging diagnostic and management difficulties. This thoughtful analysis looks at both Spitz-like melanomas as well as atypical Spitz tumors. Although the majority of Spitz nevi behave benignly, the authors correctly state that the biological potential of atypical Spitz tumors has not been characterized sufficiently.

D.C. Whitaker, M.D.

Comparison Between Lentigo Maligna Melanoma and Other Histogenetic Types of Malignant Melanoma of the Head and Neck
Cox NH, for and on Behalf of the Scottish Melanoma Group (Cumberland Infirmary, Carlisle; Univ of Glasgow, Scotland)
Br J Cancer 73:940–944, 1996   2–31

Background.—Whether the prognoses for lentigo maligna melanoma (LMM) and melanoma of other histogenetic types differ significantly is not known. This important question was investigated in a study of head and neck malignant melanomas registered with the Scottish Melanoma Group (SMG) between 1979 and 1992.

Methods and Findings.—Of 953 invasive cutaneous malignant melanomas registered with the SMG, 595 were studied to determine prognostic factors. Fifty-two percent were LMM, 25% were superficial spreading melanoma (SSM), and 23% were nodular melanoma (NM). The incidence of all types increased between 1979 and 1992. Patients with LMM and with NM were significantly older than those with SSM, their mean ages being 73, 68, and 57 years, respectively. Melanomas on the face were more frequent in women, with 90% of LMMs occurring at this site. Melanomas on the scalp, neck, and ears were more frequent in men. Kaplan-Meier estimates of the probability of survival were determined. Tumor thickness, Clark level of invasion, ulceration, histogenetic type of melanoma, and number of mitoses were prognostically significant in a stepwise analysis. In a proportional hazards model, however, tumor thickness was the dominant risk factor.

Conclusions.—Significant anatomic subsite differences occur between the sexes and for histogenetic melanoma type. However, after controlling for tumor thickness, the prognosis for invasive LMM is comparable to that of other histogenetic types.

▶ Melanomas of the head and neck are among the most difficult to treat because of the surgeon's desire to obtain high cure rates yet minimize potential disfigurement. This article provides significant evidence that depth of invasion is the most important diagnostic variable, regardless of tumor type. From the surgeon's standpoint, this simplifies matters and allows us to focus on the treatment plan and develop a prognosis based primarily on that variable.

D.C. Whitaker, M.D.

Large Congenital Melanocytic Nevi and the Risk for the Development of Malignant Melanoma: A Prospective Study

Marghoob AA, Schoenbach SP, Kopf AW, et al (State Univ of New York, Stony Brook; New York Univ)
Arch Dermatol 132:170–175, 1996   2–32

Background.—Studies have suggested that patients with large congenital melanocytic nevi are at increased risk for the development of malignant melanoma (MM). The magnitude of this risk was further explored.

Methods.—Ninety-two children with large congenital melanocytic nevi were followed up prospectively for a mean of 5.4 years. The patients were 54 girls and 38 boys, aged a median of 3 years. A control group consisted of subjects from the general population matched for age, sex, and length of follow-up.

Findings.—Malignant melanoma developed in extracutaneous sites in 3% of the patients. The cumulative 5-year life-table risk for MM development was 4.5%. Malignant melanoma development would be expected in 0.013 of the 92 control subjects. The standardized morbidity ratio was a highly significant 239.

Conclusions.—The risk for MM is significantly increased in children with large congenital melanomas. Such children should be continuously surveyed for the development of cutaneous and noncutaneous primary MM.

▶ This article is useful in that it further quantifies the risk of patients with LCMN having melanoma develop. It also points out that not all melanomas in these patients develop at epidermal sites of the integument. The authors remind us that there is no evidence that dermabrasion or destructive procedures prevent or reduce the risk of melanoma. In fact, total surgical removal of LCMN will not entirely prevent the development of melanoma.

D.C. Whitaker, M.D.

Malignant Melanoma in Italy: Risks Associated With Common and Clinically Atypical Melanocytic Nevi
Carli P, Biggeri A, Giannotti B (Univ of Florence, Italy)
J Am Acad Dermatol 32:734–739, 1995   2–33

Background.—The incidence of cutaneous malignant melanoma (MM) is increasing in white populations. Although epidemiologic studies have been carried out to determine risk factors for MM, these have been performed on light-skinned Northern European populations. This study used a case-control method to examine risk factors for MM in an Italian population.

Subjects.—All participants were residents of Florence, Italy. The controls consisted of 109 randomly selected healthy adults and the cases consisted of 106 patients with MM diagnosed between 1990 and 1992. The risk factors examined included common melanocytic nevi (CMN), large nevi, clinically atypical nevi (CAN), phototype, exposure to sunlight, sunbathing habits and history of sunburn.

Findings.—Large numbers of CMN were associated with an increased risk for MM in this Mediterranean population. Tendency to freckle and light-skinned phototype were also associated with an increased risk. Multivariate analysis indicated that the most significant independent variable associated with MM was large number of CMN.

Conclusions.—The total number of common melanocytic nevi on the entire body surface was the most important risk factor for cutaneous melanoma in this Mediterranean population.

▶ These authors conclude that the total number of commonly acquired nevi is the best predictor of risk for cutaneous melanoma in the Italian population. Moreover, they question the value of dysplastic nevi as a clinicopathologic entity and marker for melanoma. They recommend that more studies should be done of purely clinically atypical nevi, regardless of histologic features as potentially important markers of melanoma risk.

D.C. Whitaker, M.D.

Ultraviolet Irradiation Induces Acute Changes in Melanocytic Nevi

Tronnier M, Smolle J, Wolff HH (Med Univ of Lübeck, Germany; Univ of Graz, Austria)

J Invest Dermatol 104:475–478, 1995   2–34

Background.—Ultraviolet (UV) light is believed to be involved in the malignant transformation of human melanocytes. Some of the changes induced by UV radiation resemble melanoma in situ. The histologic and immunohistochemical changes induced by in vivo UV irradiation of melanocytic nevi were investigated.

Methods.—The study included 14 patients with melanocytic nevi measuring larger than 5 mm. Half of each nevus underwent irradiation with double the patient's minimal erythema dose. The irradiated and nonirradiated sides of the nevus were compared histologically and in immunohistochemical studies for the presence of HMB-45 antigen and proliferating cell nuclear antigen. Quantitative image analysis was performed.

Results.—In the irradiated portions of the nevi, there was a significant increase in suprabasally located melanocytes after 1 week. At the same time, expression of HMB-45 was dramatically increased. There was enlargement of the cytoplasm and nuclei of individual melanocytes, and a slight inflammatory infiltrate. No significant differences of any type, however, were noted in nevi excised 2 or 3 weeks after UV exposure.

Conclusions.—Melanocytic nevi exposed to UV light may temporarily show some histologic and immunohistochemical features of melanoma. These changes could pose problems in the dermatopathologic examination of pigmented lesions that have been exposed to sunlight, with possible overdiagnosis of melanoma. It remains to be determined whether the morphologic and histologic changes observed are caused by keratinocyte-derived factors and/or direct damage of melanocytes by UV.

▶ Interesting and important results in this study lead one to several questions concerning our understanding of categorization and therapy of melanocytic lesions. First of all, as a Mohs' surgeon, I am concerned that a single dose of UV light could have such a profound effect on staining patterns for HMB-45, especially because it is one of the stains used for frozen section preparation tissue specimens and the Mohs' surgical approach to melanoma. The second important point that is brought forth by this article is that when you biopsy a lesion (i.e., after sun exposure) may have a significant impact on what the pathologist's interpretation will be with increased likelihood of a "malignant" diagnosis, which may lead to significantly more aggressive therapy. I certainly have seen clinically that nevi change after a week of intense UV exposure and as such make it a point not to see my patients immediately after prolonged concentrated sun exposure. Instead, I advise them to come in one month after their "vacations" for their follow-ups.

D.J. Papadopoulos, M.D.

Influence of Sun Exposure After Childhood on the Development of Nevi: A Study in Monozygotic Twins

Roudil F, Grob J-J, Gouvernet J, et al (Hôpital Sainte-Marguerite, Marseille, France; Hôpital Timone, Marseille, France)
Eur J Dermatol 5:477–480, 1995

2–35

Background.—Sun exposure in childhood plays the main role in development of melanocytic nevi and melanoma. Evidence suggests an age-dependent response of the melanocytic system to sun exposure. Whether the effect of sun exposure on nevi development is limited to the first years of life has not been established. This question was investigated in a study of adult monozygotic twins.

Methods.—Twenty-eight pairs of monozygotic twins older than 30 years participated in the study. Physical examinations were performed, and a history of sun exposure was obtained.

Findings.—As expected, the intrapair correlation for nevus density was good. However, a 20% difference in the number of nevi was observed in most twins, which was attributed to different exposure to environmental factors after childhood. The risk of having more nevi was 2 times higher in the twin who was more sun-exposed between the ages of 15 and 30 years.

Conclusions.—The effect of sun exposure on nevi development is apparently not limited to the first years of childhood. The intrapair differences in nevi number on never-exposed areas observed in this study suggests a systemic effect of sun exposure or other yet unidentified environmental risk factors for nevi development.

▶ This study of twins is interesting because the findings show a higher density of nevi both in exposed and never exposed sites for the twin who had greater total sun exposure. The authors theorize that a possible systemic influence from sun exposure stimulates development of nevi in non-exposed areas. Most investigators may not support this theory, but it suggests an additional dimension to the risk of sun exposure.

D.C. Whitaker, M.D.

Basal Cell and Squamous Cell Carcinoma

Clinical and Histopathological Characteristics of Basal Cell Carcinoma in Japanese Patients

Kikuchi A, Shimizu H, Nishikawa T (Keio Univ, Tokyo)
Arch Dermatol 132:320–324, 1996

2–36

Objective.—Basal cell carcinoma (BCC), the most common skin malignancy, is less common in blacks and Asians than in whites. The few large studies of BCC in Japan have not addressed the histopathologic features. The clinical and histopathologic findings in a large series of Japanese patients with BCC were analyzed.

Methods.—The study included 243 Japanese patients with BCC. Factors analyzed included the color of the tumors, the patients' ages, the tumor sites, the histopathologic patterns, and the incidence of tumor recurrence and metastases. The findings were compared with those in other races.

Results.—The sample was about equally divided between men and women; the average age was 59 years. Three fourths of the BCCs had brown to glossy black pigmentation, particularly along their borders—the so-called black pearly appearance. In addition, three fourths of tumors were found on the head and neck, and 54% had a solid histopathologic pattern. One to 10 years after tumor excision, there were just 5 tumor recurrences and no metastases.

Conclusions.—The clinical and histologic features of BCC differ between races. In Japanese patients, lesional hyperpigmentation is a characteristic feature of BCCs. Larger studies will be needed to confirm the histologic characteristics and differences between races, including aggressive features.

▶ In the 1990s, we live in a diverse society, and physicians everywhere see patients who are far removed from their country of origin. Therefore, it is important for Western physicians to recognize that a large percentage of non-white patients will have pigmented or black BCC. These lesions can be clinically confused with malignant melanoma, and this underlines the need for physicians to establish diagnosis via biopsy before treatment.

D.C. Whitaker, M.D.

The Risk of Skin Cancer in Renal Transplant Recipients in Queensland, Australia

Bavinck JNB, Hardie DR, Green A, et al (Univ Hosp Leiden, The Netherlands; Queensland Inst of Med Research, Brisbane, Australia; Univ of Queensland, Australia)
Transplantation 61:715–721, 1996   2–37

Background.—Research has shown that renal transplant recipients have an increased risk of skin cancer. In Queensland, Australia, where exposure to sunlight is excessive, skin cancer is a major problem. A large series of renal transplant recipients living in Queensland underwent long-term follow-up.

Methods.—The retrospective study included 1,098 patients who had undergone transplantation 9 to 25 years earlier. The influence of immunosuppressive treatment on the development of skin cancer was determined in a subgroup of these patients. Immunosuppressive treatment consisted of cyclosporine alone or combined with prednisolone, azathioprine alone or combined with prednisolone, or cyclosporine plus azathioprine with or without prednisolone.

Findings.—According to life-table analysis, the cumulative incidence of skin cancer progressively increased from 7% after 1 year of immunosuppression to 45% after 11 years and 70% after 20 years. In a multivariate analysis, the risk of skin cancer did not differ between patients treated with long-term cyclosporine or azathioprine with or without prednisolone and those treated with cyclosporine plus azathioprine with or without prednisolone.

Conclusions.—This cumulative incidence of skin cancer is the highest ever reported. The increased risk of skin cancer is probably independent of the immunosuppressive agents used; rather, it appears to result from immunosuppression per se.

▶ This article is of special interest to dermatologists and physicians who manage the cutaneous problems of renal transplant patients. On the basis of follow-up data from 1,098 renal transplant recipients, they calculate a life-table analysis showing 7% cumulative incidence of developing a skin cancer after 1 year of immune suppression and 70% after 20 years of immune suppression. They also conclude that no difference exists in the skin cancer incidence of those patients receiving long-term cyclosporine versus long-term azathioprine. This is contrary to some initial reports, which suggested that patients receiving cyclosporine would have a lower incidence of skin cancer than patients receiving long-term azathioprine.

D.C. Whitaker, M.D.

▶ My practice involves skin cancer management for a number of transplant patients including renal, liver, and heart. Overall the renal patients seem to do better. I believe this in part is related to the length of overall experience with renal transplants, i.e., better donor selection (or at least less hurried perhaps in part related to dialysis availability) and thus less immunosuppressive therapy.

H.T. Greenway, M.D.

Intraoperative Radiation Therapy and Mohs Micrographic Surgery on an Outpatient Basis
Siegle RJ, Houser S, Nag S, et al (Arthur G James Cancer Hosp, Columbus, Ohio; Ohio State Univ, Columbus)
Dermatol Surg 21:975–978, 1995   2–38

Background.—The reported outcomes of intraoperative radiation therapy (IORT) for certain diseases are encouraging. It has been associated with increased disease control, longer survival, and acceptable complication rates. Although IORT is usually delivered while the patient is under general anesthesia, using this therapy on an outpatient basis in patients undergoing Mohs micrographic surgery for a cutaneous malignancy is possible. The treatment of one such patient is described.

Case Report.—Man, 55, was treated for recurrent squamous cell carcinoma on the right lateral neck. Recurrent disease was characterized by a rapidly growing soft-tissue mass that opened centrally and drained. Outpatient Mohs micrographic surgery was planned. The tumor was cleared in all fields except the area of the spinal accessory nerve, which was spared. Intraoperative radiation therapy was administered to the area of nerve containing possible residual tumor. No complications occurred. Forty-two months after the procedure, the patient is doing well, with no signs of recurrence or lymphadenopathy.

Conclusions.—Intraoperative radiation therapy is an effective adjunct to surgery in selected outpatients with superficial soft-tissue neoplasms. Patients undergoing Mohs surgery for tumors who are at high risk of recurrence or in whom vital structures cannot be sacrificed are candidates for IORT. The use of this adjunct in outpatient settings is also limited to those centers with access to a radiotherapy department.

▶ Spinal accessory nerve function was preserved using Mohs' surgery, intraoperative external beam radiation therapy, and postoperative radiation therapy. This case report is evidence that IORT has a role in the surgical treatment of certain cutaneous tumors. This report should encourage dermatologic surgeons to discuss IORT with a radiation therapist and consider it as adjunctive therapy in certain cases in which anatomic and functional preservation is critical.

D.C. Whitaker, M.D.

DNA Ploidy in Nonmelanoma Skin Cancer
Robinson JK, Rademaker AW, Goolsby C, et al (Northwestern Univ, Chicago)
Cancer 77:284–291, 1996   2–39

Background.—Basal cell carcinoma (BCC) and squamous cell carcinoma (SCC) are a major public health problem. Patients with SCC in the head and neck region usually die of locoregional recurrence, and patients with BCC of the head and neck have cosmetic and functional changes associated with its treatment. Flow cytometry can facilitate prognostication in patients with nonmelanoma skin cancer.
Methods.—Specimens were obtained from 40 consecutive patients with head and neck nonmelanoma cancers for prospective analysis. The patients then received follow-up for 4 years. A modified Vindelov procedure was used to prepare samples from frozen specimens.
Findings.—Metastasis to regional lymph nodes was significantly correlated with DNA aneuploidy or tetraploidy and histology of well-differentiated SCC. Direct tumor extension below the adipose tissue was correlated with an S-phase exceeding 4.1 and a proliferative fraction of more than 5.5. No recurrences were observed at the site of surgical resection.
Conclusions.—Measuring well-differentiated SCC DNA ploidy and BCC and SCC proliferative capacity or S phase is useful in predicting a

tumor's biologic proclivity for locoregional invasion or metastasis of non-melanoma skin cancer. When aggressive tumors are identified at the time of surgery, adjunctive treatment may be initiated in an attempt to prevent lethal metastasis.

▶ Risk for metastases in the head and neck are hard to predict. These findings suggest that flow cytometry and DNA ploidy may turn out to be predictors of such high-risk tumors.

D.C. Whitaker, M.D.

Lymphocyte Counts of Patients Who Have Had Skin Cancer
Czarnecki D, Meehan CJ, McColl I, et al (Austin Repatriation Med Centre, Heidelberg West; Skin and Cancer Found Inc, Melbourne, Australia)
J Am Acad Dermatol 34:772–776, 1996   2–40

Background.—Studies of lymphocyte counts in patients with skin cancer have yielded inconsistent findings, possibly because the patients studied did not comprise homogeneous groups. Lymphocyte counts in patients with skin cancer were determined to see whether any abnormalities were associated with the number of cancers removed and whether lymphocyte counts could help identify patients at risk of developing large numbers of cancers.

Methods.—One hundred twenty patients with histologically confirmed skin cancer were studied. These patients were otherwise apparently healthy. Ninety-six patients had 3 or more skin cancers, and 24 had 1 skin cancer. Total lymphocyte count, CD4 counts, and CD8 counts were determined by standard flow cytometry.

Findings.—Eighty-four patients had only basal cell carcinomas (BCCs) removed. In this homogeneous group, women had a significantly greater CD4 cell count than men. Also, patients with 20 or more BCCs had significantly lower lymphocyte counts, and those with 1 BCC had a significantly greater CD4/CD8 ratio than those with multiple BCCs.

Conclusions.—In this homogeneous group of patients with BCC, differences were found between men and women and between other patient subgroups. However, the range of lymphocyte counts was great, thus making it impossible to establish a threshold below which patients had a worse prognosis. Determining lymphocyte count does not reliably predict which patients have a larger number of skin cancers.

▶ Often it is not very interesting to review studies that find no significant difference. However, this finding is useful because it is counterintuitive to what most of us would expect. Perhaps additional studies will uncover differences, but for now it appears that lymphocyte counts do not predict risk for nonmelanoma skin cancer.

D.C. Whitaker, M.D.

Beneficial Effect of Low-Dose Systemic Retinoid in Combination With Topical Tretinoin for the Treatment and Prophylaxis of Premalignant and Malignant Skin Lesions in Renal Transplant Recipients

Rook AH, Jaworsky C, Nguyen T, et al (Univ of Pennsylvania, Philadelphia)
Transplantation 59:714–719, 1995   2–41

Background.—Aggressive squamous cell carcinomas and other skin neoplasia are a frequent occurrence in renal transplant recipients. There is evidence to suggest that high-dose systemic retinoids may be useful in chemotherapy and chemoprophylaxis for these patients; however, high-dose systemic retinoid treatment is associated with serious toxicity. Studies have also found that topical retinoid—particularly tretinoin—has antitumorigenic effects. A combination of topical tretinoin and low-dose etretinate was evaluated for the treatment of dysplastic skin lesions in renal transplant recipients.

Methods.—Eleven renal allograft recipients took part in the study. All had too many skin lesions—including actinic keratoses, squamous cell skin cancers, and warts—to be treated by excision within a short time. Seven patients elected treatment with 0.25% tretinoin cream, applied nightly to the involved areas, plus oral etretinate, 10 mg/day. The other 4 received tretinoin only. All patients were followed up by monthly clinical examination; 8 had at least 6 months' follow-up.

Results.—At 3 months, 9 of the 11 patients had at least a 25% decrease in the number of neoplastic growths. By 6 months, 6 of 8 patients had at least a 50% decrease, including 2 of 3 patients receiving tretinoin only. Four patients received combination therapy and 3 received tretinoin alone for at least 9 months; 3 and 2 patients, respectively, showed a significant decrease in their rate of new squamous cell cancers. Whereas epidermal specimens were almost completely devoid of Langerhans' cells at the start of treatment, the density of these cells increased greatly and in proportion to the duration of therapy.

Conclusions.—In patients with renal transplant, long-term topical tretinoin—with or without low-dose oral etretinate—appears effective in suppressing the development of new tumors and reducing the number of existing lesions. Both regimens reduce the number of actinic keratoses and warts, and the combination regimen decreases the recurrence rate of new squamous cell cancers. No serious adverse effects are noted. This type of therapy should be evaluated in a double-blind, placebo-controlled trial.

▶ The authors have found at least short-term benefit with a combination of topical tretinoin and low-dose retinoid. The cutaneous management of patients with organ transplants is a very difficult and chronic task. Higher dose retinoids tend to be very poorly tolerated, particularly by graft recipients. This is an encouraging finding that may turn out to have clinical utility.

D.C. Whitaker, M.D.

DNA Repair Capacity for Ultraviolet Light-Induced Damage Is Reduced in Peripheral Lymphocytes From Patients With Basal Cell Carcinoma

Wei Q, Matanoski GM, Farmer ER, et al (Johns Hopkins School of Hygiene and Public Health, Baltimore, Md; Johns Hopkins School of Medicine, Baltimore, Md)

J Invest Dermatol 104:933–936, 1995   2–42

Objective.—Basal cell carcinoma (BCC) is the most common skin cancer among white people in the United States. Sunlight exposure, red hair, and fair skin are risk factors. A mechanism for this malignancy is suggested by the observation that the autosomal recessive disease xeroderma pigmentosum, characterized by deficient DNA repair capacity, leads to ultraviolet radiation-induced development of multiple skin tumors. The results of a clinic-based, case-control study of BCC, examining the DNA repair capacity in the presence of sunlight, chemical carcinogens, and medical radiation, are reported.

Methods.—The DNA repair capacities were compared between 88 patients with BCC, aged 20 to 60 years, and 135 control patients who had nonmalignant, nondysplastic skin diseases using a host-cell reactivation assay. The assay uses T-lymphocytes isolated from peripheral blood and stimulated with phytohemagglutinin-protein fraction and transfected with damaged or undamaged plasmid containing a reporter gene encoding a bacterial enzyme, chloramphenicol acetyl transferase. The ratio of expression of damaged plasmid to expression of undamaged plasmid is an estimate of cellular DNA repair capacity.

Results.—The patients with BCC were more likely than controls to have fair skin, skin lesions, a high tendency to burn, had multiple severe sunburns, red hair, blue eyes, multiple medical radiation exposures, and a significantly lower DNA repair capacity, particularly for those with red hair. The patients with BCC at highest risk had a 10% to 28% decreased DNA repair capacity.

Conclusion.—Decreased DNA repair capacity, present in patients with BCC, is a mechanism for the development of sunlight-induced skin neoplasm.

▶ This interesting study further establishes the role of sunlight as an agent that causes decreased DNA repair capacity in patients with BCC. It was interesting to see that BCC patients with red hair and previous exposure to chemicals and medical radiation showed a reduced DNA repair capacity. One wonders what this capacity would be in melanoma, and whether this marker could be used to identify other variables that may have an impact on this disease in terms of prognosis and/or treatment.

D.J. Papadopoulos, M.D.

Frequent p53 Accumulation in the Chronically Sun-Exposed Epidermis and Clonal Expansion of p53 Mutant Cells in the Epidermis Adjacent to Basal Cell Carcinoma

Urano Y, Asano T, Yoshimoto K, et al (Univ of Tokushima, Japan)
J Invest Dermatol 104:928–932, 1995   2–43

Background.—In different types of tumors, alterations of the p53 tumor-suppressor gene are the most frequent type of genetic change. Basal cell carcinoma (BCC) is among the tumors showing p53 mutations, but it is unknown whether p53 mutation represents an early or late event in carcinogenesis. Immunohistochemical and DNA studies were performed to evaluate p53 expression in precursor lesions of BCC.

Methods.—Specimens of BCC and adjacent normal skin were obtained from Japanese patients. Immunohistochemical studies were performed using 2 different anti-p53 antibodies of CM1 and DO7. Thirteen samples of normal skin with typical sun exposure that showed epidermal CM1 staining were further screened for p53 gene mutations in epidermal DNA using polymerase chain reaction–single-strand conformation polymorphism analysis.

Results.—Immunohistochemistry frequently detected p53 expression in areas adjacent to facial BCCs, as well as in normal sun-exposed epidermis. Clusters of cells expressing p53 were sometimes found in the skin adjacent to BCCs, but not in the normal sun-exposed tissue. Also, p53 expression was reduced in normal epidermis with low levels of sun exposure. In 10 of 13 cases with epidermal CM1 staining, DNA studies showed no p53 mutations in exons 2 to 10 of the gene. However, the remaining 3 specimens showed a missense C to G transversion at a codon 249 dipyridimine site. None of the BCCs in these patients showed the codon 249 mutation.

Conclusions.—Increased p53 expression is noted in normal epidermis from around BCCs, and some of these tissues show a p53 mutation. Exposure of skin to ultraviolet light may lead to epidermal p53 exposure, and clonal expansion of p53 mutants may occur in the epidermis adjacent to BCCs. The mutant p53 clones could provide a molecular explanation for the high risk of new skin cancers in patients with BCC.

Ultraviolet Light Induces Expression of p53 and p21 in Human Skin: Effect of Sunscreen and Constitutive p21 Expression in Skin Appendages

Pontén F, Berne B, Ren Z-P, et al (Univ Hosp, Uppsala, Sweden)
J Invest Dermatol 105:402–406, 1995   2–44

Purpose.—Ultraviolet (UV) irradiation induces epidermal accumulation of p53 protein in the epidermis, and p53 has been suggested to play a key role in skin carcinogenesis. Previous studies have shown that the p21 molecule enacts cell cycle arrest to act as a downstream effector of wild-type p53. Expression of p53 and p21 in sun-exposed human skin was studied, including the effects of sunscreen.

Methods.—Eight healthy volunteers underwent UVA + UVB irradiation of untanned skin. Some areas were treated with sunscreen before irradiation. Punch biopsy specimens were obtained at various intervals before and after irradiation, and immunohistochemical studies were performed to quantify and assess the distribution of p53 and p21. Studies of skin exposed to natural sunlight were performed as well.

Results.—Irradiation induced p53 in epidermal cells within 4 hr after irradiation, with p53 levels returning to approximately normal levels after 120 hours. P53 expression peaked at 4 hr in suprabasal cells but not until 48 hours in basal cells. The epidermal pattern of p21 expression was comparable to that of p53. The mesenchymal cells of the upper dermis produced p21 but not p53 in response to irradiation, suggesting a different pathway of p21 induction.

Irradiation-induced p53 and p21 expression were almost nonexistent in type 5 skin and in areas treated with sunscreen. In additional studies, p53 was completely absent from skin that was never exposed to natural sunlight. In contrast, some demarcated areas of anagen hair follicles and sebaceous glands showed p21 reactivity, as did scattered epithelial cells. The findings suggested that p21 could play a physiologic role by stopping the cell cycle in epithelium in the terminal differentiation stage. Studies in archival skin tissues showed a more dispersed p53 staining pattern in samples obtained in the summertime than in those obtained in less sunny seasons. Normal epidermis showed intense areas of p53 staining, mainly in sun-exposed areas; this suggested possible clonal proliferation of p53 mutated keratinocytes.

Conclusions.—Both p53 and p21 appear to be involved in the response of human skin to UV exposure. The disperse pattern of p53 staining noted in this study is a common reaction of epidermis to UV radiation, a reaction that is inhibited by sunscreen and by natural or acquired skin pigmentation. Skin exposed to UV radiation may carry a high load of primary mutations in the p53 genome. This theory implies the evolution of highly efficient mechanisms by which skin can overcome the harmful effects of sunlight exposure.

▶ These 2 articles look at how sunlight affects tumor suppressor genes p53 and p21 and their pattern of staining in normal, photo-exposed, and photo-damaged skin and in basal cell carcinoma. These suppressor genes are constantly at work protecting the epidermis from ultraviolet-induced DNA damage. Their increased presence may suggest an increase in susceptibility toward the development of skin cancer. It is interesting that sunscreen and skin pigmentation-type 5 nearly eliminated expression of p53 and p21 in the first study. This is important work because we may finally be in a position to quantitatively assess sun damage and the protection afforded by many different prophylactic and therapeutic compounds applied to the skin.

D.J. Papadopoulos, M.D.

Other Tumors

Merkel Cell Carcinoma of the Skin: Imaging and Clinical Features in 93 Cases

Eftekhari F, Wallace S, Silva EG, et al (Univ of Texas MD Anderson Cancer Ctr, Houston)
Br J Radiol 69:226–233, 1996   2–45

Introduction.—The uncommon skin tumor Merkel cell carcinoma (MCC) tends to occur on the head and neck in older adults. Before metastases occur, surgery is potentially curative; for patients with metastatic disease, radiotherapy and chemotherapy may be used. The natural history, diagnosis, and treatment of MCC were described in a review of 93 cases.

Patients.—The patients (71 men and 22 women; median age, 70 years) were seen at 1 cancer center during a 13-year period. The tumor was found in the head and neck region in 64 patients, the extremities in 21, and the trunk in 10. Seventy-five percent of patients had metastases sometime during their disease course, including 38 patients with regional lymph node metastases and 32 with distant metastases. A history of other skin cancers was noted for 30% of patients.

Treatment and Outcomes.—Of 81 patients who underwent surgical excision of their primary lesions, 34 had surgery plus radiotherapy, 18 had surgery plus radiotherapy plus chemotherapy, and 5 had surgery plus chemotherapy. Twenty-six patients underwent regional lymph node dissection. Patients with regional metastases survived for a median of 34 months and those with distant metastases for 25 months. For patients without metastatic disease, 5-year survival was 63% and 10-year survival 53%.

Imaging and Pathologic Findings.—Ten patients underwent imaging studies of the primary sites and 7 of metastatic sites. In the primary lesions, sonography revealed hypoechoic nodules growing from the dermis into the subcutaneous tissues. Minimally enhancing soft tissue nodules, sometimes associated with lytic bone erosion, were noted on CT scans. Sonography showed metastatic lesions as moderately hypoechoic, whereas CT showed them as target shaped, with or without ring enhancement. The tumors could appear as blister-like, wartlike, or pea-shaped lesions (Fig 11). They measured 0.5–5.0 cm in diameter and were usually not ulcerated.

Conclusions.—A large series of patients with MCC was reviewed. The primary skin lesions are clinically apparent. Sonography or CT may provide valuable information about the depth of invasion of primary tumors; imaging studies are essential to identify regional and distant metastases. Abdominal and pelvic CT may be indicated for patients in whom chest CT shows regional lymph node metastases.

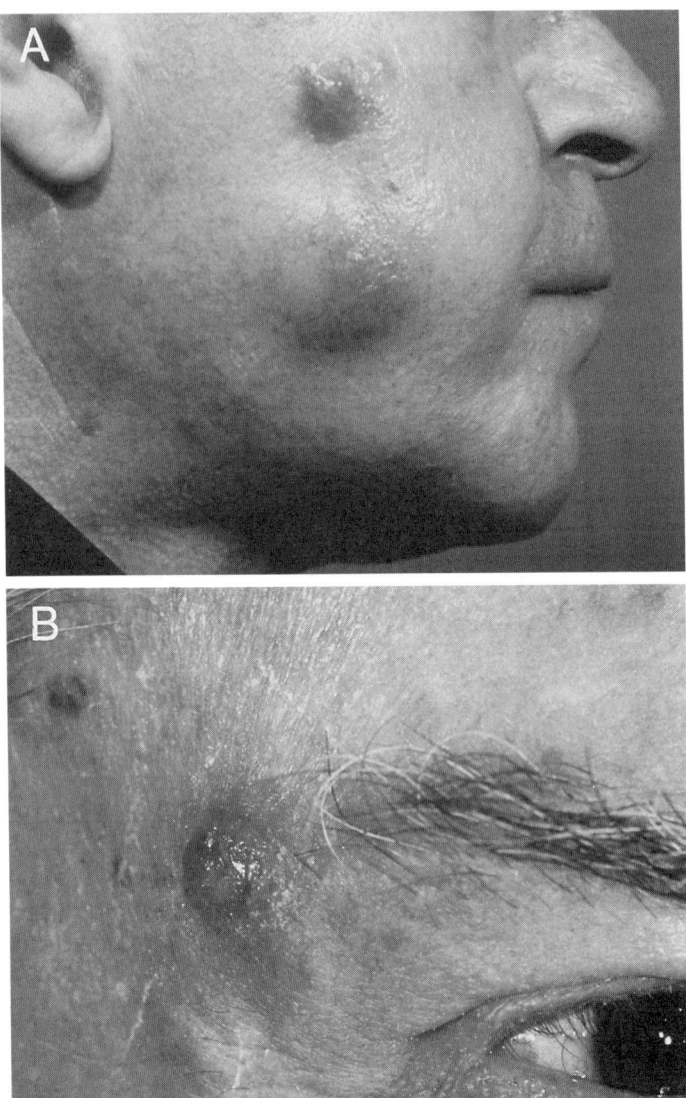

FIGURE 11.—Gross appearance of Merkel cell carcinoma in different patients. **A,** 2 lesions in the cheek, the upper one blister-like; **B,** single, erythematous, raised nodule lateral to the eyebrow. (Courtesy of Eftekhari F, Wallace S, Silva EG, et al: Merkel cell carcinoma of the skin: imaging and clinical features in 93 cases. *Br J Radiol* 69:226-233, 1996.)

▶ The important question addressed in this study is what comprises appropriate workup. It was concluded that body CT is probably only useful if regional adenopathy is present. Because the majority of MCC occurs on the head and neck, it may be appropriate to limit imaging studies to these sites unless other positive findings are demonstrated.

D.C. Whitaker, M.D.

Cutaneous Angiosarcoma of the Head and Neck: A Therapeutic Dilemma
Morrison WH, Byers RM, Garden AS, et al (Univ of Texas, Houston)
Cancer 76:319–327, 1995   2–46

Introduction.—Angiosarcomas of the head and neck, usually arising in the dermis of the scalp and upper part of the face, extend much further transdermally than their clinical appearance suggests. This makes them difficult to treat surgically. Wide-field electron-beam radiation is a rational treatment approach for patients with angiosarcomas of the face and scalp because the involved dermis and a wide margin can be treated while avoiding radiation to the brain and other normal tissues. The results of this approach in 14 patients are reviewed.

Patients.—The patients were treated by electron beam radiation over a 19-year period. All had dermal angiosarcoma of the head and neck, with primary tumors located in the scalp and forehead in 11 patients and in the upper face in 3. Multiple foci of disease were present in 11 patients. In addition to radiation, treatment included chemotherapy in 10 patients and surgery in 7. Only limited surgery was performed in patients with smaller tumors; none of the patients underwent total scalp resection.

A multiple-field electron-beam technique was used for radiation therapy. For the 6 surgically treated patients who had no macroscopic disease in the treatment field, a median radiation dose of 60 Gy was given over a median time of 40 days. For the remaining 8 patients, who did have clinically apparent disease, a radiation dose of 55 to 75 Gy was given over a median time of 44 days.

Results.—Radiation therapy controlled the disease in 5 of 6 patients who had clinically detectable disease when treated, though only 2 were disease-free at follow-up. Five of the eight patients with macroscopic disease at the time of radiation therapy had recurrences: 2 within the irradiated field and 3 at the margin of the irradiated field. The 5-year actuarial rate of disease control above the clavicles was 24% for patients with clinical disease at the time of radiation therapy and 40% for those without clinical disease. Overall 5-year actuarial distant metastasis rate was 63%. Five-year actuarial survival rate was 13% for patients with clinical disease versus 50% for those without.

Conclusions.—Radiation therapy is an effective treatment for patients with local cutaneous angiosarcoma, especially after surgical resection of macroscopic disease. For patients with distinct areas of limited disease, excision of clinically evident tumor can be followed by moderate-dose, very wide-field radiation. The prognosis is poor for patients with diffuse, multifocal disease, though radiation therapy can still control local disease in some of these patients. Effective systemic therapies for cutaneous angiosarcoma are needed.

▶ As the subtitle of this article indicates, angiosarcoma always presents a therapeutic dilemma. It nearly always tends to have extensive subclinical spread, and cures of angiosarcoma by any and all means are rare. The authors recommend specific parameters for moderate doses of radiation. This may be helpful in controlling local disease but it is of course not curative.

D.C. Whitaker, M.D.

Chondroid Syringoma of the Head and Neck: Clinical Management and Literature Review
Chen AH, Moreano EH, Houston B, et al (Univ of Iowa, Iowa City)
Ear Nose Throat J 75:104–108, 1996   2–47

Background.—Benign, mixed epithelial tumors are relatively rare cutaneous lesions that occur most often in the head and neck area. Histologically, these lesions are very similar to pleomorphic adenomas of salivary gland origin. Optimal surgical treatment involves removing a cuff of normal tissue rather than simply shelling out the tumor. One patient with a chondroid syringoma in the nasofacial groove is described.

Case Report.—Woman, 60, consulted her local physician because of a 1-year history of an asymptomatic mass in the left nasofacial crease, which had been growing. No tenderness, epiphora, or visual acuity changes occurred. On excisional biopsy, a gross specimen of 1.5 × 1 × 1 cm was removed. Mucoepidermoid carcinoma was diagnosed histologically, and she was referred to the authors' clinic. The patient's histologic slides were reviewed. The tumor was multilobulated, well circumscribed, surrounded by a fibrous connective tissue capsule, and contained many variably sized, partially branching lumina lined by a cuboidal luminal cell layer and a flattened-to-cuboidal peripheral cell layer. Occasional ducts were lined by stratified squamous keratinizing epithelium and separated by a variably fibrous, fibromyxoid and chondroid stroma, along with epithelial cell aggregates and single cells. No cytologic atypia or mitotic activity was evident. The tumor extended to the resection margin. Incompletely excised chondroid syringoma was diagnosed, and the nasofacial mass was excised again. The second specimen was noted to include scar and foreign body giant cell reaction with no residual tumor.

Conclusions.—Because of the rarity of chondroid syringoma, it is frequently not considered in the differential diagnosis of subcutaneous head and neck tumors. Surgical removal with a small cuff of normal tissue is the treatment of choice. When the diagnosis of chondroid syringoma is considered before surgery, the surgeon can plan for an adequate excision, minimizing the possibility of recurrence.

▶ These authors point out that chondroid syringoma, while benign, are lobulated in character. Therefore the tumor should be excised with a cuff of normal tissue rather than simple shelling out in order to avoid recurrence. The authors also note that on histopathologic examination this tumor may be mistaken for tumors of salivary gland origin.

D.C. Whitaker, M.D.

3 Reconstruction

Introduction

Dermatologic reconstructive surgery continues to evolve. My friend Dr. Terry Davidson of the Head and Neck Surgery Department at the University of California, San Diego, discussed our specialties evolution in this area at our 13th "Superficial Anatomy and Cutaneous Course" this past summer. Terry has helped with the reconstructive portion of this course since its inception as well as many other dermatologic surgery continuing education courses. Terry noted the assistance of other specialties such as his and the great work and leadership of our own pioneers such as Drs. Ted Tromovitch and Sam Stegman (Sam taught us to use our "smart fingers" in reconstructive planning as well as our brains) who are no longer with us. Dr. Neil Swanson, the previous editor-in-chief of this text, continued to lead us as he moved westward (Michigan to Oregon). The growth in leadership in dermatologic reconstructive surgery has been exponential. The quality of teaching and in results and outcomes is at a level where our speciality is clearly the leader. Fortunately, we can now assist in teaching our other colleagues who have been so helpful in the past.

Refinements in nasal reconstruction continues as we seek the perfect cosmetic and functional result. Anatomy knowledge and principles must be understood and adhered. The use of the nasalis muscle in flap reconstruction demonstrates our movement in myocutaneous thinking; there are several articles in this volume which assist us in our nasal reconstructions.

Skin grafts are well mastered by ourselves and collagues. The timing of application may be important as noted in 2 articles on the use of delayed grafts, especially in certain areas such as the lower extremities.

Finally, 1 option in reconstruction is to allow healing by granulation. We are aware of certain defects such as those in the inner canthus where the results achieved in this manner may exceed various surgical attempts such as flaps or grafts. Two articles focus on this but I am cautious in this time of "managed care" that we focus on what is best for the patient in each individual case and not put any primary or secondary gain ahead of this. Long ago I learned from Dr. Frederic Mohs the value of granulation healing in specific locations, but Dr. Mohs was also a great believer in "nip and tuck guiding reconstructions" if this were best for the patient. I hope that we continue to do what is best for the patient in each and every instance.

Hubert T. Greenway, M.D.

Flaps

Island Inner Canthal and Glabellar Flaps for Nasal Tip Reconstruction

Morrison WA, Donato RR, Breidahl AF, et al (St Vincent's Hosp, Melbourne, Australia)

Br J Plast Surg 48:263–270, 1995   3–1

Introduction.—Several different techniques have been used for surgical reconstruction of the nasal tip and upper lip. A technique that used inner canthal and glabellar island flaps based on the terminal branches of facial vessels for the reconstruction of the nasal tip, alae, and upper lip was described.

> *Anatomy and Technique.*—The facial artery passes upward and forward across the mandible and buccinator before it goes up the side of the nose and ends at the medial palpebral fissure, where it supplies the lacrimal sac, and anastomoses with the dorsal nasal branch of the ophthalmic artery. It is consistently possible to locate the angular artery, which originates at the facial artery and extends into the inner canthal region. In most cases, this artery is easily palpable throughout its course, particularly just inferior to the inner canthus.
>
> For patients who undergo nasal tip reconstruction, the course of the artery is palpated and marked, and a template of the defect is made. The donor area may be the inner canthal region or the glabellar region, but part of the flap must lie close to or preferably over the angular artery. The flap is elevated at the supraperiosteal level to ensure that the vascular supply is included. The angular vein can be seen at the inferior limit of the canthal flap, and the angular artery is found medial to it. The incision is extended along the nasal cheek junction toward the alar to develop the vascular pedicle; the precise incision depends on the defect. The island flap is raised and transposed into the defect, and then the pedicle is positioned underneath the alar groove incision. Small donor sites may be closed directly, whereas larger defects may require a graft or flap.

Results.—In an experience with 12 patients, no flap failures occurred. There were 2 cases of superficial necrosis that healed without tissue loss. The donor artery was palpable preoperatively in all but 2 patients. The flap donor site was the inner canthal region in 8 cases, the glabellar region in 2, and both in 2. Eleven of the 12 flaps were used to repair defects of the nasal tip and alae, including the nasal lining. The largest flap in the series was used to reconstruct the alar base and part of the upper lip.

Conclusions.—Good results are reported with inner canthal and glabellar flaps for reconstruction of the nasal tip. These flaps provide a good amount of well-vascularized tissue of the right color, texture, and thickness. They also offer a wide arc of rotation and a satisfactory donor defect in a single-stage procedure.

▶ Reconstruction of defects that involve the tip and areas on the distal third of the nose may pose the greatest challenge as we seek to restore cosmesis and retain function. As evidenced by other articles in this section, we continue to seek to improve our results. The angular artery and vein can provide appropriate vascular supply and offer an alternative to forehead flaps in certain instances. The importance of anatomy is again presented! Attention must also be paid to the donor site lest one create a problem in that area.

H.T. Greenway, M.D.

The Rintala Flap Revisited
Chiu LD, Hybarger CP, Todes-Taylor N (Kaiser Permanente Med Ctr, Oakland and San Rafael, Calif)
Plast Reconstr Surg 94:801–807, 1994   3–2

Applications.—The Rintala flap is an alternative means of closing substantial defects of the nasal tip or dorsum, particularly when there is upper columellar loss. A midline rectangular sliding flap is created, thereby excising compensatory triangles bilaterally either at the medial canthal level or just above the brow. Tip rhinoplasty and incisions in the alar crease can widen the coverage of the flap. Bilateral cheek advancement flaps and small full-thickness skin grafts may supplement the Rintala flap if a large lesion extends over the nasal tip and dorsum.

> *Technique.*—After the tumor is resected and the margins confirmed, the nasal dorsum is undermined into the glabellar and brow region at the level of the periosteum to include the procerus and glabellar muscles. Undermining extends laterally in the nasolabial area to the midpupillary line on both sides and inferiorly into the columella. The distal end of the flap includes the superior margin of the defect. Two tips are left distally for use in constructing the upper columella. After the flap is raised, excessive dorsal hump is reduced and a tip rhinoplasty done as indicated. Removal of intercrural soft tissue is followed by rejoining the domes with buried sutures and narrowing and stabilizing the tip. The flap is draped over the nose and tacked to the dorsal periosteum. Suspension sutures in the supratip and dorsal areas prevent tenting of the flap and reduce tension at the distal suture line. The tip and upper

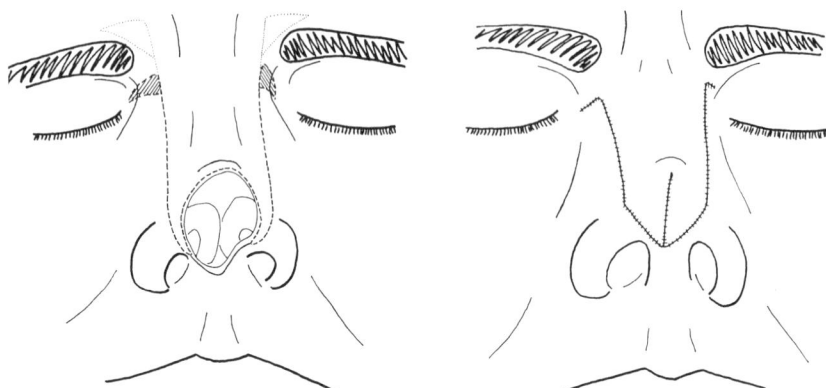

FIGURE 4.—**Left,** outline of Rintala flap (*heavy dotted line*) and Burow's triangles (*shaded area*). Note inclusion of superior wound margin to create bilateral flap tips used to reconstruct tip and columellar areas. Alternatively, a longer flap can be constructed by extending incisions superiorly and placing Burow's triangles at suprabrow level (*fine dotted line*). **Right,** after flap is positioned and tip is reconstructed. (Courtesy of Chiu LD, Hybarger CP, Todes-Taylor N: The Rintala flap revisited. *Plast Reconstr Surg* 94:801–807, 1994.)

columella are repaired by approximating the distal flap tips (Fig 4). A supratip defect is filled by medially rotating the cephalad margins of the lower lateral cartilages and, if necessary, with bilateral cheek flaps released by alar crease incisions. Burow's triangles are excised once the correct flap site is ascertained.

Advantages.—A Rintala flap was used in 15 patients who had skin cancer to repair large nasal tip defects, mainly central tip defects of 2 cm or greater. The flap design is comparatively simple and is easily executed by single-stage closure. Excellent nasal symmetry and color match are achieved. All flaps have remained viable, and there have been no complications. Defects as large as 4 cm may be closed in a single stage.

▶ Nasal tip reconstruction may be both challenging and difficult. The authors use this flap as an alternative to the forehead flap in defects of 2 cm or greater. The reduction of any dorsal nasal hump, and the use of tip rhinoplasty and suspension sutures are noteworthy. Interesting is the lack of complications and disadvantages noted by others. My problem has been the change in shape of the tip when I have used this flap for large defects; I'm sure this problem occurs less often in older patients. Revisions noted in Figure 4 may offer improvements.

H.T. Greenway, M.D.

The Peng Flap: The Flap of Choice for the Convex Curve of the Central Nasal Tip

Rowe D, Warshawski L, Carruthers A (Univ of BC, Vancouver, Canada)
Dermatol Surg 21:149–152, 1995   3–3

Introduction.—Repair of the central nasal tip presents a distinct surgical challenge because of several difficulties: matching skin thickness, avoiding deforming the nasal alae, and the convex curve. A pinch modification of the Peng flap that has provided excellent cosmetic results with minimal complications was described.

> *Surgical Technique.*—The Peng flap uses bilateral rotating arms taken from the lateral sides of the wound. With the pinch modification, the distal rotating arms, harvested from the superior sulcus of the alar groove, are extended all the way to the surgical defect to minimize advancement and thus reduce the length of the flap needed (Fig 1). A 30-degree wedge of tissue is removed from the proximal portion of the defect to facilitate placement of the proximal arms, harvested from the lateral sides of the nose. Bilateral excision Burow's triangles may be required at the proximal lateral edge to enable advancement (Fig 2). Closure extends from the Burow's triangles to the distal end of the defect with 2 lateral sidewall sutures.

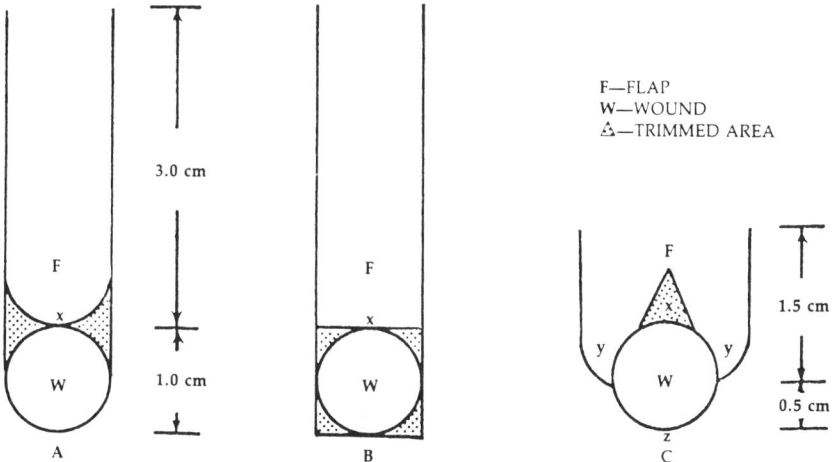

FIGURE 1.—Comparison of the "pinch" modification of the linear advancement flap to the traditional method, for 1.0-cm defect. **A** and **B**, traditional method: flap of 3.0–3.5 cm in length is needed to cover the 1.0-cm defect. **C**, "pinch" modification: flap of only 1.5–1.8 cm is needed to cover the same 1.0-cm defect because the flap moves only 0.5 cm (Reprinted by permission of the publisher from Rowe D, Warshawski L, Carruthers A: The Peng flap: The flap of choice for the convex curve of the central nasal tip. *Dermatol Surg* 21:149–152, copyright 1995 by Elsevier Science Inc.)

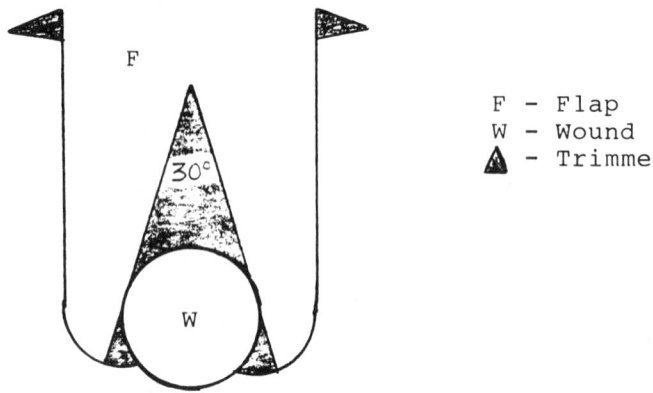

F — Flap
W — Wound
▲ — Trimmed Area

FIGURE 2.—The arms of the flap should extend as far down the distal defect as possible. A 30-degree wedge of tissue should be removed superior to the wound. Bilateral Burow's triangles should be excised to facilitate advancement. (Reprinted by permission of the publisher from Rowe D, Warshawski L, Carruthers A: The Peng flap: The flap of choice for the convex curve of the central nasal tip. *Dermatol Surg* 21:149–152, copyright 1995 by Elsevier Science Inc.)

Discussion.—Because there is minimal advancement needed, there is minimal tension on the nose tip, which reduces necrosis and shape changes in the nares. Although some distortion of the nares may occur with the repair of large defects, the symmetry of the distortion makes it aesthetically acceptable. Because the flap is wider and shorter than traditional flaps, flap survival is improved. The convex curve of the nasal tip is reproduced, which produces excellent cosmetic results.

▶ Reconstruction of the central nasal tip after skin cancer removal continues to be a most challenging area in a majority of these cases. The authors' modifications of Dr. Vincent Peng's flap for this area continues to improve our knowledge and technique as we reconstruct with "like tissue," which in this case is tissue from the distal two-thirds or sebaceous nose. Although some consider the forehead pedicle flap as the best approach, the Peng flap may be less traumatic while offering excellent results in a one stage procedure.

H.T. Greenway, M.D.

Nasal Tip Repair With Axial Flap of Nasal Muscle
Martire L Jr, Colares JH, dos Reis JM, et al (Sao Paulo, Brazil)
Aesthetic Plast Surg 19:527–530, 1995   3–4

Background.—Options for repairing the tip of the nose include a cutaneous flap of the lateral pedicle, which dislocates all cutaneous nasal covering through rotation and V-Y, and a myocutaneous flap created from the transverse part of the nasal muscle through advancement in the island to the nasal tip region. A new procedure was developed using principles similar to those of the cutaneous transplant and the myocutaneous flap.

Technique.—The surgeon marks the flap from the distal border to the affected region, up to the back of the nose. The marking is about twice as high as the vertical diameter of the lesion, and the apex corresponds to the middle vertical line of the damaged area. The inferior part is positioned just above the nasal handle (Fig 1, A). The surgeon then incises the flap and displaces it by joining the osteocartilaginous skeleton to its myocutaneous counterpart, without completely freeing it from its muscular origins (Fig 1, B), as rotating the transplant permits the proximal part of the muscle to stay in place. The surgeon makes an incision to withdraw the skin superficially to the base and in the furrow of the handle to avoid

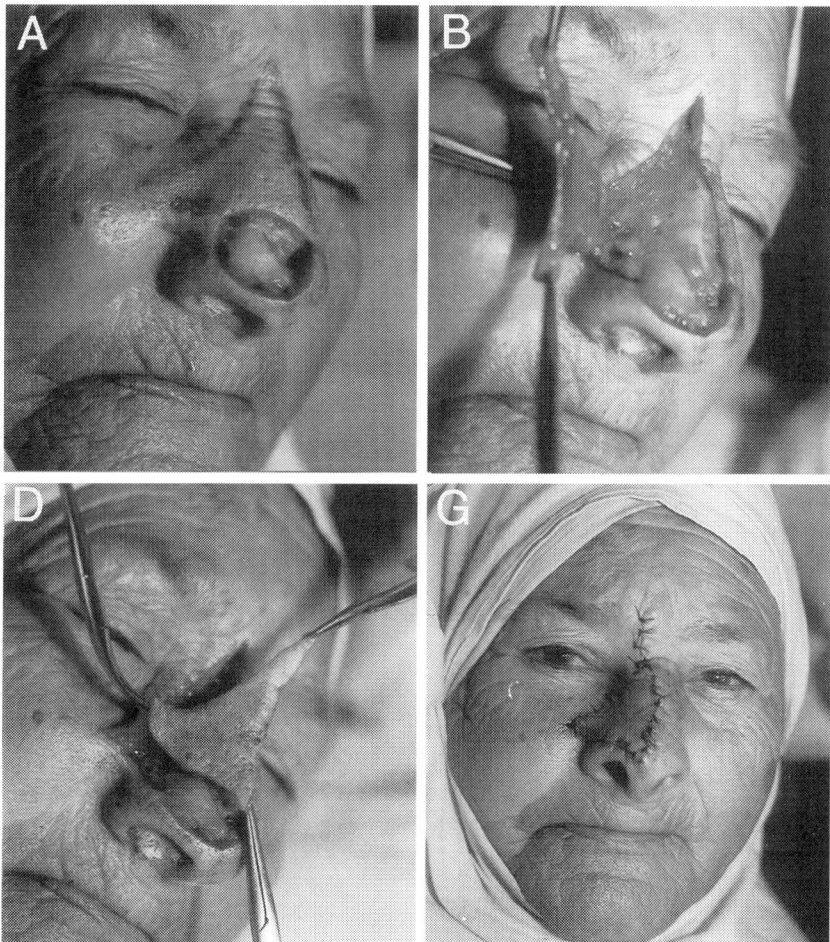

FIGURE 1.—Photos depict steps in our method of nasal tip repair using an axial flap of nasal muscle. (Courtesy of Martire L Jr, Colares JH, dos Reis JM, et al: Nasal tip repair with axial flap of nasal muscle. *Aesthetic Plast Surg* 19:527–530, copyright 1995 by Springer-Verlag.)

cutaneous redundancy and folding. The superior and lateral parts of the flap move in the V-Y direction. The transplant as a whole turns on its axis according to the needed repair (Fig 1, D). The outcomes of this procedure have been satisfactory (Fig 1, G).

Conclusions.—The technique described is useful for repairing substantial nasal tip losses. The advantages of this technique over previous methods are that it enables correction of deformities larger than 2 cm and of damage to the brim of the nose.

▶ We are increasingly doing more and larger myocutaneous flaps to repair nasal defects. These are simple and appropriate in their utilization. A clear understanding of the local anatomy and respect of the free margin of the alar rim is essential. Also, vertical, instead of horizontal, planes of undermining, which are necessary to perform these flaps, make it imperative that meticulous hemostasis be achieved before suturing. Suturing of these flaps must be done in ways to create eversion. Also, I feel that these flaps do not require a significant number of subcuticular sutures, as they frequently exhibit very little tension as a result of proper vertical undermining.

D.J. Papadopoulos, M.D.

Esthetic Refinements in Forehead Flap Nasal Reconstruction
Quatela VC, Sherris DA, Rounds MF (Univ of Rochester, NY; Mayo Clinic, Rochester, Minn)
Arch Otolaryngol Head Neck Surg 121:1106–1113, 1995   3–5

Objective.—To identify refinements in forehead flap nasal reconstruction that offer improved esthetic and functional results. The outcome of intervention was evaluated for 32 patients who had various nasal defects and had undergone forehead flap nasal reconstructive surgery in a university hospital between July 1987 and May 1994. The esthetic and functional results of the nasal reconstructions were evaluated subjectively by 3 otolaryngologists.

Interventions.—Currently accepted techniques of paramedian forehead flap nasal reconstruction were modified. These modifications included flap harvest and contouring, W-plasty closure of the superior forehead donor site, and creation of soft-tissue triangles. Open-structure rhinoplasty principles were incorporated into the cartilaginous reconstruction of the nasal tip and columella. Cartilage grafts placed at the nasal rim were used to reconstruct the alar rim.

Results.—The nasal subunits commonly reconstructed included the ala in 27 patients, the sidewall in 22, the dorsum in 18, and the tip in 15. Esthetic results were judged average to excellent. Functional results were either improved or much improved compared with preoperative breathing. Unplanned surgical revisions were performed for 2 patients. Dermabrasion was selected by 47% of patients. Postoperative intradermal injection of triamcinolone acetonide was required for 5 patients, and preoperative tissue expansion was required for 3. Neither infection, hematoma, airway obstruction, nor flap or graft loss occurred.

Conclusions.—Combination of the techniques used can result in functional and esthetically pleasing nasal reconstruction. Excellent nasal reconstruction can occur with a vascular lining, increased structural support, proper contouring of the soft-tissue envelope, and minimal donor site morbidity. After secondary flap insert, revision procedures are rarely necessary. Local epidermal turn-in flaps were not too bulky for inner lining reconstruction.

▶ Although this year's volume includes a number of nasal reconstruction procedures that, in some cases, may actually decrease the need for a forehead flap, it is in our patients' interest to be aware of the current indications and refinements, even if we personally do not perform this procedure. This is true in my practice, although my friend and colleague Ramsey Mellette, M.D., from Colorado, has presented his experiences with the forehead flap at our cadaver "Superficial Anatomy and Cutaneous Surgery" course for the past 2 summers. Clearly, this procedure is within the abilities of the experienced and advanced dermatologic surgeon. Practicing on cadaver material under the direct guidance and supervision of someone like Dr. Melette is certainly the way to begin. Thanks Ramsey!

H.T. Greenway, M.D.

Early Division of Pedicled Flaps Using a Simple Device: A New Technique
George A, Cunha-Gomes D, Thatte RL (Lokmanya Tilak Municipal Gen Hosp, Sion, Bombay, India)
Br J Plast Surg 49:119–122, 1996   3–6

Background.—The 2-staged flap is a safe and effective technique for a wide variety of plastic surgery procedures. However, the conventional technique requires 3 weeks before division of the pedicle flaps. A new technique has been developed that reliably allows early division of pedicle flaps by progressively reducing the blood flow across the flap.

Surgical Technique.—A device with 2 opposing V-shaped steel plates (Fig 1) is applied with 1 plate on either side of the bridge of the flap pedicle on the 5th postoperative day (Fig 2). Compression is increased by tightening the device's screws by 1 to 2 mm every 12 hours until the device is fully tightened by the 10th day and a deep linear groove is created in the flap, which is ready for division.

Methods.—The device was used on a variety of flaps (abdominal, superficial external pudendal artery, cross leg, groin, and medial arm flaps) in 20 patients.

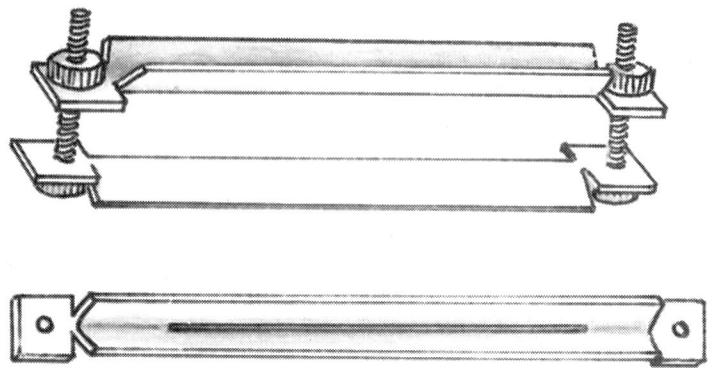

FIGURE 1.—A line diagram of the assembled device. The upper plate has a slit at the apex. (Courtesy of George A, Cunha-Gomes D, Thatte RL: Early division of pedicled flaps using a simple device: A new technique. *Br J Plast Surg* 49:119–122, 1996.)

Results.—Division of the flaps occurred on the 9th postoperative day in 8, on the 10th day in 4, on the 11th day in 2, and on the 12th, 13th, and 14th day in 1 each. Three devices were removed before division because of signs of ischemia. However, these 3 flaps were divided after 21 days and

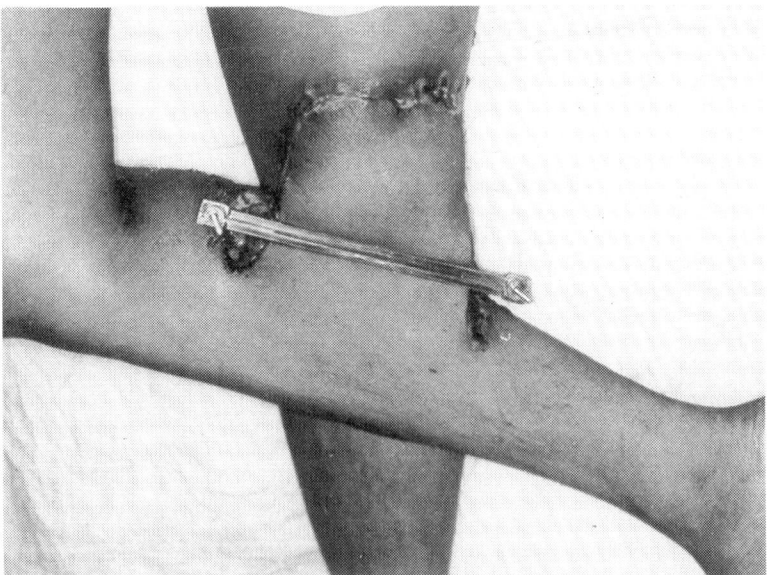

FIGURE 2.—The device applied to the bridge segment on the 5th postoperative day. (Courtesy of George A, Cunha-Gomez D, Thatte RL: Early division of pedicled flaps using a simple device: A new technique. *Br J Plast Surg* 49:119–122, 1996.)

used successfully. There were no flap losses. At follow-up 1 to 8 months after surgery, all 20 flaps were successfully settled.

Conclusions.—The device can facilitate the early division of a variety of pedicle flaps and is reliable, simple, and safe. The technique can be easily applied in a variety of clinical applications without a need for expensive monitoring equipment. The early discharge from the ward can substantially reduce costs.

▶ At times reconstruction of the nose and ear is best accomplished with pedicle flaps. Often the downside to the patient is the 3-week period required until flap division. This simple occlusion device (although not evaluated on facial flaps in this article) may offer a significant reduction in this waiting period. I suspect that the damage to the defect site, the so called "zone of trauma" may play a more important role than some realize in allowing an occlusion clamp such as this to work.

H.T. Greenway, M.D.

The Chondrocutaneous Helical Rim Advancement Flap of Antia and Buch
Ramsey ML, Marks VJ, Klingensmith MR (Geisinger Med Ctr, Danville, Pa; Westmoreland Head & Neck Surgery, Greensburg, Pa)
Dermatol Surg 21:970–974, 1995   3–7

Background.—Up to 4% of skin cancers occur at the helix, hence cutaneous surgeons commonly see patients with defects of the helix. The chondrocutaneous helical rim advancement flap originally described by Antia and Buch is a single-stage procedure that provides a broad pedicle with sufficient blood supply to promote flap survival. It is simpler and more convenient than other helix repair techniques, reducing the risk of flap-tip necrosis while offering equal or better cosmetic results. The technique and results of the chondrocutaneous helical rim advancement flap are reported.

> *Technique.*—The technique uses a series of incisions made along the area of the helical defect inferiorly into the lobule. If necessary, incisions can also be made superiorly along the helical sulcus into the helical crus. This creates a broad-based, well-vascularized flap, maximal movement of which is ensured by extensive undermining of the postauricular skin. In closing the defect, precise approximation and wound-edge eversion are essential to prevent notching of the helical rim. Subtle modifications are available to improve results in special situations, such as an M-plasty to remove redundant skin in the postauricular area or placement of the Burow's triangle in the lobule.

Experience.—The authors report very good results with use of the chondrocutaneous helical rim advancement flap in 47 patients. None of their patients had flap necrosis caused by ischemia, and none had infection. Two patients had postoperative hematomas, but the flaps healed without problems after the coagulated blood was removed.

Conclusions.—Defects of the helical rim can be well handled using the chrondrocutaneous helical rim advancement flap of Antia and Buch. This is a "simple and elegant" flap that is effective in repairing many different types of helical rim defects, particularly in patients with large, loose lobules.

▶ This article briefly presents a diagrammatic and photographic illustration of the helical rim advancement flap. This is a very useful reconstructive technique for marginal defects of the ear. Dermatologic surgeons should understand and be able to apply the technique appropriately.

D.C. Whitaker, M.D.

The Postauricular Cutaneous Advancement Flap for Repairing Ear Rim Defects

Goldberg LH, Mauldin DV, Humphreys TR (Baylor College of Medicine, Houston)
Dermatol Surg 21:28–31, 1995   3–8

Background.—The ear rim is the auricular structure most frequently affected by skin tumors. Attempts to repair the ear rim after excisional surgery, however, are confounded by the complex anatomy of the ear and its closely adherent anterior skin. Methods of closing the defect include excision of cartilage or transfer of skin from another site. A postauricular cutaneous advancement flap, which allows closure of the defect with the use of the relatively loose skin of the posterior ear, was described.

Methods.—Twelve men (average age, 74 years) underwent excision of single tumors of the ear rim followed by closure with a postauricular cutaneous advancement flap. The flap was created by using curved Metzenbaum scissors to undermine the postauricular skin between the subcutaneous fat and the perichondrium. "Dog ears" were removed along the helical rim, and the postauricular skin was advanced anteriorly. Subcutaneous absorbable sutures (5-0) were used to approximate the defect edges, and running nylon cutaneous sutures (6-0) were used to close the skin.

Results.—Cosmetic results were excellent. Rim defects after excision ranged in size from 7 × 8 to 15 × 40 mm, and the average length of closure after dog-ear removal was 36 mm. Complications occurred in only 1 patient, who experienced superficial necrosis at the flap rim (Fig 8).

Discussion.—The postauricular advancement flap offers the cosmetic advantages of perfect color match and preservation of a smooth helical rim, ear size, and ear shape. The technique also offers ease of execution, preservation of flap vascularity, and a low rate of complications. Superficial necrosis in 1 patient in this series resulted from tight cutaneous sutures.

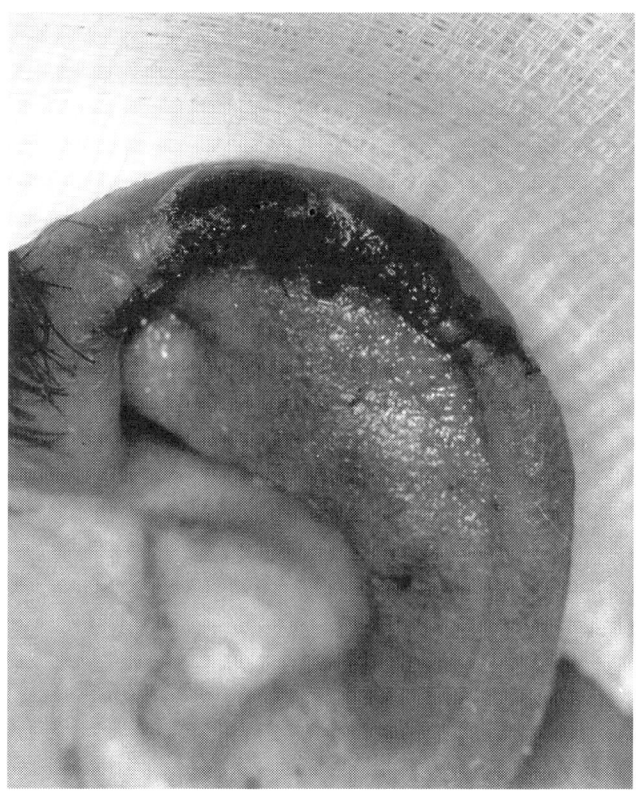

FIGURE 8.—Superficial skin necrosis along the suture line that may occur with excess skin tension. (Reprinted by permission of the publisher from Goldberg LH, Mauldin DV, Humphreys TR: The post-auricular cutaneous advancement flap for repairing ear rim defects. *Dermatol Surg* 21:28–31, copyright 1995 by Elsevier Science Inc.)

▶ As we saw from another article this year, the helix of the ear is not only the most common site on the ear for skin cancer, it also is a poor area for healing by granulation. Appropriate reconstruction, therefore, is normally indicated. Clearly, the postauricular skin differs from that of the anterior surface by being much less adherent (anatomy, again, is the basis for our understanding). Although I have tried this advancement flap, I often encounter superficial skin necrosis, as seen in Figure 8, in part no doubt related to the pull of the underlying cartilage. I recall that a number of years ago, Neil Swanson, M.D., the previous Editor-in-Chief of this series, wrote an article on the use of a bipedicle advancement flap mainly along the forehead and temple area. Perhaps helical rim defects might benefit from Dr. Swanson's flap, and I will consider it.

H.T. Greenway, M.D.

The Versatility of Double-Z Rhomboid Plasty

Ardenghy M, Hochberg J, Fuzii V, et al (Sao José do Rio Preto, São Paulo, Brazil; West Virginia Univ, Morgantown)
Ann Plast Surg 32:506–511, 1994   3–9

Objective.—The surgical technique of double-Z rhomboid plasty, including indications for the procedure, was reviewed in a study of 25 patients treated over a period of 2 years.

> *Surgical Technique.*—A rubber sponge model was used to compare the distortions that result from different methods of closure of a rhomboid defect (Fig 1). Imaginary relaxing skin tension lines (RSTL) were drawn over the flat surface of the model and surgical instruments used to create rhomboid defects. The first step in the surgical procedure is an outline of the RSTL of the affected anatomical region. A rhomboid, with 2 of its sides parallel to the RSTL, is marked around the skin lesion. Two 60-degree equilateral Z-plasties are generated on the opposite sides of the rhomboid, with care taken that 1 of the limbs of each Z-plasty is in continuity with the sides of the rhomboid parallel to the RSTL. All limbs of the Z-plasty and the rhomboid sides are of equal length; tip angles of the flaps are 60 degrees.

A rhombic shape wound remains after excision of the tumor. The initial procedure is reassessed and adjustments made if necessary. At this point the double-Z-plasty flaps are incised subcutaneously and elevated. The 4 triangular-shaped flaps created are then transposed as in a regular Z-plasty.

Results.—All patients had primary skin neoplasms with safe margins. Cosmetic results were judged good to excellent; no major distortions or asymmetries were noted and most scars were well oriented and of good quality. No recurrences have been reported after 2 years of follow-up. The procedure is indicated in cases of defects located near anatomical landmarks, for areas where only small flaps may be designed, when excessive tension prohibits primary closure, and when skin defects are across joints requiring covering.

Discussion.—The double-Z rhomboid plasty is a versatile method that minimizes distortion and is easy to understand and execute. Several factors contribute to good results: accurate orientation of the rhomboid defect and flaps in relation to RSTL; equal limb size, angles, and thickness of the flaps; and undermining beyond all incisions.

▶ The understanding of the use of the rhomboid flap and its many variations and adaptations (such as the 30-degree transposition Webster flap) for defect reconstruction remains a basic tenet we teach as part of our cadaver workshop, "Superficial Anatomy and Cutaneous Surgery Course," each year. The double rhomboid variation described here may be most useful in many

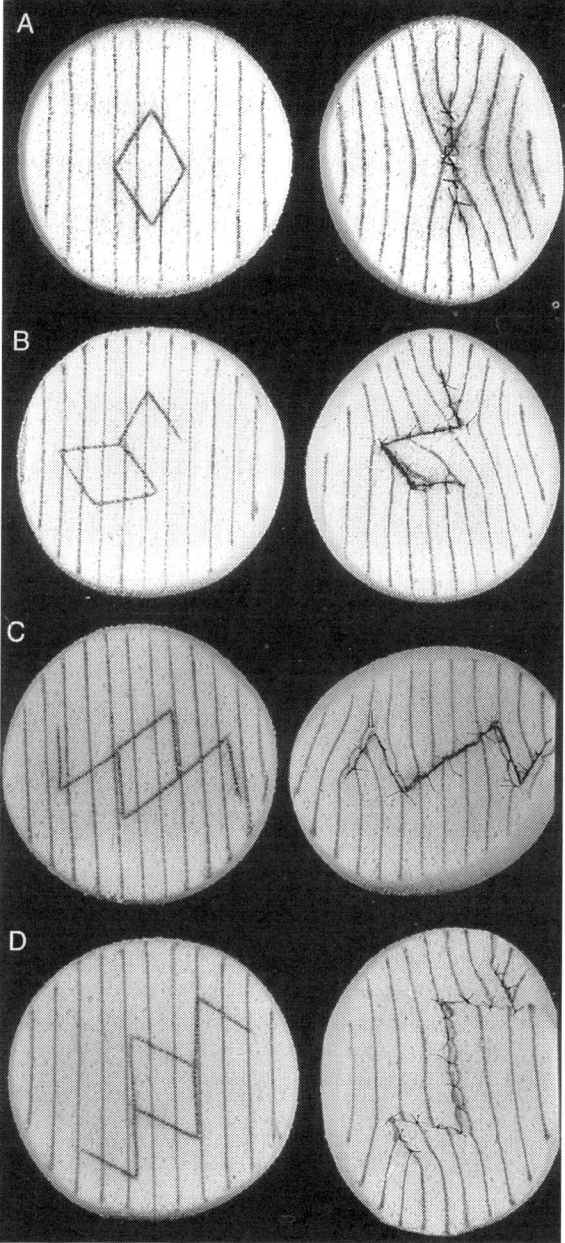

FIGURE 1.—Study of different methods of closure of a rhomboid defect in a rubber sponge model. **A**, direct closure: The suture line is parallel to the relaxed skin tension lines (*RSTL*) with significant distortion, vertical elongation, and horizontal narrowing. **B**, single rhomboid (Limberg flap): the main suture lines are perpendicular to the RSTL with deformation limited to the donor side area. **C**, the double-Z rhomboid (described by Cuono): the central suture line is oblique to the RSTL with significant vertical narrowing. **D**, the double-Z rhomboid (modification by Katoh): the central suture line is parallel to the RSTL with vertical elongation and horizontal narrowing. (Reprinted with permission from Ardenghy M, Hochberg J, Fuzii V, et al: The versatility of the double-Z rhomboid plasty. *Ann Plast Surg* 32:506–511, 1994.)

areas including the nose, temple, cheek, forearm, and dorsum of the hand. In addition to using visualization and thought processes, I also palpate the surrounding tissue with "smart fingers," as my friend Sam Stegman, M.D., taught me years ago, to help maximize results.

H.T. Greenway, M.D.

Upper Lip Reconstruction Using a Modified Perialar Crescentic Advancement Flap
de Fontaine S (Univ Hosp Erasme, Brussels, Belgium)
Eur J Plast Surg 19:69–72, 1996   3–10

Background.—The principles of aesthetic units and subunits should be observed in reconstruction of the upper lip. Scars are less noticeable if placed along the unit borders. A modified cheek advancement flap technique, which can be performed in keeping with these principles, was described.

Technique.—Cheek flap advancement with perialar crescent excision is diagrammed in Figure 1. The original defect is converted into a subunit defect such that the scar may be placed in the alar crease, the philtrum, or along the border of the upper lip. To permit flap advancement, the perialar crescent and a skin triangle must be resected. The vermilion border should be resected such that closure brings skin in contact with mucosa. The flap is dissected superficial to muscle. No muscle is transposed into an orbicularis muscle defect. Mucosal excess is apparent after flap elevation and advancement; it should be removed in the commissure, not in the upper lip, to hide the scar. Advancing mucosa into a triangular skin defect created at the lower end of the philtrum reforms the Cupid's bow. The total height of the normal philtrum is transferred to the af-

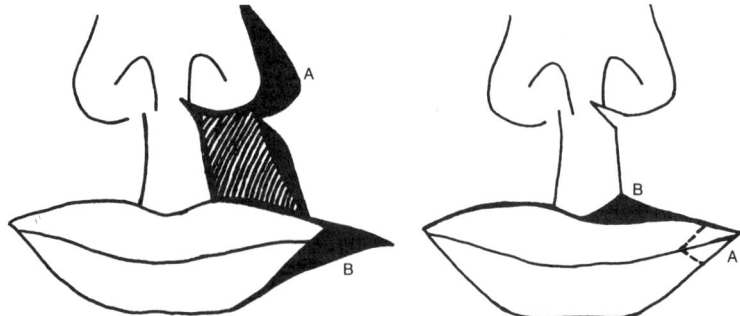

FIGURE 1.—**Left,** diagram of cheek advancement flap with perialar crescent excision (*A*) and triangular skin excision parallel to the vermilion border of the lower lip, near the oral commissure (*B*). **Right,** diagram of mucosal advancement with mucosal resection in the oral commissure (*A*) and Cupid's bow reconstruction (*B*). (Courtesy of deFontaine S: Upper lip reconstruction using a modified perialar crescentic advancement flap. *Eur J Plast Surg* 19:69–72, copyright 1996 by Springer-Verlag.)

fected side, with a skin triangle then excised partly from the skin of the medial upper lip and partly from the lower end of the cheek flap.

Discussion.—This technique provides a functional and esthetic means of reconstructing large upper lip defects. Use of the subunit approach lets correctly located flap scars mimic the normal borders of the upper lip. The cheek advancement flap described adheres to these principles and provides a good color and texture match. The inferior resection parallels the vermilion border of the lower lip, thereby leaving a minimally visible scar. Removing the excess mucosa laterally as a triangular resection in the commissure eliminates a vertical scar in the lip margin and vertical secondary retraction. Reconstruction of the Cupid's bow is also permitted.

▶ Aesthetic unit and subunit reconstruction may offer superior results. Perialar crescent excision and triangular skin excision, parallel or commissure associated, seem of benefit in selected patients. The upper lip lies within the "passport" portion of the face, and reconstruction must be tailored in each case.

H.T. Greenway, M.D.

The Submental Island Flap
Sterne GD, Januszkiewicz JS, Hall PN, et al (West Norwich Hosp, Norfolk, England)
Br J Plast Surg 49:85–89, 1996   3–11

Introduction.—Twelve elderly patients requiring facial or intraoral reconstruction were treated with the submental island flap (Fig 1). This axial pattern flap, introduced in 1993, offers a reliable source of well-matched skin and does not have the disadvantages of flaps that use skin of the anterior neck in facial reconstruction.

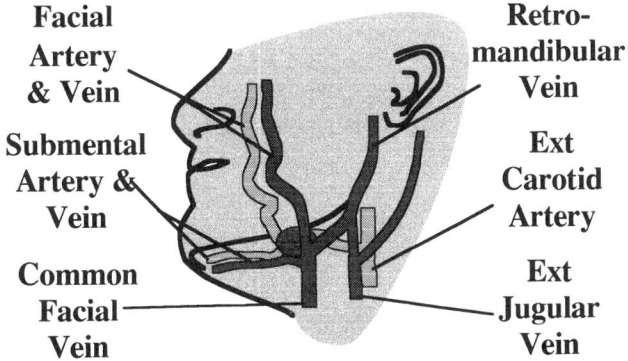

FIGURE 1.—The vascular anatomy of the submental island flap. (Courtesy of Sterne GD, Januszkiewicz JS, Hall PN, et al: The submental island flap. *Br J Plast Surg* 49:85–89, 1996.)

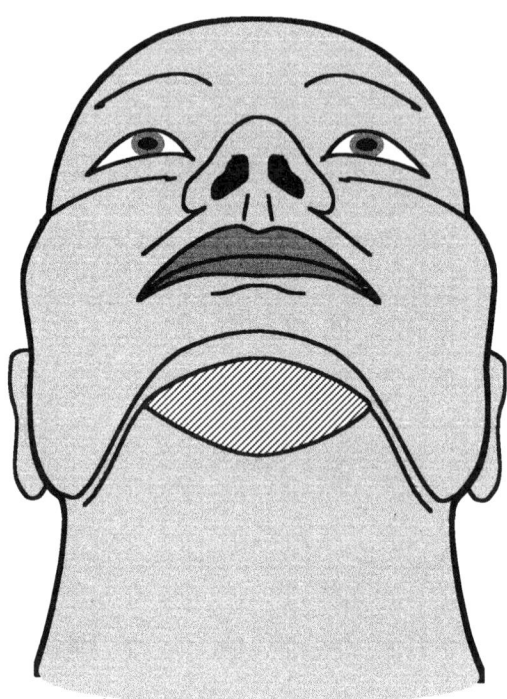

FIGURE 2.—The markings of the submental skin paddle, with optional extensions for additional pedicle dissection drawn on both sides. At operation, the incision is extended from the flap border on the ipsilateral side. (Courtesy of Sterne GD, Januszkiewicz JS, Hall PN, et al: The submental island flap. *Br J Plast Surg* 49:85–89, 1996.)

Surgical Technique.—With the patient under local or general anesthesia, the flap is planned and surface marking applied (Fig 2). In raising the flap, it is important to identify and preserve the marginal mandibular branch of the facial nerve. The flap pedicle is

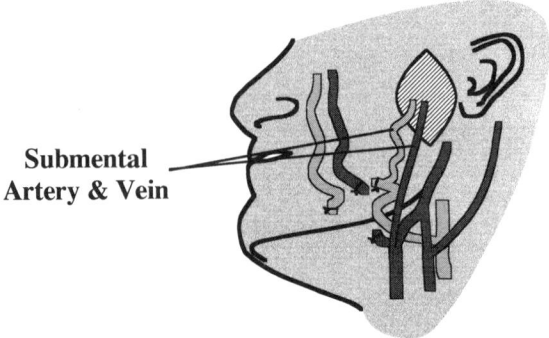

Submental Artery & Vein

FIGURE 3.—Elongation of the pedicle by division of the facial artery and vein distal to the origin of the submental artery. (Courtesy of Sterne GD, Januszkiewicz JS, Hall PN, et al: The submental island flap. *Br J Plast Surg* 49:85–89, 1996.)

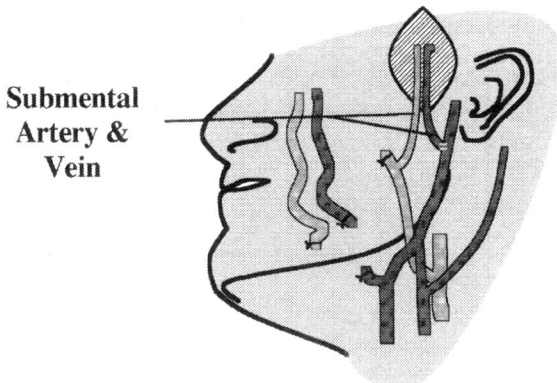

Submental Artery & Vein

FIGURE 4.—Elongation of the pedicle by division of the facial artery and vein distal to the origin of the submental artery, and division and anastomosis of the common facial or submental vein. (Courtesy of Sterne GD, Januszkiewicz JS, Hall PN, et al: The submental island flap. *Br J Plast Surg* 49:85–89, 1996.)

then dissected, if necessary, and the facial artery traced proximally. Downwards retraction on the submandibular gland reveals the submental artery. After the margins of the flap are incised, the flap is raised and a large skin paddle is produced.

Additional dissection can increase the length of the pedicle. By dividing the facial vessels distal to the origin of the submental artery, 1–2 cm of pedicle length are added (Fig 3). The taut submental or common facial vein then can be divided and anastomosed to a suitable vein near the recipient site (Fig 4). Dividing the

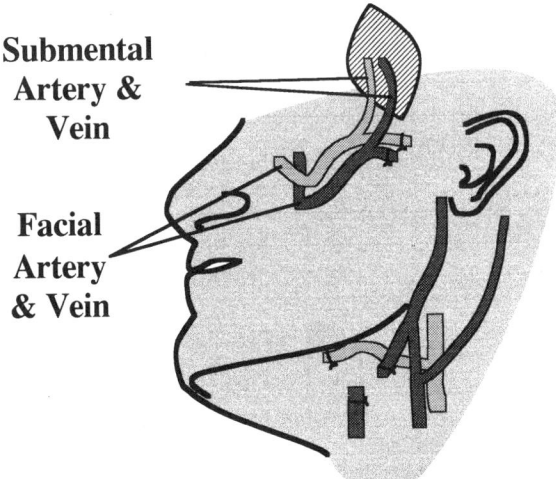

Submental Artery & Vein

Facial Artery & Vein

FIGURE 5.—Raising the flap in a reverse flow manner by dividing the facial vessels proximal to the origin of the submental artery. (Courtesy of Sterne GD, Januszkiewicz JS, Hall PN, et al: The submental island flap. *Br J Plast Surg* 49:85–89, 1996.)

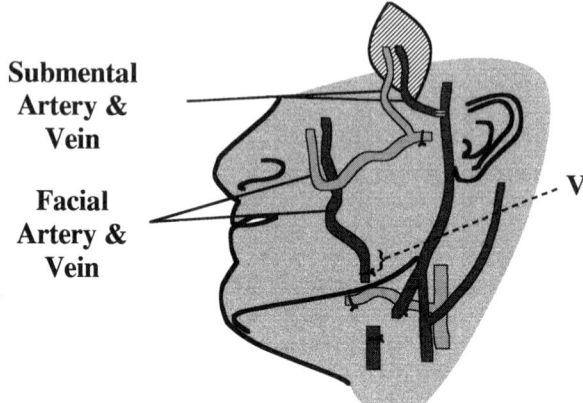

Submental Artery & Vein

Facial Artery & Vein

V

FIGURE 8.—Anastomosis of submental vein to allow orthograde venous return. The position of the constant valve in the facial vein is marked with a V. (Courtesy of Sterne GD, Januszkiewicz JS, Hall PN, et al: The submental island flap. *Br J Plast Surg* 49:85–89, 1996.)

facial vessels proximal to the origin of the facial artery and raising the entire flap can achieve even further pedicle advancement (Fig 5).

Results.—The mean age of the patients was 72 years and the maximum paddle width was 15 × 6 cm. Elderly patients are most suited for the submental island flap because of their abundance of lax tissue in this area. Flap raising and insetting required a mean period of 30 minutes; the mean postoperative stay was 9 days. All donor sites healed well. Two patients had marginal mandibular nerve palsy, a complication that can be avoided by identifying and preserving this nerve before the flap is raised. The only patient to receive a reverse flow flap eventually lost the flap. To prevent loss, a separate venous anastomosis should always be performed (Fig 8) in such cases. There was also 1 partial flap loss.

Discussion.—The submental island flap is useful for reconstruction after excision of intraoral malignancy, although its use would not be recommended when established nodal disease in the neck is present. This flap is raised easily and rapidly, offers a good skin match in color and texture, and leaves a well-hidden donor site.

▶ In addition to the seemingly straightforward indications and reliability of this flap, especially in elderly patients who may have an abundance of lax submental tissue, I found this article interesting for 2 reasons. First, to avoid the complication of damaging the marginal mandibular branch of the facial nerve, the authors rightly suggest it be identified so as to be protected. Second, it was helpful to recognize a constant valve in the facial vein (see Fig 8), which can be a problem with raising the flap in a reverse flow manner. Anatomy again can be a key to success, or a trail to problems!

H.T. Greenway, M.D.

Skin Grafts

Conchal Bowl Skin Grafting in Nasal Tip Reconstruction: Clinical and Histologic Evaluation

Rohrer TE, Dzubow LM (Boston Univ; Univ of Pennsylvania, Philadelphia)

J Am Acad Dermatol 33:476–481, 1995   3–12

Purpose.—Defects of the distal nose are commonly managed with full-thickness skin grafts taken from the periclavicular, preauricular, or post-auricular area. However, skin from these sites may not provide a good cosmetic match, largely because it lacks the highly sebaceous nature of the skin of the distal nose. The conchal bowl was evaluated as a site of donor skin to repair defects of the nasal tip.

> *Technique.*—The skin of the conchal bowl has a more "pebbled" appearance than the skin at other commonly used donor sites, and also contains more sebaceous glands. It is readily available and often provides a better color match for the skin of the distal nose. Either full-thickness or composite grafts can be harvested and used. The full-thickness grafts provide excellent results in patients with superficial defects, such as those produced by Mohs micrographic surgery. The harvest and suture techniques are the same as those used for other full-thickness grafts. The graft is harvested just above the perichondrium, which is left behind to cover the carti-lage; healing by secondary intention is allowed to occur. The donor site cartilage may be removed or perforated to permit healing. The cosmetic results are best when the graft used is slightly smaller than the defect to be covered.

Discussion.—Skin grafts from the conchal bowl provide excellent cover for defects of the skin of the distal nose. The conchal bowl is a reliable source of donor skin that provides a better cosmetic match than skin from the periclavicular, preauricular, and postauricular areas. The relative thin-ness and small size of conchal bowl skin grafts are limiting factors.

► The achievement of an excellent texture, contour, and color match on the tip of the nose with skin graft reconstruction can be a challenge. This is especially true for anything less than a shallow defect. As we see so often, anatomy can be the key as we seek to replace with "like tissue." The authors are to be commended, especially for their discussion that reviews perichondrial cutaneous grafts and the possible advantages when the peri-condrium is included in the donor graft. The knowledge that the skin in the conchal bowl has both a "pebbled" surface and contains many sebaceous glands may contribute to an enhanced result.

H.T. Greenway, M.D.

The Use of Full-thickness Skin Grafts for the Repair of Defects on the Dorsal Hand and Digits

Gloster HM Jr, Daoud MS, Roenigk RK (Mayo Clinic and Found, Rochester, Minn)

Dermatol Surg 21:953–959, 1995

3–13

Background.—Sun-induced malignancies commonly occur on the dorsal surface of the hand, but this area is not amenable to second-intention healing or primary closure after excision because wound contraction or tension can limit flexibility. Although the adjacent skin is of poor quality for use as a local flap, full-thickness skin grafting (FTSG) from other sites can produce a durable and cosmetically acceptable graft that preserves hand function. The effectiveness of FTSG in repairing surgical defects of the dorsal hand was examined.

Methods.—The results of repair of 21 dorsal-hand defects in 19 patients were evaluated retrospectively via review of written and photographic interviews and personal interviews (available for 12 patients). The patients underwent FTSG repair after Mohs micrographic surgery for excision of cutaneous squamous cell carcinoma on the dorsum of the hand or digits.

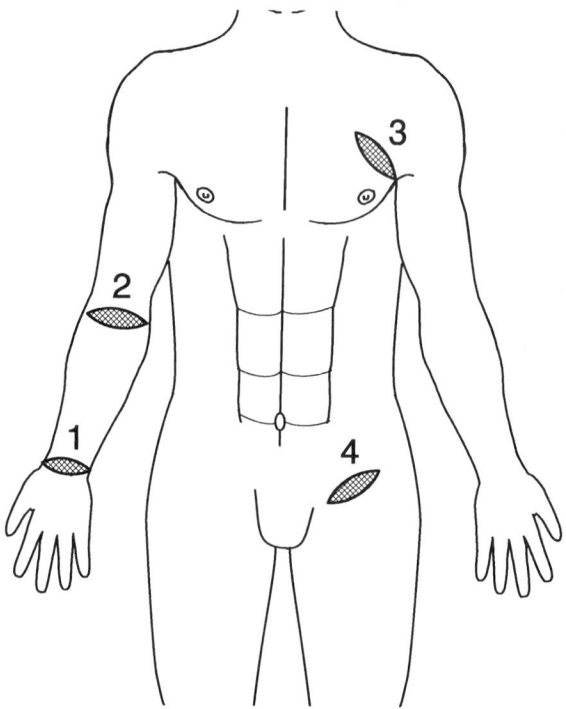

FIGURE 4.—Typical donor sites for FTSGs on the dorsum of the hands and digits include the (*1*) volar wrist, (*2*) antecubital fossa, (*3*) anterior axillary fold, and (*4*) inguinal fold. (Reprinted by permission of the publisher from Gloster HM Jr, Daoud MS, Roenigk RK: The use of full-thickness skin grafts for the repair of defects on the dorsal hand and digits. *Dermatol Surg* 21:953–959, copyright 1995 by Elsevier Science Inc.)

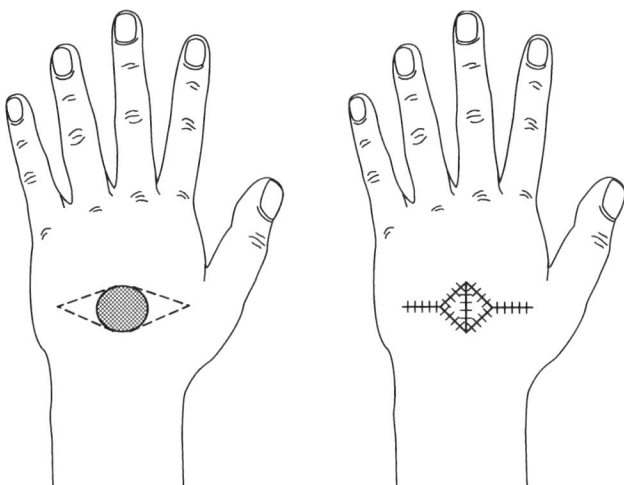

FIGURE 5.—Burow's grafts provide excellent tissue match to surrounding skin because donor skin is harvested from tissue adjacent to the defect. (Reprinted by permission of the publisher from Gloster HM Jr, Daoud MS, Roenigk RK: The use of full-thickness skin grafts for the repair of defects on the dorsal hand and digits. *Dermatol Surg* 21:953–959, copyright 1995 by Elsevier Science Inc.)

The anterior axillary fold was used as the donor site for 80% of grafts, and the antecubital fossa was used for 20%.

Results.—Patient and physician evaluations of the FTSGs were satisfactory. Functional impairment of the hand caused by graft contracture did not occur, nor did graft failure, hematoma, seroma, infection, or nerve damage.

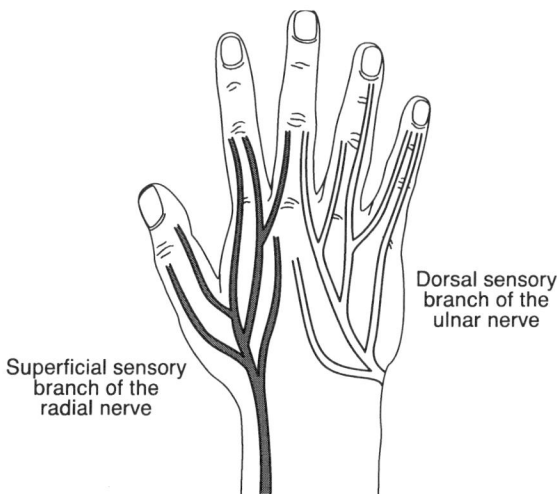

FIGURE 6.—Dorsal sensory branches of radial and ulnar nerves are superficial at the level of the wrist and are therefore vulnerable to injury. (Reprinted by permission of the publisher by Gloster HM Jr, Daoud MS, Roenigk RK: The use of full-thickness skin grafts for the repair of defects on the dorsal hand and digits. *Dermatol Surg* 21:953–959, copyright 1995 by Elsevier Science Inc.)

Discussion.—Repair of defects larger than 1 cm on the dorsum of the hand or 0.5 cm on the dorsum of the digits may be satisfactorily repaired with FTSG, which prevents wound contracture in up to 80% of instances. Typical donor areas for dorsal hand defects are shown in (Figure 4). Inguinal grafts are more apparent when used on the hand than are upper-extremity grafts; volar wrist grafts may produce a "suicide scar." Burow's grafts provide a superb tissue match (Fig 5). Superficial dissection to harvest volar wrist grafts must avoid damage to the palmar sensory branch of the median nerve (Fig 6). Grafts may fail over large areas of exposed tendon unless synovium or paratenon is present. The hand should be immobilized for at least 5 days after surgery, although splints may need to be removed earlier in older patients. The splint should flex the interphalangeal joints 10 degrees, extend the wrist 30–45 degrees, and flex the metacarpophalangeal joints 70–80 degrees. Alcohol should be prohibited perioperatively because of its potent vasodilatory effects. Aspirin, nonsteroidal anti-inflammatory drugs, and warfarin should also be avoided. Functional impairment caused by contracture of FTSGs is unlikely but can be prevented by slightly oversizing the graft and stretching the recipient defect to better anticipate its true surface area.

▶ This is an excellent review of the authors' experience and one is impressed by the total lack of postoperative complications in their series. Although this is our treatment of choice in many similar instances, on occasion we have also used split-thickness skin grafts on the dorsum of the hand and have been impressed with the results and durability. Anatomy again plays an important role (see Fig 6) in terms of possible nerve injury. Postoperative dressings and care are most important.

H.T. Greenway, M.D.

Freehand Technique to Harvest Partial-Thickness Skin to Repair Superficial Facial Defects
Snow SN, Stiff M, Lambert D, et al (Univ of Wisconsin, Madison; Ohio State Univ, Columbus)
Dermatol Surg 21:153–157, 1995   3–14

Background.—Most facial surgeons use local skin flaps or Wolfe-type full grafts for repair of facial defects. Good results can be obtained with partial-thickness grafts from the periauricular region to repair superficial defects at certain facial sites. The results of a freehand-scalpel technique for skin graft harvest were reviewed.

Technique.—In the freehand technique, a Telfa pad is used to create a template of the skin defect. A number 15 scalpel blade and the pencil-grip hand position is used to access the dermis with a beveled or vertical outline incision. The sebaceous glands are cut by slicing the graft at the level of the upper-reticular dermis; the initial cutting angle is similar to that used in micrographic surgery, but a more blunted-vertical angle is used once the desired dermal plane is reached. This angle helps stabilize the dermis as the graft is cut and ensures a fairly even dermal thickness. The graft averages 1 mm in thickness. After the graft is placed on the recipient site, a bolster is tied in the usual fashion.

Results.—This freehand graft technique was used to cover facial defects in 65 patients, including nose, ear, and forehead sites. There were 3 cases of postoperative hematoma that resulted in partial graft necrosis, but no grafts were lost. There were a few problems with persistent erythema, hypopigmented grafts, and late subgraft folliculitis. The experience suggested that a very good take and skin match could be expected in over 90% of cases.

Conclusions.—Skin grafts harvested in freehand fashion from the preauricular cheek and subauricular nose are very useful to provide cover for superficial facial defects. This technique expands the choices of potential donor sites, allows the surgeon to create a graft of the needed shape and depth, does not require specialized instrumentation, and achieves wound repair with good appearance and function. The authors use freehand partial-thickness skin grafts rather than conventional full-thickness skin grafts for almost all superficial facial defects.

▶ The freehand harvest of partial- or split-thickness skin for grafts has been described for a number of years with a variety of skin graft knives (Ferris Smith, Cobbett, Watson, etc.). The authors feel they can obtain acceptable results freehand with a number 15 or 10 blade. Their results speak for themselves, but I prefer and recommend consideration of those knives that allow thickness settings to obtain a more uniform donor, available in both power and non-power styles. Having said this, I have on occasion obtained split-thickness skin for facial defects from the same donor sites described through the utilization of a Personna® stainless steel sterilized razor blade and found the results acceptable. Interestingly, we refer to this instrument as a "number 5" in order to separate it from a "number 10 or 15 blade," as the majority of this work is done under local anesthesia.

H.T. Greenway, M.D.

Delayed Full-Thickness Grafting of Lower Leg Defects Following Removal of Skin Malignancies
Coldiron BM, Rivera E (Univ of Cincinnati, Ohio; Univ of Illinois, Chicago; Indiana Univ, Indianapolis)
Dermatol Surg 22:23–26, 1996   3–15

Background.—When skin cancers are removed from the lower leg, it is sometimes difficult to close the wound, particularly in distal areas where the skin is taut. If the wound cannot be closed primarily or with a local flap, a skin graft is performed. Full-thickness grafts are generally preferred over split-thickness grafts, but they may not survive the immediate post-operative period. Delayed grafting is described as an alternative approach to the management of lower leg wounds.

Methods.—Thirteen patients whose wounds could not be closed primarily or with a local flap underwent Mohs micrographic surgery to remove skin cancers from the lower legs. Many had diseases that would have reduced the chances of a successful immediate graft. After 10 to 21 days of healing by granulation, the wounds were covered with a full-thickness graft from the ipsilateral inguinal crease. For large grafts, both inguinal creases were used. After donor site closure, the graft was defatted and the wound was lightly curetted. Oral antibiotics were given on the day of the graft. After 10 to 14 days of bolstering, all sutures were removed. The edges and base of the graft were approximated with stainless steel staples. The patients were instructed to keep the limb elevated for 5 days and to keep the graft site dry.

Results.—Take was 100% in 11 of 13 grafts, 70% in 1, and 60% in 1. At a follow-up of 2 and 6 months, all patients were free of recurrent tumor, with good graft stability and sensation.

Conclusions.—A delayed full-thickness skin graft can be a very helpful procedure for wounds of the distal leg. A delay of the graft enhances the chances of a successful full-thickness graft, which has several advantages over split-thickness grafts. It also avoids the need to hospitalize the patient for elevation of the extremity.

▶ The authors delayed reconstruction for a period of 10 to 21 days and believed, as have others, that this enhanced graft survival. I also have found this to be beneficial, especially with full thickness grafts such as those in this case. The donor was the inguinal crease, an acceptable area. I have, however, seen problems from this site when used on the face related to hair growth in the graft. Split thickness skin grafts also work well over the lower legs.

H.T. Greenway, M.D.

Success of Delayed Full-Thickness Skin Grafts After Mohs Micrographic Surgery

Thibault M-J, Bennett RG (Univ of California, Los Angeles; Univ of Southern California, Los Angeles)
J Am Acad Dermatol 32:1004–1009, 1995   3–16

Objective.—There is yet no recent clinical study that has systematically investigated the clinical factors that may affect the success of full-thickness skin grafts after Mohs micrographic surgery. The factors that may affect outcome of full-thickness skin grafts after Mohs micrographic surgery were examined retrospectively.

Methods.—In 117 patients who had a full-thickness skin graft after Mohs micrographic surgery, patient variables (age, sex, diseases, medications, and smoking), tumor variables (tumor type and anatomical location), and skin graft variables (size, donor site, delays in days before skin graft placement, and complications) were correlated with skin graft success. Skin grafts were placed on wounds between the same day of and up to 8 days after surgery. Daily wound dressing and topical antibiotics were performed during the delay between surgery and graft placement.

Findings.—Delay of skin graft placement by more than 1 day correlated significantly with subsequent skin graft success. Necrosis occurred in 32% of patients who received skin graft 1 day after surgery, compared with only 3.7% of patients who received the skin graft between 2 and 8 days after surgery. Skin graft necrosis occurred more often in men (25%) than in women (8.6%).

Conclusion.—It is proposed that full-thickness skin graft placement should be performed after a delay of 2 to 8 days after Mohs micrographic surgery, particularly in men. The delay allows for elaboration of granulation tissue in the recipient site, resulting in adequate vascularity on the surfaces to be grafted. In addition, lower bacterial count induced by daily wound dressing and topical antibiotics during the delay favors graft success. Delayed application of the graft may eliminate bleeding and hematoma formation.

▶ Delayed skin grafting plays a very useful role in dermatologic surgery and Mohs micrographic surgery. This paper is important in that it defines what these authors feel is the optimal period to perform the graft. The graft could be performed with a longer delay, but it might be necessary to excise excess granulation tissue to achieve optimal conformation of the graft to the defect.

D.C. Whitaker, M.D.

Use of Dermagraft, a Cultured Human Dermis, to Treat Diabetic Foot Ulcers

Gentzkow GD, Prendergast JJ, Iwasaki SD, et al (Advanced Tissue Sciences Inc, La Jolla, Calif; Endocrine-Metabolic Associates, Atherton, Calif; Diabetes and Metabolic Ctr of Florida, Orlando)
Diabetes Care 19:350–354, 1996   3–17

Background.—Diabetic foot ulcers are typically treated with debridement and moist wound dressings, with special shoes to reduce pressure. However, cultured human dermis has recently been developed as a wound-healing tool. Neonatal dermal fibroblasts are cultured onto a bioabsorbable mesh, which then forms a living tissue with normal dermal matrix proteins and cytokines. The ability of a cultured human dermis, Dermagraft, to improve the healing of diabetic foot ulcers was evaluated in a controlled, prospective, multicenter, randomized, single-blind study.

Methods.—Fifty patients with full-thickness diabetic ulcers were randomly assigned to 4 treatment groups: 1 piece of Dermagraft applied weekly for 8 weeks (group A); 2 pieces of Dermagraft applied every 2 weeks for 8 weeks (group B); 1 piece of Dermagraft applied every 2 weeks for 8 weeks (group C); or no Dermagraft (control group). All 4 groups were also given standard care, including debridement, dressings, and pressure relief. Efficacy was evaluated by comparison of the percentage of patients achieving complete wound closure and 50% wound closure at week 12, time to complete wound closure and 50% wound closure, and the percentage of change in wound area and volume each week.

Results.—At week 12, complete wound closure was achieved in 50% of group A, 21.4% of group B, 18.2% of group C, and 7.7% of the control group. At week 12, 50% wound closure was achieved in 75% of group A, 50% of group B, 18.2% of group C, and 23.1% of the control group. Decreases in wound area and wound volume were significantly greater in the groups treated with Dermagraft, with a clear dose-response pattern. The time to complete and 50% wound closure was significantly faster in group A than in the control group. There were no recurrences in the 11 patients with completely healed ulcers, with an average follow-up of 14 months. There were no adverse treatment effects.

Conclusions.—Dermagraft treatment resulted in significant improvements in the rate and time of complete or 50% closure and in the reduction in volume of diabetic foot ulcers in a dose-dependent manner. The lack of recurrence may also indicate an improved quality, as well as rate, of healing.

▶ The ability to culture neonatal dermal fibroblasts on a bioabsorbable polyglactin mesh for clinical use is a tremendous achievement. The aforementioned study provided pilot evidence, and future work will determine its effectiveness when compared with multiple other treatment modalities, including porcine grafts and human allografts. Although cost is a factor, the ability to successfully treat this problem in this group of patients is highly desirable.

H.T. Greenway, M.D.

Secondary Intention Granulation Healing

Outcome Analysis of Mohs Surgery of the Lip and Chin: Comparing Secondary Intention Healing and Surgery
Becker GD, Adams LA, Levin BC (Southern California Permanente Med Group, Panorama City)
Laryngoscope 105:1176–1183, 1995   3–18

Introduction.—Facial skin cancer is commonly treated with microscopically controlled (Mohs) surgery to minimize tissue resection and optimize cure. The wounds resulting from Mohs surgery can be surgically repaired immediately or allowed to heal by secondary intention. It has been suggested that the cosmetic results may be better with Mohs wounds on concave areas of the face than on convex areas. The predictors of wound healing were studied in a retrospective and prospective evaluation of a large group of patients with Mohs defects of the lip and chin.

Methods.—Consecutive patients with defects of the lip and chin from Mohs surgical treatment of basal or squamous cell carcinoma over a 10-year period were evaluated. Patients were followed prospectively after January 1, 1994. There were 105 patients whose wounds were allowed to heal by secondary intention and 42 patients with surgically repaired wounds. The acceptability of the final cosmetic result was documented at least 6 months after surgery.

Results.—Healing by secondary intention required 3–6 weeks, depending upon the size and depth of the wounds. With wounds of the upper lip healing by secondary intention, acceptable cosmetic results were achieved in all patients with wounds involving the lip proper only, but in only 50% of the patients with wounds encroaching within 2 mm of the vermilion. The outcome of surgical repair of upper lip wounds was acceptable for 10 of 12 patients. Among patients with wounds involving the nasolabial fold, healing by secondary intention resulted in acceptable results in 27 of 28 patients, but only 9 of the 17 patients who underwent surgical repair of these wounds had acceptable cosmetic outcomes. Seven of 8 patients with philtrum wounds had an acceptable result, including 4 of 5 patients with vermilion involvement, as did all 4 patients who had primary surgical repair. Among patients with lower lip wounds, there was vermilion distortion in 67% of those healed with secondary intention and 50% of those who had primary surgical reconstruction. Scarring and/or dimpling occurred in all patients with chin wounds healed by secondary intention and 56% of the chin wounds repaired surgically.

Conclusion.—The location of the facial wound is the primary predictor of the cosmetic outcome of healing by secondary intention. Wounds that are on the chin or involve or are close to the vermilion may be best managed with surgical repair. Other wounds may have better cosmetic results if allowed to heal by secondary intention, with revisional surgery reserved for unacceptable wound-healing results.

▶ This outcome analysis is a useful follow-up to John Zitelli's original article in 1983 on secondary intention healing of the face. The original article established that most soft-tissue wounds in this location heal in 3 to 6 weeks. These authors further point out that cosmetic outcome in secondary intention healing can be predicted in most instances.

D.C. Whitaker, M.D.

Reference

1. Zitelli JA: Wound healing by secondary intention. A cosmetic appraisal. *J Am Acad Dermatol* 9:407–415, 1983.

Healing by Secondary Intention of Auricular Defects After Mohs Surgery

Levin BC, Adams LA, Becker GD (Kaiser Permanente Med Ctr, Panorama City, Calif)
Arch Otolaryngol Head Neck Surg 122:59–66, 1996   3–19

Background.—It is generally accepted that full-thickness skin defects that result from cancer surgery should immediately be reconstructed to preserve function and minimize cosmetic deformity. As a result, few studies have evaluated the results of healing by secondary intention. However, healing by secondary intention can improve cancer surveillance, simplify wound management, and avoid the costs and complications of reconstructive surgery. The results of healing by secondary intention in patients with auricular defects after Mohs surgery were presented.

Methods.—The study included 133 patients with full-thickness auricular skin defects after Mohs surgery. One hundred twenty-six of the patients were men, and the mean age was 66 years. Defect locations included the helix, antihelix, concha, pretragal and tragal areas, lobule, and posterior aspect. Most patients had defects of a single subunit. The patient or family performed wound care at home that included daily cleansing and application of bacitracin zinc and polymyxin B sulfate ointment and a dressing. Various wound healing parameters were recorded, and the cosmetic results were evaluated at least 6 months postoperatively.

Results.—All 133 defects healed by secondary intention within 3 to 10 weeks; defects with exposed cartilage were at the longer end of the range. Few patients required postoperative analgesics, and antibiotics were used only arbitrarily. Three patients had wound infections, though none of these caused permanent sequelae. Defects of the central auricle had the best cosmetic results, often better than those of surgically repaired defects. Even defects with large areas of exposed cartilage healed well.

Conclusions.—Healing by secondary intention gives predictably good results in patients with auricular skin defects after Mohs surgery. The location of the wound is an important factor in the cosmetic results; healing by secondary intention is not necessarily contraindicated in defects with exposed cartilage. These patients do not require routine prophylactic antibiotics.

▶ During my fellowship with Dr. Fred Mohs, I learned an immense amount about secondary healing and how anatomy and location play important roles. The authors clearly demonstrate that the most common site for skin cancer on the ear, the helix (25% of patients in this study) was a poor site for secondary intention healing, and only 17 of 39 patients had an acceptable cosmetic result. The authors state emphatically that the central auricle (i.e., concha, antihelix, and posterior aspect of the auricle) heal achieves cosmetic results that are superior to surgically repaired defects, so perhaps a double blinded comparative trial might be helpful. In an arena of managed care, where less care may offer greater financial incentive to the physician, we must continue to put the patients interest first.

H.T. Greenway, M.D.

4 Aesthetic Dermatologic Surgery

Introduction

Dermatologic surgeons are increasingly being trained in performing cosmetic procedures. There has been a literal explosion of courses and seminars nationally and internationally geared at improving our skills in the mechanisms and fine art of these techniques. More and more residents applying for surgical fellowships are critically assessing programs in terms of the availability of being trained by their mentors to perform surgical hair restoration, sclerotherapy, liposuction, cutaneous laser surgery, dermabrasion and chemical peels. In addition to being informed about techniques which the field of dermatology has been instrumental in developing, it is also mandatory for us as practicing physicians to be able to inform our patients about new corrective procedures offered by our plastic surgical, ENT, and occuloplastic colleagues.

With these 2 goals in mind, we have made an attempt in this section to present innovative and interesting approaches in these areas, by authors from all over the world, in the hope that we will stimulate intra and interdisciplinary dialogue. We are all aware of the impact accelerated and more efficacious worldwide communication has had on our lives. It is our hope that this trend will lead to an enhancement in our ability to share information on a worldwide basis, especially as it pertains to aesthetic dermatologic surgery.

Diamondis J. Papadopoulos, M.D.

Surgical Management of the Aging Face

The Anterior Extension Face-Lift
Johnson CM Jr, Godin MS (Hedgewood Surgical Ctr, New Orleans, La; Med College of Virginia, Richmond)
Arch Otolaryngol Head Neck Surg 121:613–616, 1995   4–1

Rationale.—When performing face-lift surgery, it is important to confront the lateral orbital region, where redundant skin may lend a heavy or wrinkled appearance. The usual techniques entail cuts into the temporal head that can displace the hairline. The anterior temporal extension, used in conjunction with "deep-plane" face-lift methods, is a useful means of enhancing the lateral orbital area in selected patients.

> *Technique.*—The standard deep-plane rhytidectomy is modified so that the incision curves horizontally across the temporal hairline and is carried inferiorly in the preauricular crease. It rarely is necessary to incise onto or behind the tragus. Finally the incision extends about the inferior aspect of the lobule and onto the posterior auricular surface before curving gently into the postauricular hairline at the level of the inferior antihelical crus. The temporal incision may be continued anteriorly toward the lateral canthus. The flap is dissected in the neck just superficial to the platysma; subcutaneously and deep to the platysma in the midface (remaining superficial to the parotid-masseteric fascia); and subcutaneously in the temporal region up to the lateral aspect of the orbicularis oculis and zygomaticus major muscles. The skin is replaced under minimal tension after placing closed suction drains, and the extension incision is closed with interrupted vertical mattress sutures of 6–0 nylon.

Patients.—Anterior extension incisions were used in 15% of 98 patients having primary face-lift surgery in a 1-year period and in 69% of those having revision.

Results.—All but 1 of 35 patients having face-lift surgery with anterior temporal extensions were pleased with the outcome 3 months postoperatively. The exception was a patient with loose forehead skin who had a small skin fold over the line of the temporal extension incision.

Conclusion.—Anterior extension is a useful adjunct to face-lift surgery, particularly in elderly patients with hypoblastic skin and patients having revisional surgery. The procedure provides considerable control over the lateral orbital and temporal regions and results in a very natural appearance.

▶ This article makes a good point about placement of lines of incision in certain individuals. I find myself constantly reminding residents that proper placement of lines of incisions is based on many factors, not the least of which is patient age, degree of sun damage, skin texture and color skin type. Two procedures in the same anatomic area, for the same indication, performed in an identical manner in 2 individuals could have drastically different results. There are 2 things to learn from this article: 1) that you may be able, under the right circumstances, to perform surgical maneuvers that defy prior experience; and 2) that you must "pick your spots" (choose your patients carefully) when doing this. As a result of these 2 rules, you may be able to improve the quality and the breadth of your surgery.

D.J. Papadopoulos, M.D.

Subcutaneous Approach for Elevation of the Malar Fat Pad Through a Prehairline Incision
Collawn SS, Vasconez LO, Gamboa M, et al (Univ of Alabama, Birmingham)
Plast Reconstr Surg 97:836–841, 1996   4–2

Background.—The development of a deep nasolabial groove with aging is related to a lack of suspension of the cheek skin and malar fat pad. The described technique elevates the malar fat pad by way of a direct subcutaneous dissection over the lateral half of the malar fat pad, then elevates the fat pad almost vertically with interrupted sutures that are secured to the temporoparietal fascia of the prehairline incision.

> *Technique Overview.*—In standard rhytidectomy, a prehairline incision is made in the temporal area, and dissection is started in the preauricular area behind the tragus. Dissection is extended to expose the lateral half of the malar fat pad; no dissection under the malar fat pad occurs. Two interrupted sutures (4-0 nylon) are placed through the fat pad to elevate it almost vertically and at least perpendicular to the nasolabial line. After the sutures are anchored to the temporoparietal fascia of the prehairline incision, tension is applied until the nasolabial folds are corrected and the prominence of the cheeks is increased. The rhytidectomy then proceeds, including appropriate neck correction.

Results.—The described procedure was performed on 52 patients over an 18–month period; all patients showed maintained improvement in nasolabial folds and midface cheek projection for as long as 1 year (Fig 3).

Conclusions.—Vertical suspension of the malar fat pad is safe and allows the creation of a more youthful cheek and a lessening of the prominence of the nasolabial folds. No complications occurred with this technique.

▶ This technique involves more suspension anchored on the temporoparietal fascia with the malar fat pads pulled up vertically. Clear 4–0 nylon suture is used as a suspender. The authors reported 1-year follow-up results. It will be interesting to see long-term results of follow-up because it is well established that even nylon suture can be absorbed with time. Nevertheless, the authors show some excellent results at 1 year.

D.J. Papadopoulos, M.D.

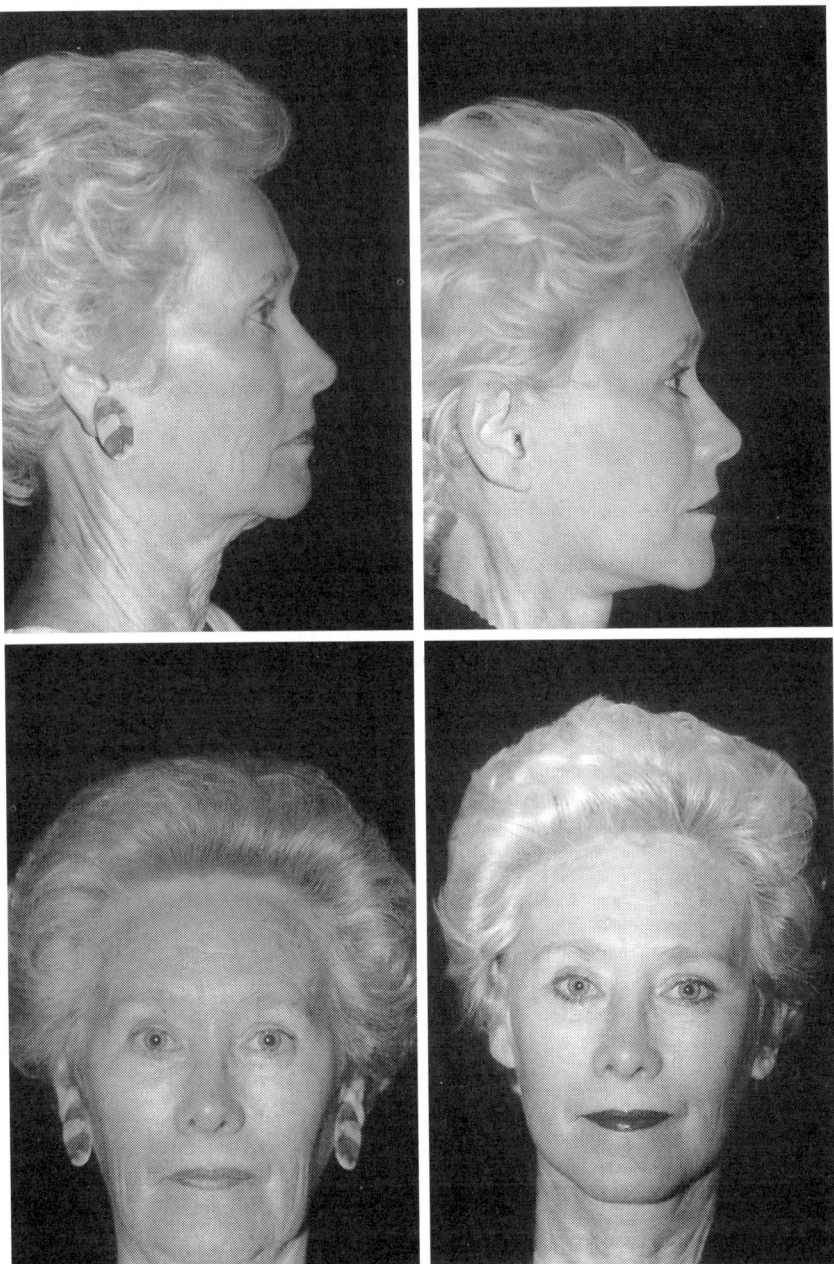

FIGURE 3.—The 60-year-old patient shown in these photographs has elevated malar fat pads and improved nasolabial folds at 1 year. (Courtesy of Collawn SS, Vasconez LO, Gamboa M, et al: Subcutaneous approach for elevation of the malar fat pad through a prehairline incision. *Plast Reconstr Surg* 97:836–841, 1996.)

Subcutaneous Incisionless (Subcision) Surgery for the Correction of Depressed Scars and Wrinkles

Orentreich DS, Orentreich N (New York)
Dermatol Surg 21:543–549, 1995   4–3

Introduction.—Subcision is a technique of subcuticular undermining that can improve the appearance of scars and wrinkles without having to incise the skin or inject an augmenting agent. The term—which is a contraction of *"subcutaneous incisionless"* surgery—consists of cutting beneath a depressed scar or contour using a tribeveled hypodermic needle (Fig 1) that is inserted under the skin through a needle puncture. The goal is to elevate the base of the defect to the level of the surrounding skin.

How It Works.—Subcision achieves its effect in 2 ways: by releasing the skin from its attachment to deeper tissues, thereby elevating it, and by inducing through controlled injury a wound healing response that leads to connective tissue formation, which augments the depressed sites.

Technique.—A 1-inch, 22-gauge disposable hypodermic B-D needle may be used in most cases, although larger needles may be helpful in treating cellulite and large, bound-down scars (Fig 6). The area to be subcised is anesthetized; the needle then is inserted a few millimeters from the depressed site and advanced beneath it, orienting the bevel upward. The needle tip is manipulated to cut under the skin surface, using the free hand as a guide and to stretch or stabilize the treated site. A lancing-type motion (Fig 2) may be used to subcise very fibrotic scars or under "crow's feet" wrinkles. Horizontal fanning and vertical movements of the needle tip also

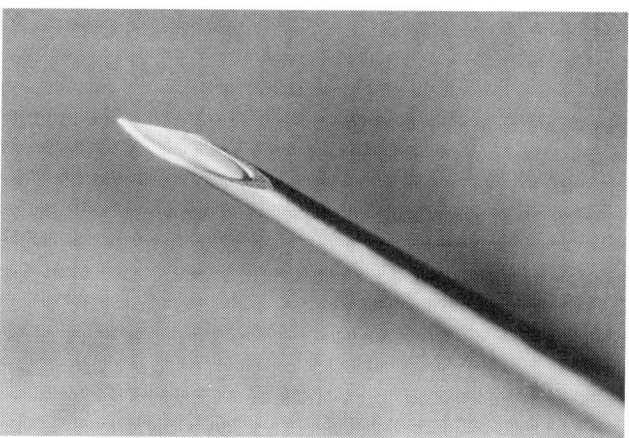

FIGURE 1.—Tribeveled hypodermic needle. Note its sharp edges. (Reprinted by permission of the publisher from Orentreich DS, Orentreich N: Subcutaneous incisionless (subcision) surgery for the correction of depressed scars and wrinkles. *Dermatol Surg* 21:543–549, copyright 1995 by Elsevier Science Inc.)

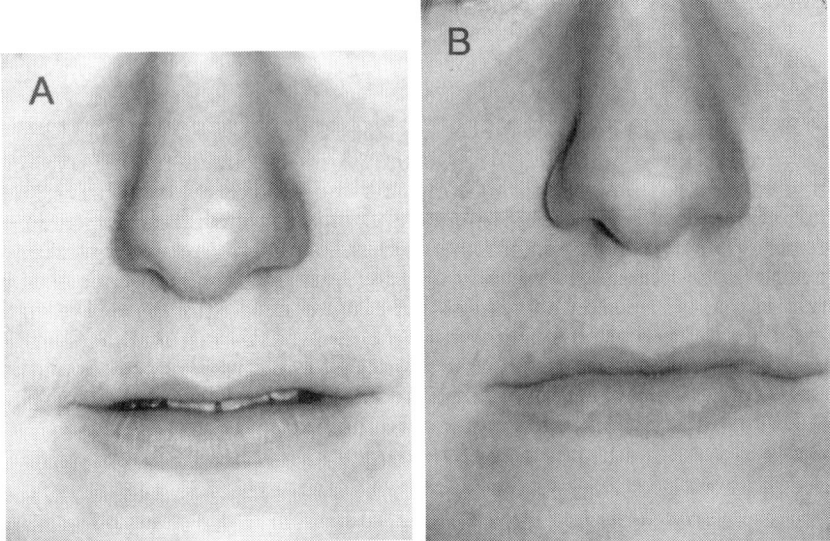

FIGURE 6.—A, a 21-year-old woman before subcision to correct a varicella scar on left tip of nose. B, 1 month postsubcision shows nearly complete correction. (Reprinted by permission of the publisher from Orentreich DS, Orentreich N: Subcutaneous incisionless (subcision) surgery for the correction of depressed scars and wrinkles. *Dermatol Surg* 21:543–549, copyright 1995 by Elsevier Science Inc.)

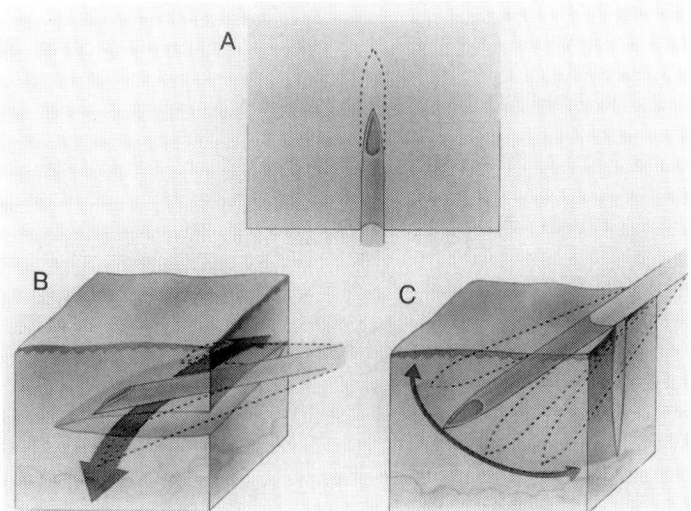

FIGURE 2.—Nomenclature. A, lancing subcision denotes inserting and withdrawing movements. B, horizontal fanning subcision denotes side-to-side movement. Note that the bevel is pointing upward. C, vertical subcision denotes cutting in a plane that is perpendicular to the skin surface. Note that the bevel is oriented vertically. (Reprinted by permission of the publisher from Orentreich DS, Orentreich N: Subcutaneous incisionless (subcision) surgery for the correction of depressed scars and wrinkles. *Dermatol Surg* 21:543–549, copyright 1995 by Elsevier Science Inc.)

may be useful. Direct manual pressure is applied for several minutes immediately after treating a site to ensure hemostasis.

Individualized Approach.—Depressed, bound-down scars usually are treated by subcision in the mid- to deep dermis to cut through the fibrous bands of scar tissue. Distensile depressed scars are managed by subcising in the deep dermis or subdermally. Subdermal subcision is appropriate for relieving facial expression lines. So-called cellulite that produces a dimpled appearance of the upper legs and buttocks is treated by subcision in the adipose layer. A majority of patients with moderate wrinkling or scarring may be adequately treated in 3 to 6 visits. Scar correction generally is permanent.

Patient Selection.—Active infection is an absolute contraindication to subcision. The deep, "ice pick" scar is best managed by punch grafting. Relative contraindications to subcision include the depressed, atrophic scar, a bleeding diathesis, and a history of keloid scarring after injury or surgery.

Complications.—Disruption of the pilosebaceous apparatus may result in localized cyst-like lesions, which respond to incision and drainage or intralesional steroid injection. Some patients may have temporary postinflammatory hyperpigmentation and should avoid solar exposure for at least a month. Excessive fibroplasia is a problem in 5% to 10% of cases. The elevated skin responds well to intralesional steroid injections.

▶ I have done this, and as a result of this article, am looking forward to doing it on bigger scars and on rhytides. It would be wonderful to be in a position where an inducer of fibroblasts to make more glycosaminoglycans or collagen could be injected immediately after this procedure, in an attempt to get even better responses.

D.J. Papadopoulos, M.D.

Suprafibromuscular Facelifting With Periosteal Suspension of the Superficial Musculoaponeurotic System and Fat Pad of Bichat Rotation: Tightening the Net
Keller GS, Cray J (Keller Facial Plastic Surgery Clinic, Santa Barbara, Calif)
Arch Otolaryngol Head Neck Surg 122:377–384, 1996   4–4

Introduction.—A facelift technique that tightens the suspensory net of the face while improving the safety of the facial nerve is described. The superficial musculoaponeurotic system (SMAS) is a complex fibromuscular suspensory "net" composed of the facial musculature and fibrous embryologic remnants. It is lined above and below by layers of fascia. The fibrofatty cheek fat, areolar tissue, subcutaneous fat, and skin are suspended on top of the net and its lining. Fat, deep fascia, the facial nerve, deep musculature, and bony structure of the face lie below the net and its lining. The net loosens and stretches in the process of aging. The technique described resuspends and fixes the SMAS net upward.

Methods.—The literature on modified composite facelift techniques was reviewed. Twenty-two fresh cadavers were dissected to identify the SMAS and develop a suprafibromuscular facelift technique. Sixty-one women and 12 men underwent this new technique.

> *Surgical Technique.*—A suprafibromuscular facelift dissection was performed in a subcutaneous plane along the mandible to within 3 to 4 cm from the lobule of the ear. A laser was used to make an incision through the SMAS at the level of the zygoma. Dissection over the malar eminence was over the periosteum and under the orbicularis. A midcheek dissection was made over the fibromuscular SMAS in the layer of areolar tissue. The fat pad of Bichat was rotated, if needed, for cheek augmentation. Suspension sutures were placed from the SMAS to the malar eminence to stabilize the elevation of the nasolabial fold, the melolabial fold, and the corner of the mouth. The malar fat pad was stabilized by a laterally directed flap of the SMAS sutured to the temporal fascia.

Results.—Patients were followed for 6 to 18 months. All patients maintained their nasolabial, melolabial, and malar fat pad corrections. In 5 patients who underwent a modified composite facelift on one side of the face and a suprafibromuscular layer lift with periosteal suspension on the opposite side, the postoperative appearance was similar bilaterally. One patient had a temporary zygomatic branch palsy on the composite facelift side of the face. Subjective comparison of the techniques indicated that the composite facelift plane seemed to experience greater postoperative swelling and longer postoperative recovery than the side that underwent dissection in the suprafibromuscular plane. No facial nerve complications developed.

Conclusion.—A side-to-side visual comparison of the sub-SMAS composite facelift and suprafibromuscular SMAS facelift showed no difference in results. Findings suggest that the SMAS facelift is safer than the composite facelift for the integrity of the facial nerve. Rotating the fat pad of Bichat can augment the submalar or malar areas without the use of a prosthetic implant. This approach also reduces the melolabial mound.

▶ We are not talking about the Internet here, but I am sure that if the results hold up for longer than 18 months of follow-up, this procedure might hit the airways in a big way. This is an innovative way to address a very difficult problem. Most corrections of the nasolabial folds, the melolabial folds, the malar fat pad, and the corner of the mouth that do not involve implants have usually resulted in a "wind tunnel" look because of over correction. By examining and clearly defining what series of anatomic events over time lead to distortion of the above-aforementioned anatomic structures and by correcting them by "tightening the net," these authors may have shared with us a way to approach these patients with these problems.

D.J. Papadopoulos, M.D.

Central Suspension Technique of the Midface
Hagerty RC (Med Univ of South Carolina, Charleston)
Plast Reconstr Surg 96:728–730, 1995   4–5

Introduction.—A technique that combines the lateral suspension of the orbicularis muscle, skin removal, and subcutaneous dissection of the nasolabial fold was developed to elevate the soft tissues of the midface and soften the nasolabial fold. The technique was described and its results in 17 patients reviewed.

> *Surgical Procedure.*—A blepharoplasty incision is placed 2–3 cm lateral to the lateral canthus, extending medially along the subciliary line to the punctum. Dissection begins through the orbicularis oculi at the incision and continues medially under the orbicularis

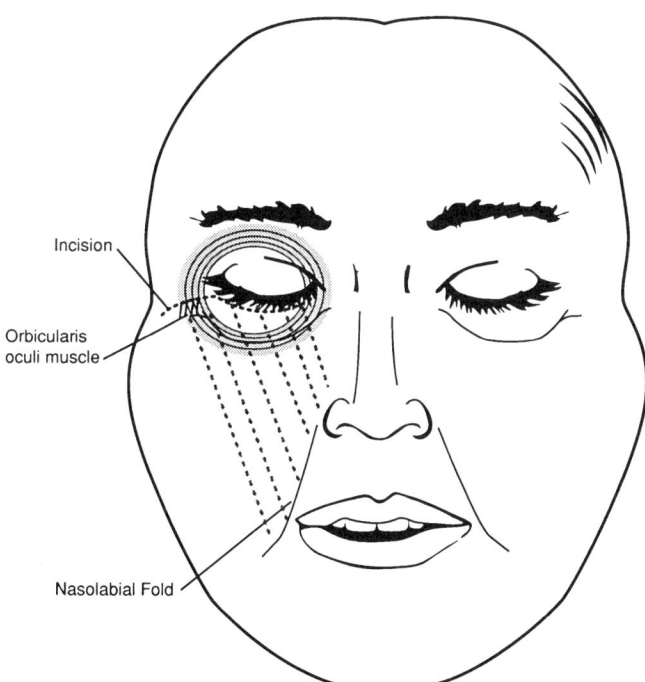

FIGURE 1.—Subcutaneous dissection extends along lateral third of inferior border of orbicularis oculi muscle to below the nasolabial crease. The submuscular dissection extends the lateral third of the orbicularis muscle. The incision through the muscle is made only lateral to the lateral canthus. (Courtesy of Hagerty RC: Central suspension technique of the midface. *Plast Reconstr Surg* 96:728–730, 1995.)

oculi muscle. At the lateral canthus, dissection continues in the subcutaneous plane above the orbicularis oculi muscle, which is elevated on the malar eminence lateral to the lateral canthus, leaving the tarsal portion in place (Fig 1). The muscle skin flap is pulled diagonally, perpendicular to the nasolabial fold (Fig 2). Without tendon incision, the inferior ramus of the lateral canthal tendon is sutured to a higher position on the orbital rim periosteum. Excess muscle and/or skin are excised lateral and medial to the lateral canthus (Fig 3). An excessive fat pad exaggerating the nasolabial crease can be suctioned conservatively. The orbicularis oculi muscle is attached to the periosteum over the lateral orbital rim laterally, and the skin is closed with sutures. Incisional tension is reduced with the application of tape and cold compresses for 24 hours.

Methods.—Seventeen patients underwent the procedure over a 1-year period. All were followed for at least 6 months.

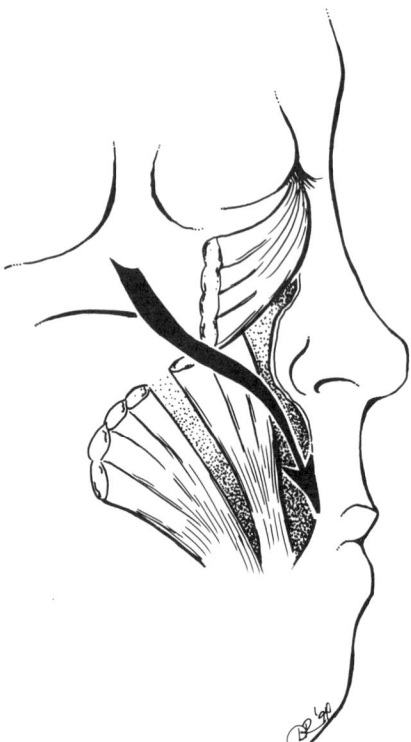

FIGURE 2.—Only skin is elevated medial to the lateral canthus. The dissection lateral to the lateral canthus includes both skin and orbicularis muscle. The vector pull is diagonal and perpendicular to the nasolabial fold that has been freed subcutaneously. (Courtesy of Hagerty RC: Central suspension technique of the midface. *Plast Reconstr Surg* 96:728–730, 1995.)

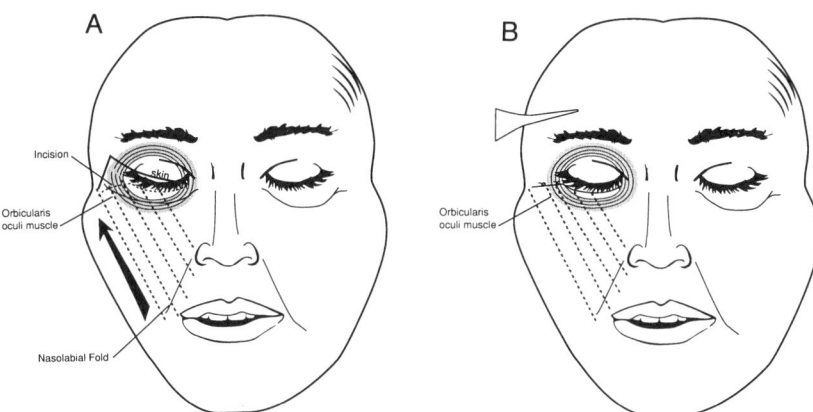

FIGURE 3.—Left: The excess orbicularis oculi muscle and skin lateral to the lateral canthus and excess skin medial to the lateral canthus are resected. **Right:** The muscle is resuspended laterally to the lateral orbital wall periosteum. (Courtesy of Hagerty RC: Central suspension technique of the midface. *Plast Reconstr Surg* 96:728–730, 1995.)

Results.—There were more dramatic results in patients with moderate nasolabial folds than in patients with heavy nasolabial folds. The lateral incision healed rapidly in most of the patients but took up to 3 months in a few. Complications included paresthesia involving the infraorbital nerve in 1 patient (which resolved in 3 months) and the development of small,

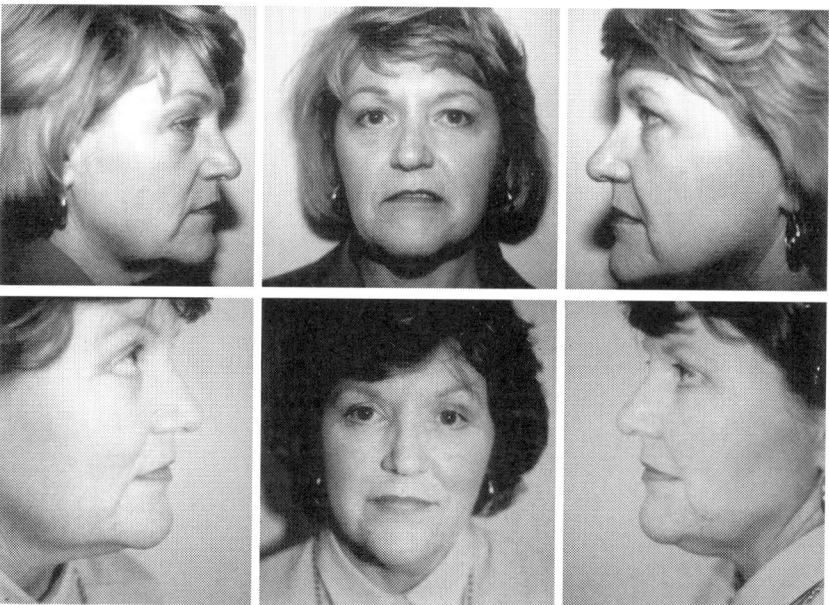

FIGURE 4.—A 47-year-old woman with premature aging showing preoperative and postoperative views after central face lift and upper eyelid blepharoplasty. (Courtesy of Hagerty RC: Central suspension technique of the midface. *Plast Reconstr Surg* 96:728–730, 1995.)

firm nodules in 5 patients (which resolved in up to 3 months). Lateral scleral show and rounded lateral eyelid were avoided by conservative resection of skin medial to the lateral canthus and the lateral canthopexy.

Conclusion.—This central suspension technique can be effective in addressing moderate nasolabial folds (Fig 4), particularly in younger patients and in older patients who have undergone a previous facelift. Its results are less dramatic than facelift techniques because it cannot resuspend the cheek pad.

▶ Here is another interesting suspension technique with no transfer of the cheek fat of Bichat. It would be interesting to see what the combination of tightening the net procedure and parts of this procedure would have on the longevity of the results. We will continue to see more of these suspension procedures, especially with the added use and benefits of endoscopy and newer suture materials.

D.J. Papadopoulos, M.D.

Transconjunctival Blepharoplasty: Further Applications and Adjuncts
Dodenhoff TG (Phoenix, Ariz)
Aesthetic Plast Surg 19:511–517, 1995   4–6

Introduction.—The use of transconjunctival blepharoplasty (TCB) has been extended, with some modifications, to patients who not only have

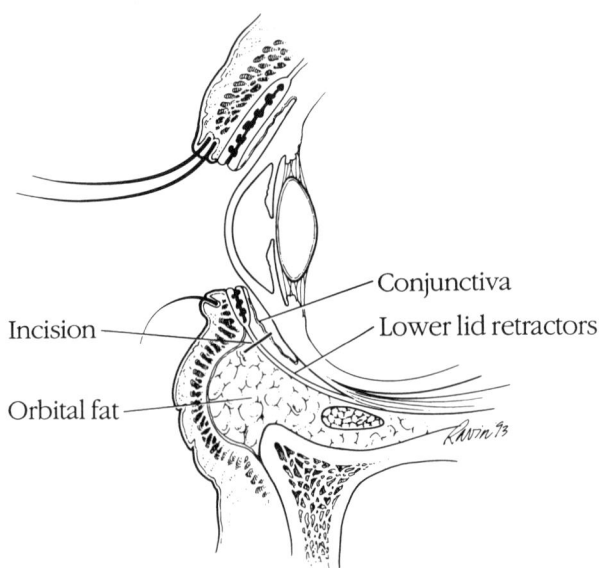

FIGURE 1.—Surgical anatomy of eyelid relative to transconjunctival blepharoplasty. (Courtesy of Dodenhoff TG: Transconjunctival blepharoplasty: Further applications and adjuncts. *Aesthetic Plast Surg* 19:511–517, copyright 1995 by Springer-Verlag).

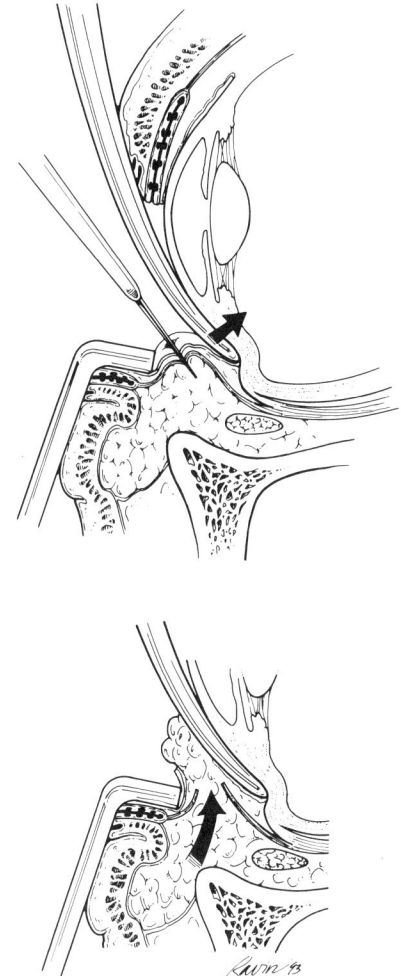

FIGURE 2.—Retractors in place; incision made with cutting electrocautery. (Courtesy of Dodenhoff TG: Transconjunctival blepharoplasty: Further applications and adjuncts. *Aesthetic Plast Surg* 19:511–517, copyright 1995 by Springer-Verlag.)

excess orbital fat, but have fine wrinkles, excess skin or orbicularis muscle relaxation or redundancy. The technique combines transconjunctival removal of fat via the Baylis technique (Fig 1) with a chemical peel, pinch excision, or lateral canthoplasty.

Surgical Technique.—The surgeon sits above the patient with the assistant on the patient's left side, if the surgeon is right-handed. The patient is sedated and then injected with epinephrine. The Baylis pyrex globe protector is used to protect the globe. The assistant retracts the lower lid with a Desmaires retractor. The

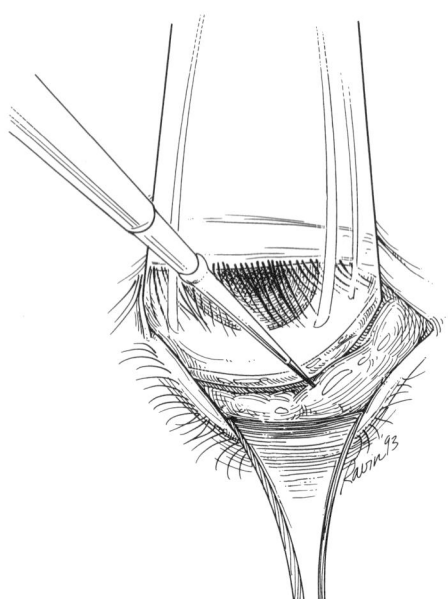

FIGURE 3.—Operative technique depicted graphically. (Courtesy of Dodenhoff TG: Transconjunctival blepharoplasty: Further applications and adjuncts. *Aesthetic Plast Surg* 19:511–517, copyright 1995 by Springer-Verlag.)

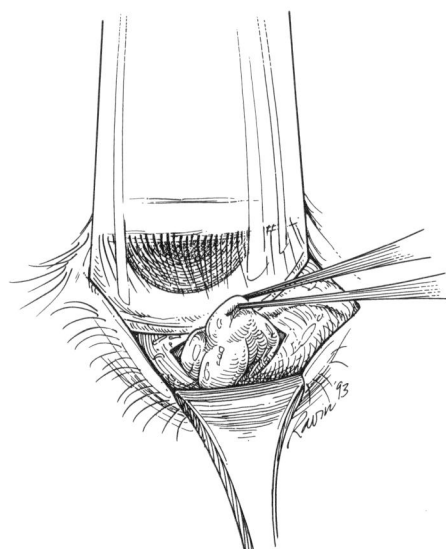

FIGURE 4.—After penetrating the conjunctiva and capsulopalpebral fascia, the excess fat bulges into the field. (Courtesy of Dodenhoff TG: Transconjunctival blepharoplasty: Further applications and adjuncts. *Aesthetic Plast Surg* 19:511–517, copyright 1995 by Springer-Verlag.)

Baylis pyrex retractor is placed into the sulcus below the orbital rim and abutting the orbital floor (Fig 2). The incision is made between the 2 retractors (Fig 3), below the lower border of the tarsal plate, and above the lowest portion of the scleral conjunctival globe/lid sulcus. When the incision is through the conjunctiva and the capsulopalpebral fascia, the retractors are rocked to produce the maximum bulge. The yellow fat will be apparent (Fig 4) and can be removed after clamping and cauterizing. The lower eyelid incision should be sutured. At this time, the pinch technique can be used to remove excess skin, a lateral canthoplasty, or a chemical peel can be performed.

Results.—From 1990 to 1993, 102 patients underwent lower-lid blepharoplasties. Of these, 86 were performed by the transconjunctival method and 16 by the standard skin-muscle flap method. Of the TCBs, 13 were performed alone, 22 had an associated skin pinch excision, 8 had a lateral canthoplasty, and 38 had a chemical peel.

Conclusions.—Transconjunctival blepharoplasty has been used for fat removal for many years. The authors have combined it with skin pinch excision, canthoplasty, or chemical peel and expanded its use to patients with excess skin and the relaxed soft tissues of aging. Combining these procedures does not significantly increase operating time and produces eyelids with an excellent appearance.

▶ Excellent article with some fine adjustments to an already proven and effective technique. The author is to be commended for his clear and detail-oriented way of writing, which makes apparent exactly what he has performed on his patients.

D.J. Papadopoulos, M.D.

Endoscopic Surgical Correction of Glabellar Creases

Matarasso A, Matarasso SL (Albert Einstein College, New York; Univ of California, San Francisco)
Dermatol Surg 21:695–700, 1995   4–7

Introduction.—The forehead is an area that is frequently used in the expression of emotions (Fig 1). The ideal proportions for this region of the face have been well characterized (Fig 4). Hyperactivity in this region can result in aesthetically displeasing configurations that may even convey unwanted emotions to the observer. In an attempt to improve this situation, a variety of temporary techniques have been proposed. There is also the classic brow-lift operation, which relies on a large scalp incision and is unpopular with patients (Fig 2). This report describes endoscopic excision of the frown muscle complex, a new technique to solve the problems of the forehead and brow area.

Brow Position-The Curtain of Emotion

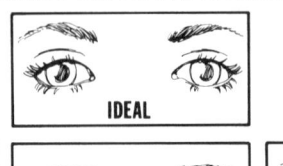

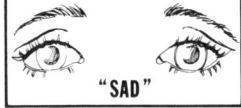
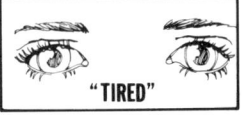
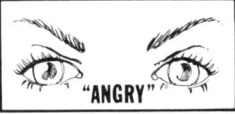

FIGURE 1.—The eyebrow reflects a diversity of emotion, whether intentional or involuntary. (Reprinted by permission of the publisher from Matarasso A, Matarasso SL: Endoscopic surgical correction of glabellar creases. *Dermatol Surg* 21:695–700, copyright 1995 by Elsevier Science Inc.)

Surgical Technique.—Surgery is performed under local anesthesia as an outpatient procedure. Preoperatively, patients are asked to animate their forehead muscles so these can be indicated on the skin, as an aid to endoscopy. The operation begins with 3-cm vertical incisions in the frontal hairline to gain access to the depressor muscles. A midline forehead optical cavity is prepared by undermining so an endoscope can be introduced. The depressor muscles are released, but their substance preserved to prevent a contour defect. Heavy sutures are used to provide external retraction. The wounds are closed with sutures or staples. A snug headband is worn for 2 or 3 weeks to minimize swelling. The procedure takes 30 to 60 minutes and patients are discharged when alert and stable.

Objective Analysis in Forehead-Brow Position

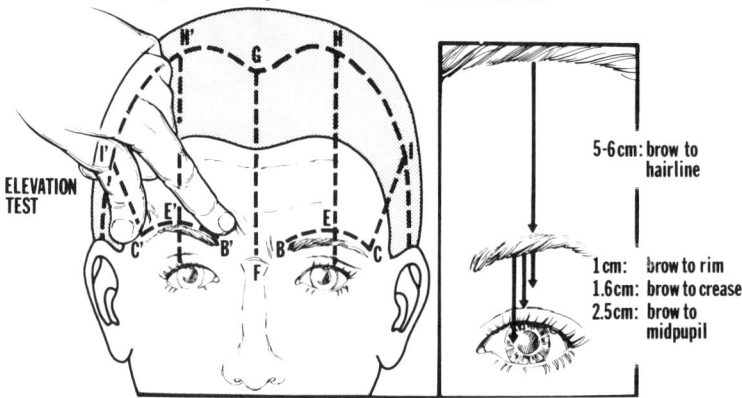

FIGURE 4.—The ideal spatial relationships of the brow have been described as well as numerical parameters (after Ellenbogen). The letters are used as reference points for brow positioning. These also vary according to age, race, gender, and cultural orientation. (Reprinted by permission of the publisher from Matarasso A, Matarasso SL: Endoscopic surgical correction of glabellar creases, *Dermatol Surg* 21:695–700, copyright 1995 by Elsevier Science Inc.)

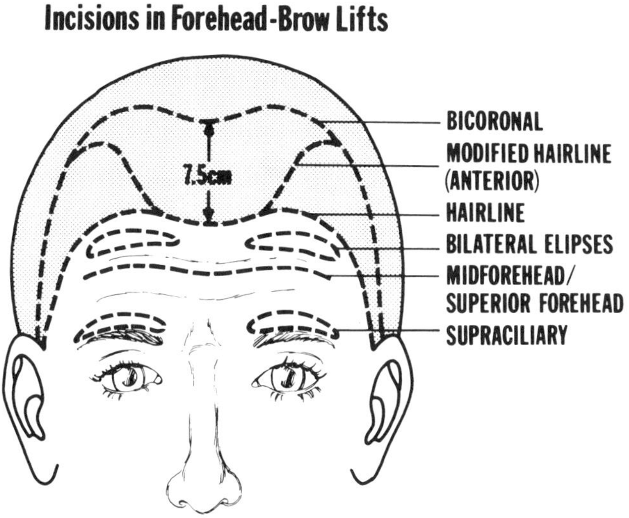

Incisions in Forehead-Brow Lifts

FIGURE 2.—The traditional incisions that were routinely considered to address the forehead-eyebrow area. All of these alternatives have been associated with transient hypesthesias, some with alopecia or abnormal scarring. (Reprinted by permission of the publisher from Matarasso A, Matarasso SL: Endoscopic surgical correction of glabellar creases. *Dermatol Surg* 21:695–700, copyright 1995 by Elsevier Science Inc.)

Patients.—This patient series consisted of 9 women and 1 man, aged 38 to 68 years, who were operated on with this technique. The available follow-up was from 6 to 20 months.

Results.—Patients were pleased with the results of this surgery. There were no cases of hair loss, permanent sensory changes, scarring, hematomas, infections, or permanent nerve injuries. Patients resumed moderate activity in 24 hours and returned to full activity in 7 to 10 days. Sutures were removed after 1 week.

Conclusions.—The introduction of endoscopic surgery permits a simpler and more cost-effective way to address esthetic problems in the forehead and brow region.

▶ A wonderful, permanent adjunct for those patients needing brow or forehead lifts, or simply as a direct one-time procedure to correct glabellar creases in younger patients.

D.J. Papadopoulos, M.D.

The Trifurcated SMAS Flap: Three-Part Segmentation of the Conventional Flap for Improved Results in the Midface, Cheek, and Neck

Connell BF, Marten TJ (Santa Ana, Calif; San Francisco, Calif)
Aesthetic Plast Surg 19:415–420, 1995   4–8

Introduction.—Although the conventional SMAS flap is useful for facelifts, it can only be advanced in 1 direction and sutured in place under uniform tension. A 3-part trifurcated SMAS flap that allows for 3 independent vectors of correction for the cheek, jowl, and neck (Fig 1) was described.

> *Surgical Technique.*—Incisions are made and skin flaps undermined under direct vision using sharp scissors dissection. Skin flaps are retracted and a line is traced over the zygomatic arch, superior to that typically used for facelifts, and then turned inferiorly and continued over the parotid gland and along the sulcus anterior to the ear. The SMAS is incised and the entire flap elevated as a single unit. The flap is shifted to determine the direction that produces the best effect on the cheek and jowl. A line is drawn parallel to the superior margin over the cut edge beneath. The SMAS is incised along this line, partially separating the superior segment. The superior segment is advanced in the direction that produces the best improvement in the upper midface and then sutured. The superior edge of the middle segment is then anchored with sutures. Gentle traction is placed on the posterior edge of the middle segment and a line is traced parallel to the posterior margin and over the cut edge beneath. The flap is transposed to a postauricular location and advanced with traction to tighten the submental region. It is sutured to the mastoid fascia. Skin flaps are advanced and trimmed and closure completed.

Patients.—There were more than 300 patients who underwent a segmented SMAS procedure during a 5-year period. The patients ranged in age from 36 to 83 years. There were 23 females for every male patient. Available follow-up ranged from 6 to 52 months.

Conclusions.—Although the conventional SMAS flap provides good results, it does not provide the separate vectors required for optimal simultaneous improvement in the midface, cheek, jowl, and neck. Separation of this flap into 3 segments improves the results.

▶ Interesting modification of the traditional SMAS flap with specific correction of 3 difficult areas, i.e., submental, mandibular line, and midcheek. Also, the posterior transposition flap is fixed to the mastoid fascia instead of the sternocleidomastoid muscle. These results are impressive, and it will be important to see what the long-term clinical results will prove to be in these patients at the 3- and 5-year mark.

D.J. Papadopoulos, M.D.

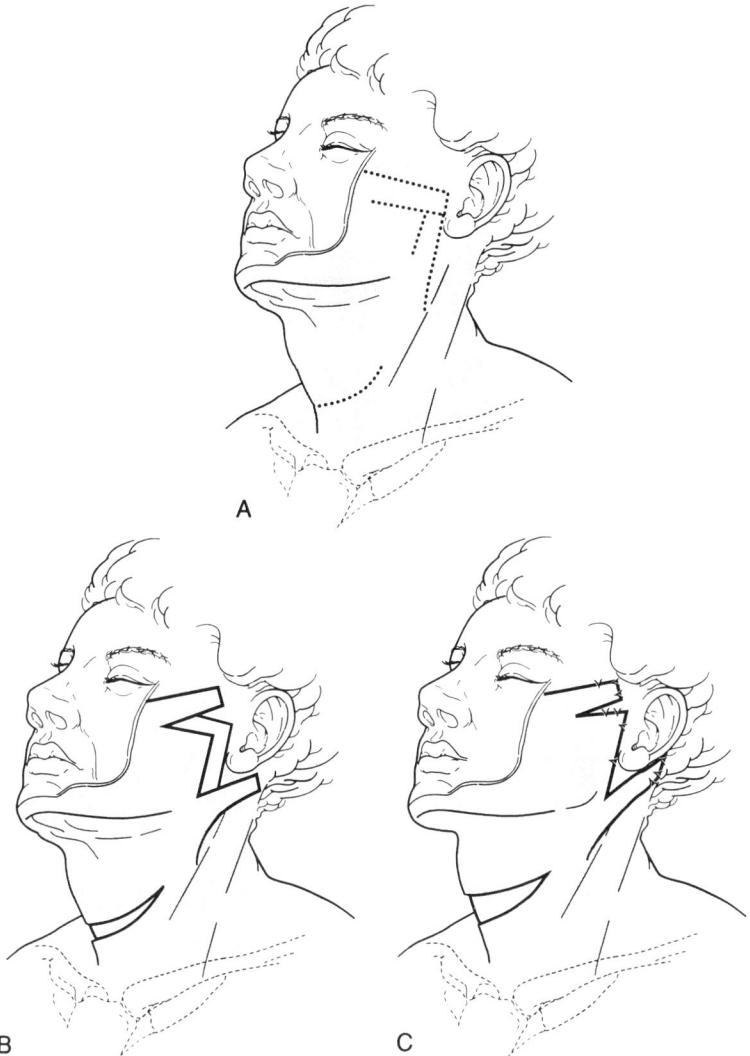

FIGURE 1.—(**A**) Plan for trifurcated SMAS flap. (**B**) The superior and posterior margins of the cheek SMAS are separated to form the malar and postauricular flaps. (**C**) Malar, cheek, and postauricular component flaps are advanced along independent vectors to produce maximum improvement in each area. (Courtesy of Connell BF, Marten TJ: The trifurcated SMAS flap: Three-part segmentation of the conventional flap for improved results in the midface, cheek, and neck. *Aesthetic Plast Surg* 19:415–420, copyright 1995 by Springer-Verlag.)

Aging of the Upper Lip: A New Treatment Technique

Hinderer UT (Clìnica Mirasierra, Madrid)
Aesthetic Plast Surg 19:519–526, 1995
4–9

Background.—Signs of aging are first evident in the periocular region, then in the perioral region. Patients worry about deep wrinkles on the upper lip, which are difficult to hide with lipstick or makeup. Decreased thickness and elasticity of involved tissues and a decrease in hypodermic fat contribute to superficial and progressively deep vertical wrinkles, elongation and flattening of the lip, a descending of the angles of the mouth, and progressive deepening of the nasolabial sulcus. A variety of techniques have been used to treat the alterations to the lip caused by aging; the author's present personal technique was highlighted.

Technique Overview.—Instead of using a silicone sheet, as the author proposed in 1970, the current (since 1992) technique interposes a layer of pretemporal areolar tissue between the skin and the orbicularis muscle. The skin is excised at the nasolabial junction on the basis of a technique described by Cardoso and Sperli in 1971. In the current technique, however, the author dissects the skin of the vermilion border and inserts a trapezoidal graft of pretemporal areolar tissue (the graft is obtained during rhytidectomy). Vicryl (Johnson & Johnson) sutures are used to fix the graft at the level of the nasolabial folds. A chemical peel is also sometimes used. A moderate compressive dressing is applied, and sutures are replaced with sterile strips on the fourth day.

Results.—This technique has provided satisfactory results for all 15 patients on which it has been performed. Moderate edema may last as long as 2 months. The author believes this technique is superior to previously used techniques. Later removal of a silicone sheet is not required, and the vermilion does not require volume expansion by lipofilling or injection of foreign material. Wrinkles caused by retraction of the fibers that join the dermis and orbicularis muscles are corrected. The vermilion is everted, producing a fuller look, and the lip is shortened, providing a concave, youthful appearance.

▶ For all those who are serious about cosmetic lip surgery, this article, with its references, is required reading as much for the historical review as for the interesting new treatment technique. It is a rich description of the different techniques used by someone who has a wide breadth of experience.

D.J. Papadopoulos, M.D.

Alar Rim Excision: A Method of Thinning Bulky Nostrils

Matarasso A (Manhattan Eye, Ear, and Throat Hosp, New York; Albert Einstein College, New York)
Plast Reconstr Surg 97:828–834, 1996
4–10

Introduction.—Rhinoplasty is usually performed as an intranasal operation with the goal of reducing or expanding the osseocartilaginous framework of the nose. Achievement of narrower nostril rims would be desirable, if it could be achieved with minimal scarring. The technique of alar thinning or alar rim excision, performed through an alar base approach is described in this article.

Background.—The borders of the nasal alar subunit approximate a triangle, with the base at the alar groove. The inferior border is the alar rim, the anterior surface is nasal skin and the inner surface is vestibular skin. Two layers of muscle, the levator labii superioris and the pars alaris musculi nasalis insert in the nasal rim. The nasal alar subunit is entirely composed of soft tissue.

Patients.—The study group for this procedure consisted of 12 consecutive patients who underwent alar rim excision to thin a bulky nostril rim via an alar base incision. The patients' ages ranged from 25 to 45 years. There were 10 females and 2 males. Nine were white; 1, Hispanic; 1, Asian; and 1 black. These cases were retrospectively reviewed.

Surgical Technique.—The alar base incisions were outlined in ink. The field was anesthetized. Traction was applied between the nostril and upper lip and the incision was made. The leading edge of the alar rim was elevated, and a triangular incision of the subcutaneous tissue was initiated and alar rim excision continued by coring. The excision extended to all borders. After debulking, the width of the alar rim depended on the 2 opposing skin surfaces. The alar rim was then repositioned and closed. The dead space created by the alar rim excision can be narrowed by several techniques. At the end of the procedure, the nose was packed with gauze and a splint applied. The sutures were removed by the third postoperative day.

Results.—Six of the 12 patients were available for follow-up. All patients were satisfied with the results. There were no complications or revisions. There was no apparent loss of function. Edema resolved during several months.

Conclusions.—For patients who are disturbed by thick nostrils, this method of internally thinning the nostril rim using an alar base groove incision is described. This method provides good results, without scarring or risking alar rim elevation.

▶ A very interesting article and an ingenious approach to thinning bulky nostrils. This article is important to us as dermatologic surgeons because it is a nice review of the local anatomy and gives us a different approach when considering reconstruction of this area. As a Mohs surgeon, I frequently have the opposite problem and must consider reshaping the vestibule with borrowed myocutaneous flap skin. Alar groove approaches may be a way to consider introduction of fillers, such as fat, to give more fullness to the rim and vestibule. This article is required reading by all those who perform nasal reconstruction, and the author is to be commended for his tremendous meticulous, sensitive, and refined description and approach to a very difficult and subtle problem.

D.J. Papadopoulos, M.D.

Use of Double Gloves to Protect the Surgeon From Blood Contact During Aesthetic Procedures
Greco RJ, Garza JR (Savannah, Ga; Pittsburgh, Pa)
Aesthetic Plast Surg 19:265–267, 1995   4–11

Introduction.—During aesthetic surgical procedures, there is increasing concern regarding the plastic surgeon's exposure to blood and the transmission of blood-borne pathogens such as HIV and hepatitis B virus. Surgical gloves are relied upon for protection from contact with blood and other body fluids; however, frank needle-stick injury has occurred to the surgeon once every 20–40 operations, and blood contact occurs in 32% of aesthetic operations in which the surgeon uses a single pair of surgical gloves. During aesthetic surgical procedures, the reduction of blood contact exposure was tested by using 2 pairs of gloves.

Methods.—In consecutive aesthetic double-gloved surgical operations, 103 pairs of gloves used by right-handed surgeons with at least 6 years of postgraduate surgical training were evaluated. The latex gloves were tested for holes by filling them with water and squeezing each finger individually as well as the palm for evidence of drops of water.

Results.—A decrease of 70% was seen in the contact rates. Perforations were seen in 26 outer gloves (12.6%) and in 10 inner gloves (4.9%) (Fig 1). All inner-glove perforations had corresponded with a perforation of the outer-glove, representing blood contact. All of the perforations stemmed from a specific event, such as a needle stick, which was remembered by the surgeons. The surgeon was exposed 8.7% of the times, whereas the assistant was exposed 3.5% of the times; the most common location of the outer-glove perforation was the left index finger (33%). Most of the perforations occurred in procedures lasting more than 2 hours.

Conclusion.—When compared with single-glove use during aesthetic procedures, double gloving had reduced the surgeon's risk of blood contact exposure by 70%. The incidence of blood contact was reduced to 9.7% with double gloving compared with 32% in the study using single gloves. Strong consideration should be given to double gloving during aesthetic surgical procedures in this era of AIDS and hepatitis B virus exposure.

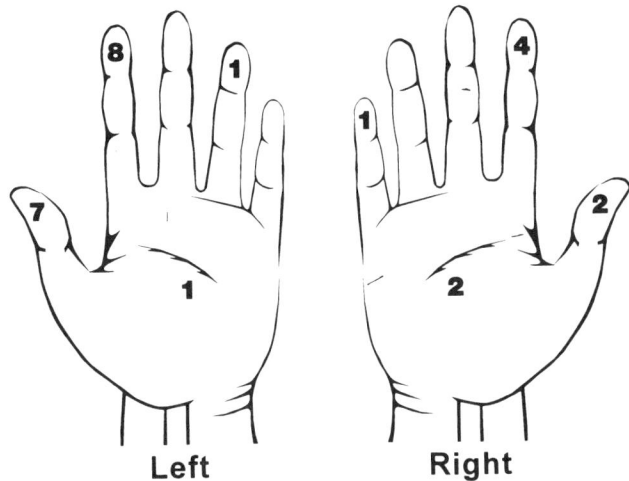

Left   **Right**

FIGURE 1.—Locations of outer-glove perforations in the study population. (Courtesy of Greco RJ, Garza JR: Use of double gloves to protect the surgeon from blood contact during aesthetic procedures. *Aesthetic Plast Surg* 19:265–267, copyright 1995 by Springer-Verlag.)

▶ This is useful information for those who perform extensive surgery in high-risk populations, i.e., renal or heart transplant recipients with skin cancers or patients with clearly documented hepatitis B or HIV infection. We routinely do this and make it a point to change gloves frequently during high-risk procedures.

D.J. Papadopoulos, M.D.

Aging Skin

The Effects of Aging on the Cutaneous Microvasculature
Kelly RI, Pearse R, Bull RH, et al (St Georges Hosp, London; Laboratories de Recherche de L'Oreal, Aulnay-sous-Bois, France)
J Am Acad Dermatol 33:749–756, 1995   4–12

Objectives.—An attempt was made to evaluate age-related structural and functional changes in the cutaneous microvasculature and to assess the role of these changes in skin color differences between young and old individuals.

Background.—There is little information to support the notion that various skin components decrease in size and number. It has been reported that wheal resorption, disappearance of diffusible dye, clearance of radio-labeled material such as sodium 22, and blister development after topical 50% ammonium hydroxide are delayed in the elderly. These changes may result in reduced thermoregulation, reduced capacity to clear antigens, and delayed development of inflammatory reactions. It has also been suggested that changes in skin color in the elderly are caused by reduced skin vasculature.

Methods.—Two groups of 13 subjects each were studied. The age range of the older group was 65 to 88 years, and that of the younger group was 18 to 26 years. In vivo capillaroscopy with fluorescein angiography, and laser Doppler flowmetry were used to compare degree of skin pigmentation, erythema, and number of visible telangiectases. The forehead and the ventral aspect of the forearm were studied.

Results.—In the skin of older subjects, dermal papillary loops were significantly reduced compared with skin of younger patients. In the forehead and forearm skin of older patients, there was increased volume fraction in horizontal vessels. No significant differences between young and old skin were shown by laser-Doppler studies. Hyperemic responsiveness seemed to be more rapid in the older subjects. A hand-held color reflectance meter showed that the skin color in older subjects was significantly darker and redder, especially in men.

Conclusions.—Chronologic aging and photoaging result in substantial loss of dermal nutritional vessel density and surface area for exchange. Evaluation of blood flow vasodilatory responsiveness indicated little evidence of changes in cutaneous vascular aging as a major factor in reduced thermoregulation and other physiologic deficiencies.

▶ This is interesting information that we, as dermatologic surgeons, intuitively have assessed in our clinical practices. What is confounding is that, despite this article's data and our clinical observations, older patients generally heal with less scarring than younger patients for similar procedures in similar anatomic locations. This probably relates to alterations in ground substance and fibroblast activity as a function of age. It will be interesting to see how the decrease in cutaneous microvasculature with aging has an impact on fibroblast numbers and function (i.e., production of ground substance and collagen types). By knowing this information, we might be able to intervene at critical times during the wound healing process to achieve less surgical scarring.

D.J. Papadopoulos, M.D.

Two Concentrations of Topical Tretinoin (Retinoic Acid) Cause Similar Improvement of Photoaging but Different Degrees of Irritation: A Double-Blind, Vehicle-Controlled Comparison of 0.1% and 0.025% Tretinoin Creams
Griffiths CEM, Kang S, Ellis CN, et al (Univ of Michigan, Ann Arbor)
Arch Dermatol 131:1037–1044, 1995   4–13

Background.—Photoaging can be effectively treated using topical tretinoin (all-*trans*-retinoic acid). It is not yet clear, however, whether irritation is responsible for all or only part of the favorable treatment effect. Similarly, the concentration of tretinoin needed to maximize clinical response with minimal side effects is not yet known, nor have the effects of long-term treatment on components of the cutaneous immune system been established. These questions therefore were addressed in the present study.

Patients and Methods.—Ninety-nine photoaged patients (44 to 81 years old) completed this 48-week double-blind study. Of these, 32 were randomly assigned to once daily treatment with 0.1% tretinoin cream, 35 to 0.025% tretinoin, and 32 to vehicle treatment. Topical or systemic retinoids had not been used by any patient for at least 6 months before study enrollment. Medications were applied to the entire face and forearms, the amount of which was increased as long as side effects such as erythema and scaling were tolerable. Histologic characteristics, keratinocyte expression of HLA-DR and intercellular adhesion molecule-1, numbers of epidermal Langerhans' cells and epidermal and dermal T lymphocytes, and vascularity (as determined by dermal endothelial cell area) were evaluated at baseline, at 2 and 4 weeks of treatment, and monthly thereafter until study completion.

Results.—Statistically significant overall improvement in photoaging of the face was observed with both 0.1% and 0.025% tretinoin, as compared with vehicle treatment. Clinically or statistically significant differences were not observed between the 2 medication concentrations. Both concentrations of tretinoin resulted in comparable statistically significant epidermal thickening after 48 weeks, at 30% and 28% for 0.1% and 0.025% tretinoin, respectively, compared with an 11% decrease for vehicle. Similar increases in vascularity also were noted with use of each concentration of tretinoin, of 100% and 89%, respectively, compared with a 9% decrease for vehicle treatment. Irritant side effects, including erythema and scaling, were significantly greater with the 0.1% concentration compared with 0.025% tretinoin. Comparisons between the tretinoin and vehicle treatments did not reveal any significant changes in any of the immunologic markers.

Conclusions.—Comparable clinical and histologic changes occur in patients treated with either 0.1% or 0.025% tretinoin, even though the incidence of irritation is significantly greater with the higher concentration. Mechanisms other than irritation thus appear to govern tretinoin-mediated repair of photoaging.

▶ Although this is important information for us to use in clinical practice, we must always remember that not all patients are going to benefit from this observation. It is my belief that in patients with very sebaceous skin (who strictly adhere to treatment) 0.025% tretinoin cream has minimal therapeutic effect. In these patients, I have frequently found that using medication on a twice a day basis may be necessary for a period of time. Also, the use of 8% to 10% glycolic acid cleansers, once during the day, may help these patients get a more therapeutic effect from the use of their tretinoin cream.

D.J. Papadopoulos, M.D.

Effects of A-Hydroxy Acids on Photoaged Skin: A Pilot Clinical, Histologic, and Ultrastructural Study

Ditre CM, Griffin TD, Murphy GF, et al (Hahnemann Univ, Philadelphia; Univ of Pa, Philadelphia)
J Am Acad Dermatol 34:187–195, 1996   4–14

Introduction.—Previous studies have indicated that α-hydroxy acids (AHAs) can improve photoaged skin. More information is needed about the mechanisms of action of AHAs on the epidermal and dermal compartments. A clinical and microanalytic study of the effects of AHAs on photoaged human skin is reported.

Methods.—The study sample comprised 17 white patients with moderate to severe photoaged skin. They were randomized to apply a 25% concentration of AHA lotion, containing either lactic acid, glycolic acid, or citric acid, on one forearm twice daily. On the other forearm, the patients applied a placebo lotion. Treatment continued for an average of 6 months, during which regular measurements of forearm skin thickness were performed. After treatment, biopsy specimens from the AHA- and placebo-treated arms were obtained.

Results.—Skin thickness increased by about 25% in the arms treated with AHA lotion, from a mean of 11.5 to 14.3 mm. This change was apparent by comparative pinching. On histologic analysis of biopsy specimens, the mean epidermal thickness was greater in AHA-treated skin. Papillary dermal changes were noted as well, including increased thickness, increased acid mucopolysaccharides, improved quality of elastic fibers, and increased density of collagen. No inflammatory changes were present. Electron microscopy showed a reduced number of desmosomes and tonofilament aggregation on the AHA-treated arms.

Conclusions.—Topical application of AHA lotions appears to improve the epidermal and dermal components of photoaged skin, with no signs of inflammation or a wound healing process. Increased skin thickness is readily apparent, and significant improvements in the histologic and electron microscopic findings are noted as well.

▶ This is an excellent study that substantiates to a certain degree what we have all seen in clinical practice...that AHAs do moderately improve skin texture and appearance if used properly and concomitantly with sun protection. Of interest would be what role combined therapies with long-term use of lower concentrations of AHAs with intermittent peels would have on the histopathologic picture. Hopefully, work like this will continue to advance our understanding of these interesting compounds.

D.J. Papadopoulos, M.D.

Botulinum Toxin

Cosmetic Denervation of the Muscles of Facial Expression With *Botulinum* Toxin: A Dose-Response Study

Garcia A, Fulton JE Jr (Newport Beach, Calif)
Dermatol Surg 22:39–43, 1996   4–15

Objective.—Cosmetic denervation with *Botulinum* toxin has many characteristics of the ideal cosmetic procedure: it produces quick and reversible benefits with few adverse effects. *Botulinum* toxin injection has been proposed as a treatment for frown lines. The use of *Botulinum* toxin to treat other muscles of facial expression is reported, including the effects of dose and toxin storage time.

Methods.—The experience included 183 patients: 164 women and 19 men, average age 45 years. All underwent cosmetic denervation of the muscles of facial expression using *Botulinum* toxin. The injections were performed by a standard protocol by using cooling, injection, and compression to reduce pain and bruising (Fig 2). Most patients underwent treatment of the corrugator, the lateral orbicularis oculi, and the frontalis muscles in a single session. The dose of *Botulinum* toxin needed to produce the desired effect was analyzed, as were the effects of length of storage of reconstituted toxin.

Results.—Dilution studies showed that concentrations of 10 and 20 U/mL produced the same results as a 100 U/mL concentration. Thereafter,

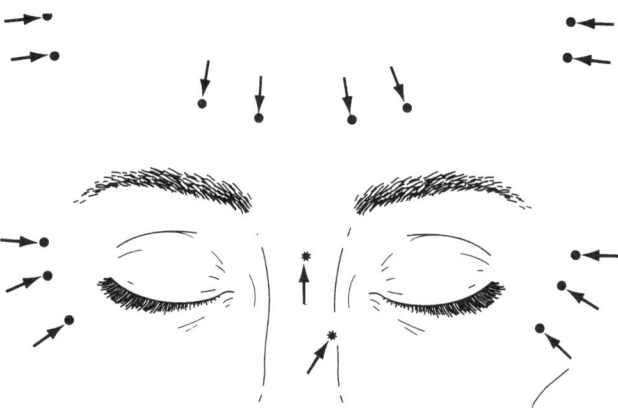

FIGURE 2.—The method of injection of Botulinum toxin. The right lateral orbicularis oculi muscle is cooled with ice. The patient is then asked to smile; the muscle mounds between the linear depressions are injected with 0.1 cc (1 U) of toxin. Meanwhile, the other side is being iced. While the left side is being injected, the right side is compressed with gauze. The corrugators are then cooled and injected, followed with the right frontalis muscle, and then the left frontalis muscle. The procerus and nasal orbicularis oculi muscles are injected last, if necessary. The progression of cooling, injection, and compression minimizes bruising. The total dosage used per session is between 15 and 20 U. A repeat session may be done at 3–6 months and again at 6–12 months. Injection sites are marked by arrows; sites marked by asterisks are given occasionally. (Reprinted by permission of the publisher from Garcia A, Fulton JE Jr: Cosmetic denervation of the muscles of facial expression with botulinum toxin: A dose-response study. *Dermatol Surg* 22:39–43, copyright 1996 by Elsevier Science Inc.)

a 10 U/mL concentration was used as the standard. The results appeared to be the same with 1-month-old solution as with freshly reconstituted toxin. Several 0.1- 0.2-cc toxin injections were sufficient to balloon out each muscle group. Results were noted within 5 to 7 days, and the improvement lasted for 12 to 15 weeks. The patients expressed great satisfaction with their results and often returned for repeat treatments (Figs 5 and 6). Patients undergoing 2 or 3 treatments had loss of muscle tone lasting up to 1 year. Side effects were minimal.

Discussion.—*Botulinum* toxin injection is a highly effective procedure for cosmetic denervation of the muscles of the face for facial rejuvenation. This treatment can be cost-effective when proper doses and dilutions are given—the authors treat 6 to 10 patients over several days with a single vial of reconstituted toxin. The temporary nature of the results can be an advantage; the more lasting results obtained with repeated treatments warrant further evaluation.

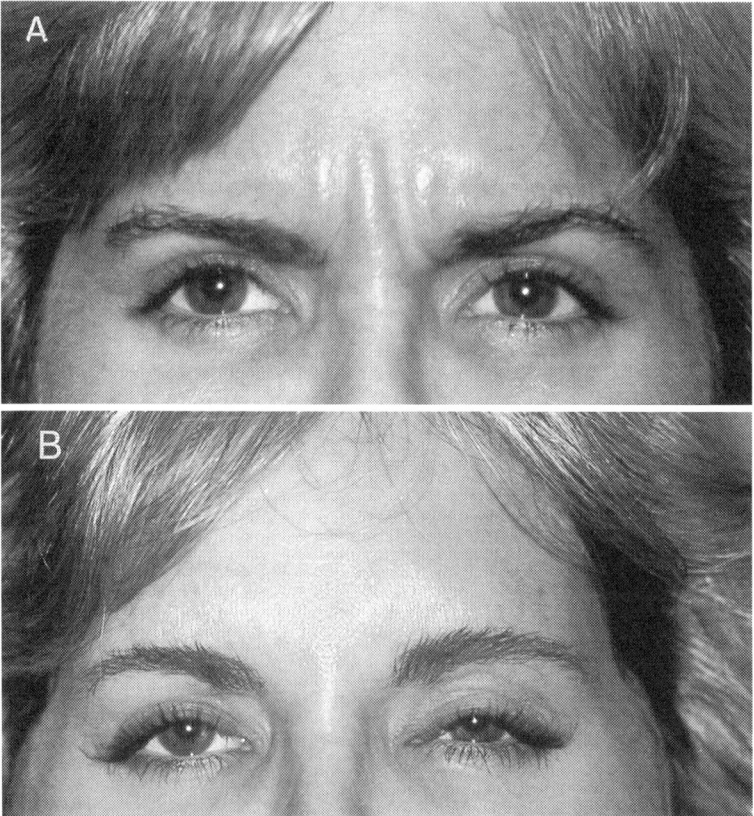

FIGURE 5.—**A**, before, and **B**, after denervation of the corrugator muscles. Note that the eyes appear to be frowning but the forehead does not. (Reprinted by permission of the publisher from Garcia A, Fulton JE Jr: Cosmetic denervation of the muscles of facial expression with botulinum toxin: A dose-response study. *Dermatol Surg* 22:39–43, copyright 1996 by Elsevier Science Inc.)

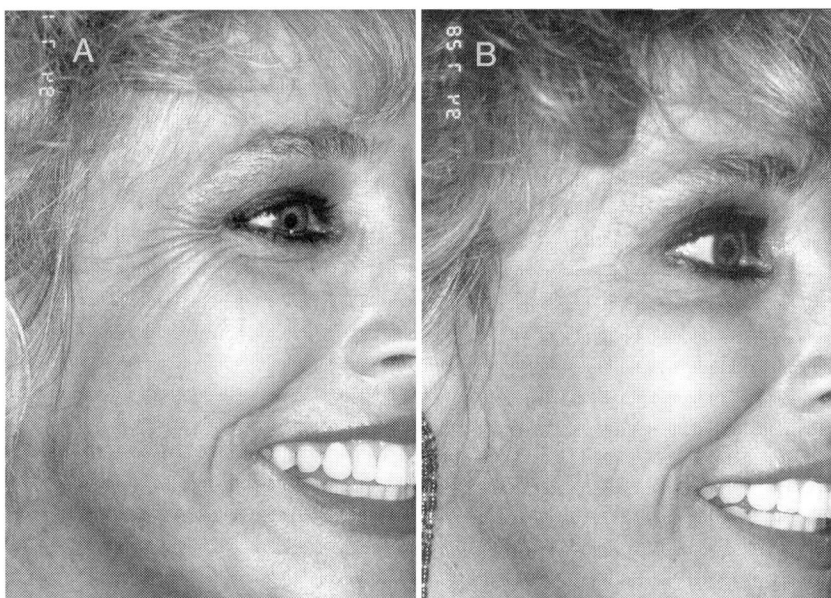

FIGURE 6.—**A**, before, and **B**, after denervation of the lateral orbicularis oculi (crow's feet). There is a diminution of the crow's feet both at rest and following attempted animation. (Reprinted by permission of the publisher from Garcia A, Fulton JE Jr: Cosmetic denervation of the muscles of facial expression with botulinum toxin: A dose-response study. *Dermatol Surg* 22:39–43, copyright 1996 by Elsevier Science Inc.)

▶ Although it is valuable for us to know that responses can be obtained with lower concentrations of *Botulinum* toxin and that the reconstituted solution is effective for 1 month, the 1 general complaint with any injection product is that it needs to be repeated too frequently. So it is with great interest that permanent loss of muscle tone was noted in some patients. How long this effect will last will be interesting to note. Another concern is that we must take great caution and alert our staff that this product needs to be reconstituted precisely.

D.J. Papadopoulos, M.D.

Liposuction

The Tumescent Technique Revisited
Bussien R, Maillard G-F (Lausanne, Switzerland)
Eur J Plast Surg 19:124–131, 1996   4–16

Introduction.—Classic liposuction was performed with a dry technique under general anesthetic without infiltration, a technique that was associated with an unacceptable rate of severe hemorrhaging. Klein's tumescent technique was developed in an attempt to perform liposuction as an outpatient surgical procedure without anesthesia. Several variations of the technique have been developed. The advantages and disadvantages of these techniques were considered.

Solutions.—A 50% hypotonic solution of NaCl was thought to have an osmotic effect, but it was found to be weak. The osmotic balance governs the distribution of water and electrolytes. Crystalloids are usually used perioperatively; isotonic or slightly hypotonic liquids are preferred to physiologic liquids, which may cause water intoxication and salt intolerance postoperatively. Lactated Ringer's solution, because of its similarity to the interstitial compartment conditions, is recommended as the infiltration solution.

Local Anesthetics.—Lidocaine is the most commonly used local anesthetic. It can have toxic reactions, either immediately (which causes rapid and total collapse and often death before treatment is begun) or delayed (5 to 30 minutes after injection with a progression in stages that allows effective treatment). Therefore, the usual maximal dose is 7 mg/kg of lidocaine (Klein's solution). However, care should be taken with lidocaine injections in patients with severe hepatorenal disease, in whom lidocaine may accumulate. Bupivacaine can increase lidocaine's length of action, and the combination reduces the toxicity of both. The combination of lidocaine and epinephrine causes vasoconstriction, which causes the anesthetics to be retained at the infiltration site, but the effects on bleeding are controversial. Because bicarbonate neutralizes acids, it may reduce injection pain by opposing lidocaine's acidity. A concentration of 5 mEq/l is recommended.

Temperature.—Cold infiltration fluids can induce hypothermia, cause shivering, and increase the oxygen debt. Room temperature infusions are recommended.

Conclusion.—A room temperature solution of lidocaine in lactated Ringer's is recommended for local anesthesia during liposuction. Sodium bicarbonate 8.4% in a 5-mEq/l is useful to adjust, but not to completely counteract the solution's acidity. Further study is needed to determine the effects of epinephrine in the solution.

▶ Whereas my close friend, my liposuction mentor (along with Dr. Patrick Lillis), and certainly one of "immortal status" (as labeled by Dr. Larry Field), Dr. Jeff Klein, is recognized for his Klein formula in this review, he certainly is otherwise given less respect and significance than his contributions warrant. This in part appears to be related to his status as a "surgeon dermatologist" who was "researching the possibility of outpatient surgery without the aid of an anesthetist," and Jeff's formula "nowdays is used so frequently that it cannot be considered anymore as a harmless office procedure." All dermatologic surgeons should read this to see how some of our plastic surgeon colleagues wish to portray dermatologic surgeons. Take heart, Jeff Klein, the head of our plastic surgery division at Scripps Clinic continues to oppose my liposuction practice, but didn't hesitate to send his head nurse to borrow my "Klein pump" when his inferior equipment didn't work!

H.T. Greenway, M.D.

Superficial Liposuction
Bolivar de Souza Pinto E, Erazo I PJ, Prado Filho FSA, et al (São Paulo, Brazil)
Aesthetic Plast Surg 20:111–122, 1996   4–17

Introduction.—Despite criticisms against its use, liposuction has advanced in the world of plastic surgery. Reported is the experience of 12 years of superficial liposuction. Concerns about superficial and deep aspiration and skin retraction are addressed.

Methods.—A conventional liposuction machine with a maximum vacuum pressure of 400 mm Hg is used for most surgeries. Modified cannula are used that provide greater ease in making tunnels, permit safe undermining of the cellulite areas and safe separation of the cross fibers, and allow fat injections. Syringes are used for small procedures and liposuction in isolated areas. Most procedures are performed under general anesthesia. Patients are given one midazolam tablet orally 1 hour before surgery. The area to be liposuctioned undergoes infiltration that is initiated in the deep layer toward the superficial. Well-performed infiltration is crucial for good results.

  Surgical Techniques in Diverse Regions.
  Submental Region.—An incision should be made medially in the underchin region and a number 3 cannula should be worked superficially and carefully to avoid damage to the mandibular branch of the facial nerve and the m. platisma.
  Breast.—Liposuction performed in the medial and lateral quadrants improves conditions for conventional surgery, particularly for correction of axial extensions of the breast. This approach decreases the length of the scar in large-reduction mammoplasties.
  Abdomen.—A cutting pinto cannula number 4, then number 6 is used for the lower abdomen. The orifices should face downward to make various criss-cross tunnels and thus avoid depressions. Treatment of the areolar layer is performed with a perforating tip cannula number 4, keeping the orifice of the cannula turned down. A slender cannula number 3 is then used in the layer directly below the skin for fine refinement and to empty the entire areolar layer. In the absence of muscular flaccidity, the retraction of the skin will allow a good contour with no change in circulation. The miniabdomen surgical procedure is recommended for patients with excess skin. A musculature plication can be performed through a small skin incision through the lower ellipse of removed skin.

Dorsal Region.—The upper, middle, and lower dorsal regions are treated separately. The upper region is treated through an incision made in the transitional region from the cervical column to the thorax, using a number 6 cannula with perforating cutting tips. The middle region is treated using criss-cross tunnels in a fan shape through an incision made at the lumbar column level or thorax-lumbar transitional region. The lower region is treated through an incision in the lumbosacral region.

Upper Limbs.—The best results are obtained using skin retraction. A number 4 cannula is used initially, and a number 3 cannula is used for refinement.

Lower Limbs.—Unlike preparation for other regions, patients should be seated for demarcation to avoid depressions. A number 3 cannula should be used.

Outer Face of the Thigh.—This area must be worked carefully for good results.

Saddle Bags.—A number 4 or 5 cannula should be used for the deep layer. A number 3 cannula with defined tips should be used for the superficial portion. Lipodystrophy of the haunches provides a long-lasting, harmonious, and gratifying result.

Inner Face of the Thigh.—This area is difficult to treat because of less tension, more skin flaccidity, and more restricted access and mobilization because of its important anatomical structures. For this reason, superficial liposuction with number 3 and 4 cannulas is used, even for the gigantic lipodystrophies of this region. A second surgery is performed 6 months later to perform classic dermolipectomy to treat cutaneous retractions. This approach gives better results.

Anterior Face of the Thigh.—In this location, only the most exaggerated lipodystrophies should be treated. Caution should be used to aspirate as superficially as possible with a number 3 or 4 perforating cannula. The deep layer should be kept intact to prevent depressions and collapse of fat tissue, followed by intense flaccidity. Less experienced surgeons should approach this region with caution and apprehension.

Body Contour.—Patients are encouraged during initial evaluation to view the body as a whole, rather than focusing on particular parts when placed in front of a mirror. Computer images are used to help patients understand what can be achieved for them.

Lipoinjection.—Any area can be used as a donor site. Lipoinjection is used to fill depressions in the body contour, improve facial contour, and correct minimal scar depressions, facial wrinkles, body contour deformities, and big craniofacial deformities. For small corrections, the procedure can be performed under local anesthesia. Larger procedures require general anesthesia. Harvest is performed with the lipoaspirator at a pressure that never exceeds 400 mm hg vacuum. Collected fat is washed with

Ringer's lactate until it is totally clear and freed from its liquid part, then filtered and placed in a syringe for lipoinsertion.

Conclusion.—Careful treatment of deep and superficial layers of fat tissue and the use of lipoinjection to lessen irregularities can give good results. Skin does retract after judicious treatment of the fat layers. It is possible to offer patients safe and long-lasting results from superficial liposuction procedures.

▶ The authors show some impressive photography of pre- and postliposuction patients. Several points of interest in this article include:

1. The placement of tumescent local anesthesia in correct anatomic location greatly enhances their ability to perform these procedures.

2. The ability to harvest fat during a liposuction procedure, filter it, store it in the freezer at approximately 4SC for a maximum of 6 months, and subsequently to use it as a filler.

3. Their ability (as shown in the photographs) to improve cellulite significantly by suctioning fat with a number 3 cannula and then severing the trabecula between the dermis and the hypodermis with a duckbill-shaped cannula. These excellent results are no doubt the result of a broad 12-year experience.

D.J. Papadopoulos, M.D.

Viability of Fat Obtained by Syringe Suction Lipectomy: Effects of Local Anesthesia With Lidocaine

Moore JH Jr, Kolaczynski JW, Morales LM, et al (Philadelphia)
Aesthetic Plast Surg 19:335–339, 1995   4–18

Background.—Peer's cell survival theory states that the fate of a fat graft depends on the number of surviving viable cells. Fat cells harvested by syringe suction may be adversely affected by tissue trauma, desiccation, decreased vascularity, or local anesthetics. To better determine the reasons for the success or failure of transplantation of free autologous fat harvested by blunt syringe suction lipectomy, the components of the harvesting and grafting process were separately examined.

Methods.—Adipose tissue samples from 12 patients were excised during elective surgery. Samples were also obtained from 8 outpatients; 2 fat biopsy specimens each were obtained from 4 of these outpatients to compare the effects on tissue of local anesthesia with 1% lidocaine versus 1% lidocaine with 1:100,000 epinephrine. Fat obtained through lipectomy and intraoperatively was digested with collagenase to isolate the adipocytes.

Results.—Intraoperative and syringe-suction sample collection yielded nearly equal mechanical damage associated with sample handling and cell isolation (less than 6% of total cell mass). The isolated cells did not differ functionally, responded similarly to insulin stimulation of glucose trans-

TABLE 1.—Lipolysis in Fresh and Cultured Cells: Glycerol Release to the Medium (nmol/10^5 cells/h)

	Fresh cells	Cultured cells	Washed cells after culture
Control			
Basal	52.1	67.0	68.1
Epinephrine–stimulated	71.6	—	247.0
Cells exposed continuously to 0.1%			
Lidocaine before and during culture			
Basal	28.8	44.2	72.6
Epinephrine-stimulated	48.4	—	261.0

(Courtesy of Moore JH Jr, Kolaczynski JW, Morales LM, et al: Viability of fat obtained by syringe suction lipectomy: effects of local anesthesia with lidocaine. *Aesth Plast Surg* 19:335–339, copyright 1995 by Springer-Verlag.)

port and epinephrine-stimulated lipolysis, and showed the same growth pattern in culture. Lidocaine potently inhibited adipocyte glucose transport, lipolysis, and growth in culture. However, the cells could regain full function after washing, regardless of previous length of exposure to the drug (30 minutes or 10 days) (Table 1).

Conclusions.—Local anesthesia with lidocaine may halt the metabolism and growth of harvested adipocytes, but the effect persists only as long as lidocaine is present. Adipose tissue harvested through syringe lipectomy appears fully viable and functional; the method of cell harvest did not affect adipocyte metabolism.

▶ This study provides excellent and very important information that may help increase the long-term percentage of take of fat as a filler substance. Lidocaine is probably only one variable. Temperature, location of harvest, location of harvested fat, handling, blood contents, and admixture or not of adnexal structures probably and intuitively may play a role in the percentage of take.

D.J. Papadopoulos, M.D.

Blood Loss During Suction-Assisted Lipectomy With Large Volumes of Dilute Adrenaline

Samdal F, Amland PF, Bugge JF (Norwegian Natl Hosp, Oslo; Univ Hosp of Oslo, Norway)
Scand J Plast Reconstr Hand Surg 29:161–165, 1995   4–19

Introduction.—In patients in whom large volumes are removed during liposuction, excessive blood loss becomes a concern. There has been controversy over the effect of dilute adrenaline injections on blood loss. The effect of the "super-wet" technique on blood loss during suction-assisted lipectomy was discussed.

Methods.—Twenty-six patients were involved in this study. Thirteen had liposuction performed under local anesthesia, and 13 patients elected general anesthesia. All were treated preoperatively with injections of dilute adrenaline (1/1 million) in a volume equal to the volume expected in the aspirate. Hemoglobin levels were measured in all aspirates, and blood loss was then calculated.

Results.—The mean volume aspirated during this liposucton was more than 2,400 mL. Twenty-four hours after surgery, hemoglobin levels dropped from 13.1 mg/dL to 12.0 mg/dL. Approximately 16.5 mL of whole blood was removed per liter of aspirate. No differences were reported between the groups undergoing local or general anesthesia. Approximately 180 mL of additional blood was lost for sample collections.

Discussion.—There are 3 routes of blood loss during liposuction: (1) into the aspirate; (2) into the dead space; and (3) into the dressings and sponges. In this study, only a small amount was lost as a result of aspiration, and the greatest loss was due to sampling. The injection of dilute adrenaline is believed to have contributed to the low blood loss. Other types of surgery already use dilute adrenaline to decrease blood loss during surgery. Blood loss with this technique is decreased for other reasons as well. The preoperative injection of saline compresses blood vessels, which decreases bleeding. Distension of the fatty tissue itself occurs when large volumes of saline are injected. This facilitates liposuction as well. In conclusion, when large volumes of a dilute solution of adrenaline are injected before liposuction, blood loss during the procedure decreases.

▶ Here is one more article that acknowledges the benefits of tumescent liposuction. It is quickly becoming the gold standard, even in the plastic surgical community, and the hope is that this will continue.

D.J. Papadopoulos, M.D.

Effect of Syringe-Assisted Liposuction on Activation of Cascade Systems and Circulating Cells When Using the Superwet or Tumescent Technique
Samdal F, Aasen AO, Mollnes TE, et al (Inst of Surgical Research, Oslo, Norway; Univ Hosp of Oslo, Norway; Univ of Tromsø, Norway)
Ann Plast Surg 35:242–248, 1995   4–20

Background.—Although liposuction is the most common plastic surgery worldwide, few reports have addressed its systemic effects. In addition, nonfatal serious complications and several deaths associated with the procedure have been reported. The extent to which liposuction affects complement activation or other cascade systems is not known. To address this question, the effects of syringe-assisted liposuction using the superwet or tumescent technique on various components of the coagulation, fibrinolytic, plasma kallikrein-kinin, and complement systems were investigated.

Methods.—Participants included 22 patients undergoing liposuction aspiration of a volume of 1,000 mL or more. Mean aspirate volume was relatively high (2,648 mL). Plasma levels of kallikrein, prekallikrein, kallikrein inhibitor, plasmin, plasminogen, antiplasmin, prothrombin, antithrombin, complement C3 activation products, terminal complement complex, interleukin-6, and tumor necrosis factor-α were measured.

Results.— Changes in the variables with time were small and well within the normal ranges. Interleukin-6 peaks (measured in 9 patients) were on the same order of magnitude as those measured in patients having hernia repair and were lower than those measured in patients having breast reconstruction. Tumor necrosis factor-α was not detected in the 9 patients tested.

Conclusions.—The degree of surgical trauma inflicted by syringe-assisted liposuction, at least in the manner it was performed in these patients, appears to be small to moderate. No clinically significant activation of the cascade systems was detected.

▶ This is a good negative study to help us better understand why complications may occur during liposuction. The authors have published many articles and have a wide experience with tumescent liposuction. This study is an interesting look at how tumescent "superwet" technique affects the complement–clotting cascade system. The alteration in this cascade seen during "dry methods" of liposuction further establishes, in my mind, that the only way to go is wet—very, very wet.

D.J. Papadopoulos, M.D.

Effect of L-Ornithine 8-Vasopressin on Blood Loss During Liposuction
Lalinde E, Sanz J, Ballesteros A, et al (Univ of Navarra, Pamplona, Spain)
Ann Plast Surg 34:613–618, 1995   4–21

Background.—Because blood loss during liposuction can be problematic, infiltration with epinephrine before aspiration is an accepted practice. The use of epinephrine is not without cardiovascular risk, however. Thus, an alternative method of producing vasoconstriction that does not have secondary effects at the cardiovascular level is needed. L-ornithine 8-vasopressin, a synthetic polypeptide (POR 8, Sandoz Laboratories), was evaluated in this capacity.

Methods.—Participants included 20 patients undergoing liposuction of the trochanteric region for the first time (volume > 1,000 mL). Patients in group A received presurgical infiltration with chilled saline containing L-ornithine 8-vasopressin at a dilution of 0.01 IU/mL (maximum dose, 20 IU). Patients in group B underwent traditional vasoconstriction with epinephrine. An atraumatic cannula of the authors' own design was used for the infiltrations.

Results.—The only reported complications of the procedures were subcutaneous hematomas in some of the liposuctioned areas. No patient required blood or plasma transfusion. No statistically significant differences were found between the 2 treatment groups in terms of total fluid suctioned, percentage of total fat, total fat removed, loss of hemoglobin and hematocrit after liposuction, or amount of blood loss.

Conclusions.—Blood loss 72 hours after liposuction with L-ornithine 8-vasopressin did not differ significantly from blood loss occurring with epinephrine as the vasoconstrictor. However, the amounts of fat removed were high (mean total amount of suctioned fat: 2,818 mL with epinephrine and 3,125 mL with vasopressin). The authors' cannula and L-ornithine 8-vasopressin were associated with minimal blood loss, even with extraction of large volumes of fat.

▶ This article is interesting because of the novel use of L-ornithine 8-vasopressin for liposuction. Vasopressin is also occasionally used in Europe and Australia admixed to the anesthetic solution for hair transplantation procedures. Unfortunately, the authors did not give enough credit to the introduction of tumescent technique because it did not serve their purposes in this study. They basically attempted to compare the results they obtained using vasopressin with results of direct infiltration of epinephrine before liposuction. They subsequently compared their results to those with the tumescent technique and ultimately found no significant differences. (as one would expect between the tumescent technique without vasopressin.) Nevertheless, vasopressin is an important substance that we should be using more to control bleeding. More studies need to be done to assess proper variables.

D.J. Papadopoulos, M.D.

Transplantation

Long-Term Survival of Fat Transplants: Controlled Demonstrations
Coleman SR (New York)
Aesthetic Plast Surg 19:421–425, 1995   4–22

Introduction.—Although fatty tissue can be transplanted as a filler to create a lasting correction, it is not always permanent. The techniques for using fat have been modified in an attempt to guarantee permanent fatty replacement.

Methods.—Intact parcels of fatty tissue, subject to the minimum pressure and exposure, and untainted by blood, oil, or lidocaine were placed with a nutritional source in an effort to increase survival. The shadow of a nearby uncorrected crease on the same face was used as a control. Patients were photographed yearly for 6 years.

> *Case Study.*—Woman, 47, presented for correction of nasolabial folds. After anesthetic, fatty tissue was harvested from the submental region with a 3-holed blunt tipped cannula using low-pressure suction. Any fatty tissue with significant amounts of associated blood or oil was discarded. The fatty tissue was infiltrated using 16-gauge needles. The correction was maintained for 77 months of follow-up.

Results.—Follow-up was available for 6 years. During that time, no reabsorption was noted in the experimental crease, as compared with the control crease.

Conclusions.—Free transfer of autologous fat tissue remains controversial in plastic surgery. This controlled clinical study demonstrated a simple method using fat tissue that can be used to achieve long-term soft tissue augmentation with high patient satisfaction and few complications.

▶ In my heart, I want to believe that fat that has been transplanted will survive for many years, and the author here makes a good argument for technique and processing of fat as critical components in the whole procedure. The photographs presented of the 2 patients are 2 good examples of his point. Hopefully, as we get better at processing and injecting fat, we can begin to appreciate and better use this filler.

D.J. Papadopoulos, M.D.

Filler Substances—Collagen

Guidelines of Care for Soft Tissue Augmentation: Fat Transplantation
Drake LA, Dinehart SM, Farmer ER, et al (American Academy of Dermatology, Schaumburg, Ill)
J Am Acad Dermatol 34:690–694, 1996   4–23

Introduction.—Guidelines for fat transplantation address the quality of dermatologic care and discuss its scope, providing additional information to facilitate the understanding of those outside the profession.

Scope.—Fat transplantation has been used to treat lipoatrophy resulting from diseases such as acne, trauma, lipodystrophy, hemifacial atrophy, cutaneous lupus erythematosus, scleroderma, idiopathy, senescence, and postintralesional injections. Fat transplantation has also been used for cosmetic treatment of senescence, facial rytids, malar augmentation, chin augmentation, correction of defects after liposuction, and dorsal hand rejuvenation. Fat injections are not usually used to treat fine wrinkling or bound-down or nondistensible scars.

Issue.—Physician qualifications include training in fat transplantation, a residency or board certification, and a knowledge of transplantation physiology, anatomy, and complications.

Diagnostic Criteria.—Patient information should include a history, a physical examination, and selection of a donor site. The physician should verify the patient's understanding and expectations of the procedure. The diagnostics tests should be appropriate and may include clotting studies, biopsies, and imaging studies.

Surgical Treatment.—After obtaining the patient's informed consent, selecting a surgical setting, choosing an anesthesia, and deciding the volume of fat to be extracted, the fat is aspirated by syringe or removed by a machine-assisted liposuction aspirator.

After harvest, the fat is separated from other fluids and reinjected into the donor site either using the same syringe or, if machine-assisted, transferring the fat to another syringe or to an injection gun. Postoperative care consists mainly of application of ice packs to the recipient site, immobilizing the site, and providing medication. Edema, ecchymosis, discomfort, punctate scarring, and dysesthesia are expected. Occasionally, persistent edema, asymmetry, hematoma, lumping, or persistent bleeding may develop. Rarely, infection may occur. Additional fat may be frozen, and collagen may be collected for injection into fine wrinkles.

Conclusion.—These guidelines are not comprehensive, and final decisions must be made by the physician.

Guidelines of Care for Soft Tissue Augmentation: Collagen Implants
Drake LA, Dinehart SM, Farmer ER, et al (American Academy of Dermatology, Schaumburg, Ill)
J Am Acad Dermatol 34:698–702, 1996   4–24

Introduction.—Guidelines for using collagen implants address the quality of dermatologic care and discuss the scope of care, providing additional information to facilitate the understanding of those outside the profession.

Scope.—The implant, reconstituted fibrillar bovine collagen, is injected into the dermis to augment soft tissues. The implant is also available in a cross-linked version, prepared with glutaraldehyde, that shows decreased biologic degradation. The preparation comes preloaded in a syringe and is suspended in phosphate-buffered saline containing 0.3% lidocaine. Collagen implants are suitable for corns, calluses, depressed scars, wrinkles, creases, lines, dermal atrophy, angular cheilitis, and contour enhancement. Ice-pick scars, viral pockmarks, stretch marks, and loss of subcutaneous tissue usually do not respond to treatment.

Issue.—Physician qualifications include training in bovine collagen implantation techniques, a residency or board certification, and a knowledge of skin and cutaneous tissue.

Diagnostic Criteria.—Patient information should include a history, a physical examination, and notation of use of immunosuppressive therapy, bleeding disorders, history of keloids, allergic reactions to collagen, active dermatologic disease, and contraindications for implantation. The physician should verify the patient's tolerance of side effects and understanding and expectations of the procedure and should perform a skin test.

Treatment.—After obtaining the patient's informed consent, cleansing the area, and placing the patient in a vertical position, the physician pierces the skin at a 45-degree angle and injects the collagen. The non–cross-linked product is used for superficial defects, whereas the cross-linked product is used for deeper dermal filling. In some cases, the products are layered to attain maximal correction. Erythema, temporary overcorrection, whealing, bruising, and edema commonly occur after treatment. Occasionally ridging or beading or reactivation of a latent herpes simplex infection may occur. Rarely, recurrent, intermittent swelling, local necrosis, or abscess may develop. The potential risk of serious connective tissue disease as a result of collagen injection is controversial.

Conclusion.—These guidelines are not comprehensive, and final decisions must be made by the physician.

Guidelines of Care for Soft Tissue Augmentation: Gelatin Matrix Implant
Drake LA, Dinehart SM, Farmer ER, et al (American Academy of Dermatology, Schaumburg, Ill)
J Am Acad Dermatol 34:695–697, 1996   4–25

Introduction.—Guidelines for gelatin matrix implantation address the quality of dermatologic care and discuss its scope, providing additional information to facilitate the understanding of those outside the profession.

Scope.—The implant consists of a lyophilized gelatin powder, derived from pig collagen, and ϵ-aminocaproic acid. When reconstituted with the patient's serum and normal saline, the implant encourages wound healing and elevates soft tissue defects. Trauma or disease can result in loss of the dermis and subcutaneous tissue. Gelatin matrix implantation is suitable for soft, distensible scars and some nondistensible scars, creases, and furrows. Superficial wrinkles, ice-pick scars, pockmarks, stretch marks, and loss of subcutaneous tissue usually do not respond to treatment.

Issue.—Physician qualifications include training in gelatin matrix implantation techniques, a residency or board certification, and a knowledge of skin and cutaneous tissue and selection of appropriate implant components for the defect.

Diagnostic Criteria.—Patient information should include a history, a physical examination, and contraindications for implantation. The physician should verify the patient's understanding and expectations of the procedure and should perform a skin test.

Treatment.—After obtaining the patient's informed consent, outlining the skin area, and choosing a local anesthetic, if appropriate, the physician injects the implant into the papillary, mid-, or reticular dermis with a 27- to 20-gauge needle. Postoperative care may consist of application of ice packs to the site. Bruising, ecchymosis, inflammation, and swelling may be present for as long as 2 weeks. Allergic reactions are rare. Lidocaine (1%) and/or more saline may be used in place of plasma.

Conclusion.—These guidelines are not comprehensive, and final decisions must be made by the physician.

▶ These 3 articles are required reading for those interested in getting involved with soft tissue augmentation. The bibliographies provided in these guidelines of care articles are very valuable and should probably be the first step in building a foundation for effectively performing these procedures.

The committees involved should also be commended for coming together and forming these guidelines, because this is usually a very difficult practice due to individual practitioner differences in performing soft tissue augmentation.

D.J. Papadopoulos, M.D.

Chin Augmentation Using Minimally Invasive Technique and Bioplastique
Ersek RA, Stovall RB, Vazquez-Salisbury A (Texas State Univ, Austin; Univ of Texas, Austin)
Plast Reconstr Surg 95:985–992, 1995   4–26

Introduction.—Techniques for chin augmentation have been beset with problems. The use of an injectable biphasic polymer fabricated for soft

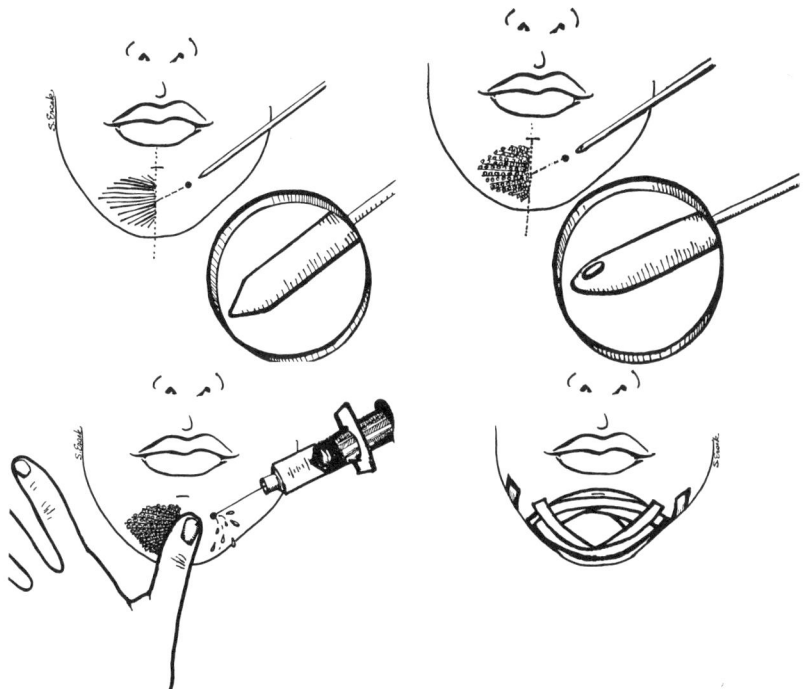

FIGURE 1.—(**Above, left**) The initial process of pretunneling in a radial fashion from a remote puncture site using the pencil-tipped pocar. By pretunneling the half opposite the entrance site, the instrument remains at or just above the level of the periosteum. (**Above, right**) Precise placement of the particles using the blunt cannula. By mimicking the path and technique of the pocar while in constant motion and with slight trigger pressure only on withdrawal, particles are evenly distributed within the highly arrayed network of tunnels well beneath the dermis. (**Below, left**) By holding digital pressure over the midline while rinsing the remote puncture site and "no man's land" with local anesthesia, retention of particles within the wound itself is prevented. (**Below, right**) Immobilization of the area from the sublabial crease to the submandibular ridge allows an even diffusion of particles within the augmentation area. (Courtesy of Ersek RA, Stovall RB, Vazquez-Salisbury A: Chin augmentation using minimally invasive technique and Bioplastique. *Plast Reconstr Surg* 95:985–992, 1995.)

tissue augmentation is described in 13 patients who underwent chin augmentation.

Methods.—The biphasic polymer consisted of solid microparticles between 100–600 µm in diameter. These inert particles were prefabricated with a textured surface and suspended in a biocompatible gel vehicle. Bioplastique, the gel polymer, was sterilized and placed in cartridges for injection. A special pencil-tipped pocar was used to establish a network of tunnels within the subcutaneous tissue of the chin (Fig 1). A newly designed cannula with an injection gun was used to implant the microparticles. Injection was done only on withdrawal and mimicked the path and technique of the pocar. Precise and even placement of the microparticles was possible. The chin was splinted with suture strips to immobilize the area. During the first postoperative week, patients were told to use digital manipulation to dissociate any palpable irregularities.

Results.—Thirteen patients received a total of 18.2 cc of Bioplastique in 14 injections. The infection rate was zero. Two patients required removal of some of the Bioplastique. This was easily accomplished, using an 18-gauge or larger needle and rotating the needle to remove particles while passing through the area of excess augmentation. Patients experienced lasting aesthetic improvement and are asymptomatic at a maximum follow-up of 60 months postoperatively.

Conclusion.—The aesthetic improvements experienced by patients occur because the particles become surrounded by a fibrous capsule, thus enhancing augmentation. It appears that Bioplastique is not susceptible to infection and provides a permanent, yet removable, soft-tissue augmentation.

▶ The authors clearly state here that the injection of this material is indicated in those patients with minor chin deficiencies, which I think is an important point to remember no matter what the material to be used is going to be. The advantages of this material are:

1. it is permanent, yet removable;
2. it is easy to use;
3. there have been no infections to date, and
4. there is no migration. It appears that this material may have great potential and might be used for other indications of soft tissue augmentation.

D.J. Papadopoulos, M.D.

PMMA Microspheres (Artecoll) for Skin and Soft-Tissue Augmentation: Part II. Clinical Investigations
Lemperle G, Hazan-Gaúthier N, Lemperle M (St Markus Hosp, Frankfurt/Main, Germany)
Plast Reconstr Surg 96:627–634, 1995   4–27

Introduction.—For long-lasting correction of wrinkles and other skin defects, Artecoll, consisting of bone cement microspheres produced by

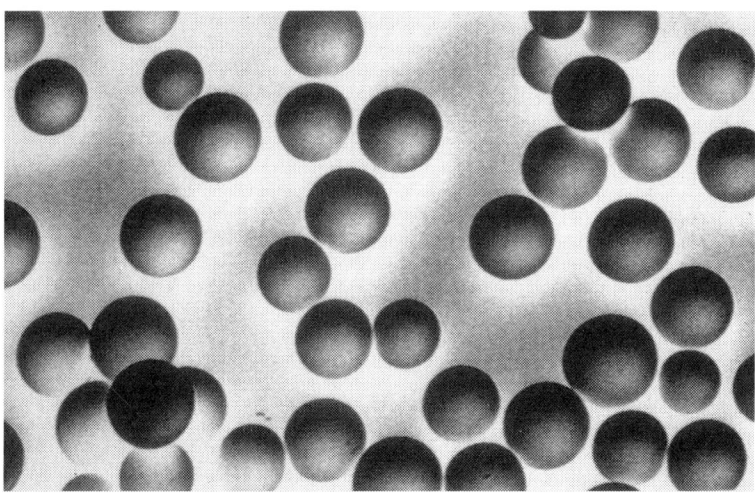

FIGURE 1.—Electronmicroscopy shows polymethyl-methacrylate microspheres at 30–40 μm diameter and an absolutely smooth surface. (Courtesy of Lemperle G, Hazan-Gaúthier N, Lemperle M: PMMA microspheres [Artecoll] for skin and soft-tissue augmentation: Part II. Clinical investigations. *Plast Reconstr Surg* 96:627–634, 1995.)

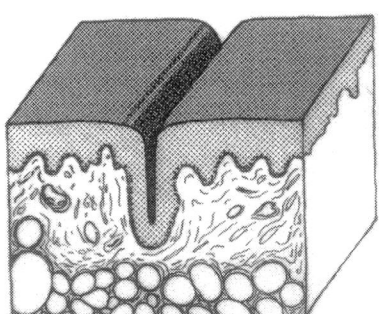 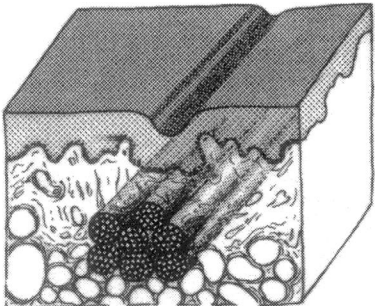

FIGURE 2.—Artecoll should be applied into a series of channels or in a fanlike manner, into the lower third of the dermis. (Courtesy of Lemperle G, Hazan-Gaúthier N, Lemperle M: PMMA microspheres [Artecoll] for skin and soft-tissue augmentation: Part II. Clinical investigations. *Plast Reconstr Surg* 96:627–634, 1995.)

TABLE II.—Patients in the Second Prospective Study

No. of patients	118
Age	26–72 years
Gender	108 females; 10 males
No. of wrinkles	200
Implantations	Performed from November 1990 through March 1992
No. of applications	292
Evaluations	Performed from March 1992 through January 1994

(From Lemperle G, Hazan-Gaúthier N, Lemperle M: PMMA microspheres [Artecoll] for skin and soft-tissue augmentation: Part II. Clinical investigations. *Plast Reconstr Surg* 96:627–634, 1995. Courtesy of Nischan T: Klinische Studie über die Biokompatibilität von PMMA-Mikrosphären in der Haut. Thesis, Johann-Wolfgang-Goethe Univ, Frankfurt/Main, Germany, 1995.)

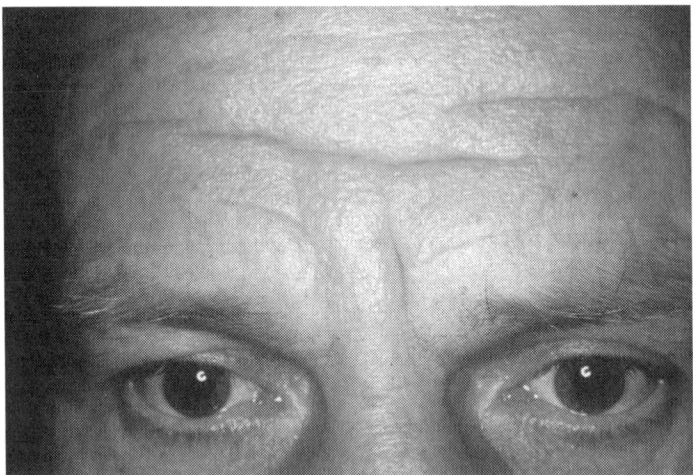

FIGURE 4.—Deep furrows and glabellar frowns. (Courtesy of Lemperly G, Hazan-Gaúthier N, Lemperle M: PMMA microspheres [Artecoll] for skin and soft-tissue augmentation: Part II. Clinical investigations. *Plast Reconstr Surg* 96:627–634, 1995.)

suspension-polymerization, is injected. The fine polymethol-methacrylate microspheres of 30–40 µm in diameter have a very smooth surface (Fig 1). Artecoll is not as easily applied as collagen and remains under the skin for many years. By means of a 27-gauge ½ -inch needle, Artecoll is implanted subdermally by 1-mL or 0.5-mL syringes (Fig 2).

Methods.—From a group of 2,000 patients who received Artecoll or Arteplast—a similar product—between 1989 and 1995, 100 patients with

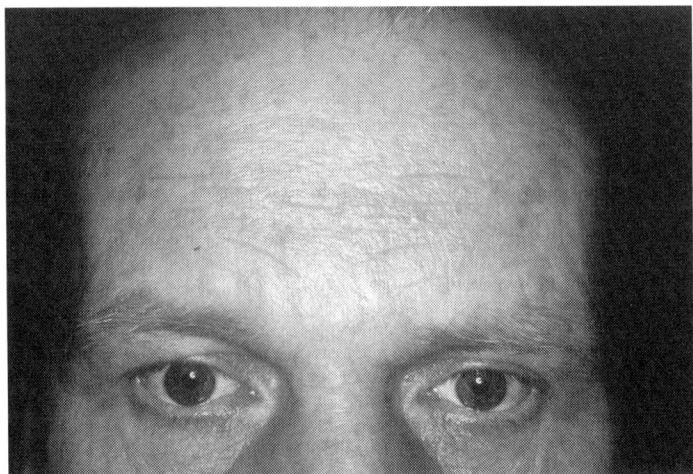

FIGURE 5.—Deep furrows and glabellar frowns 3 years after implantation of a total of 2.3 cc of Arteplast (3 injections within 4 months). (Courtesy of Lemperle G, Hazan-Gaúthier N, Lemperle M: PMMA microspheres [Artecoll] for skin and soft-tissue augmentation: Part II. Clinical investigations. *Plast Reconstr Surg* 96:627–634, 1995.)

TABLE I.—Indications for Artecoll Implantation

Main indications
   Glabellar frowns (22.5%)
   Nasolabial folds (27%)
   Perioral lines (15%)
   Depressed corners of the mouth (13%)
Other possible indications
   Lip augmentation
   Philtrum augmentation
   Horizontal chin folds
   Depressions after rhinoplasty
   Horizontal frontal furrows
   Neck folds
Limiting indications
   Firm scars and acne scars
   Single crow's feet
   Dark shadowed eyelids
   Unevenness and dimples after facelifting
   Alveolar ridge augmentation in toothless patients
Medical indications
   Enophthalmous
   Small skull defects
   Sclerodermia
   Romberg disease
   Drill holes
   Hypoplastic malar bones
   Tripod fracture of the malar bone
   Chin augmentation
   Bony defects in face and hands
   Small funnel chest
   Visible borders of solid silicone implants
   Nipple reconstruction and augmentation
   Vocal cord paralysis (?)
   Rhinolalia in cleft palate patients (?)
   Urinary stress incontinence
   Urethro–vesical reflux

(Courtesy of Lemperle G, Hazan-Gaúthier N, Lemperle M: PMMA microspheres [Artecoll] for skin and soft-tissue augmentation: Part II. Clinical investigations. *Plast Reconstr Surg* 96:627–634, 1995.)

193 implantation sites were enrolled in a prospective study, and 188 patients with 200 pairs of wrinkles were objectively reviewed (Table II). After the surgeries, patients filled out anonymous questionnaires.

Results.—Overall, 89.5% of patients were satisfied or pleased with the result of the treatment; 10.5% noted no difference or had side effects, although comparisons of the preoperative and postoperative slides did show a slight improvement. Moderate improvement was noted by 25.5% of patients; striking and lasting improvement in folds and wrinkles was noted by 64% of patients. Side effects included swelling, redness, and moderate pain, generally lasting for 2 days. Slight itching usually subsides within weeks or months.

Conclusion.—The technique is best used for patients between 40 and 50 years of age when excess skin does not justify a facelift. Indications include glabellar frowns (Figs 4 and 5), nasolabial folds, perioral lines, and depressed corners of the mouth (Table I). Other possible indications include lip augmentation, horizontal chin folds, and depressions after rhinoplasty.

Limiting indications include firm scars and acne scars, single crow's feet, and dark shadowed eyelids. Contraindications are known allergy to collagen, susceptibility to keloids, thin and flaccid skin, and atrophic skin diseases. Artecoll must be implanted subdermally, never intradermally. If the gray of the needle shines through the skin, the implant will be located too superficially. The overall complication rate is low.

▶ The authors describe a broad experience with these Plexiglas/collagen microspheres, but their argument for this material's use is not very convincing. Like all injectable materials, this one is operator dependent and, as such, complications are also, to a great degree, operator dependent. It would be difficult for me to recommend to my population of patients a nonpermanent therapy with a 10% complication rate and with 34% of the patients exhibiting palpable implants. Also, even though the Oppenheimer effect (i.e., the formation of sarcomas within capsules around plastic sheets in rats) has never been seen in humans, it would be difficult for me to believe that, upon mentioning this to my patients, they would agree to this therapy.

D.J. Papadopoulos, M.D.

Dermabrasion/Chemical Peel

Dermabrasive Scar Revision: Immunohistochemical and Ultrastructural Evaluation
Harmon CB, Zelickson BD, Roenigk RK, et al (Mayo Clinic and Mayo Found, Rochester, Minn; Univ of Minnesota Minneapolis)
Dermatol Surg 21:503–508, 1995   4–28

Background.—Facial scar dermabrasion 4 to 8 weeks after injury can eliminate all evidence of scar. The cellular and structural mechanisms by which this process occurs, however, is unclear. Wound healing after dermabrasive scar revision was investigated.

Methods.—Seven patients undergoing surgical scar abrasion 6 to 8 weeks after injury were studied. Punch biopsy specimens were obtained before and after dermabrasion, and comparative electron microscopic and immunohistochemical studies were done. The presence, location, and temporal expression of tenascin, epiligrin, cadherins, and integrin subunits were observed by monoclonal antibody staining.

Findings.—Collagen bundle density and size were increased and showed a tendency toward unidirectional orientation of fibers parallel to the epidermal surface. There was an upregulation of tenascin expression throughout the papillary dermis. In addition, α-6/β-4 integrin subunit was expressed on the keratinocytes throughout the stratum spinosum.

Conclusions.—These ultrastructural comparisons between preabrasion and postabrasion specimens illuminate the mechanisms by which primary cicatrix formation is altered by dermabrasive scar revision. Extracellular ligand expression is modified, which influences epithelial cell-cell interaction, and connective tissue is reorganized.

▶ An interesting commentary on cellular and subcellular events that occur during a procedure that we all know is beneficial for scar revision. It would be interesting to see how these events change quantitatively and qualitatively over time for similar wounds and similar locations. Also of interest would be TGF-1, 2, and 3 measurements of this material and the relative ratio changes of TGF-1:TGF-2 and 3.

D.J. Papadopoulos, M.D.

Dermabrasion for Prophylaxis and Treatment of Actinic Keratoses
Coleman WP III, Yarborough JM, Mandy SH (Tulane Univ, New Orleans, La; Univ of Miami, Fla)
Dermatol Surg 22:17–21, 1996   4–29

Introduction.—Actinic keratoses are circumscribed lesions found on sun-exposed surfaces in fair-skinned individuals. They are premalignant and may evolve into squamous cell carcinomas. The longer an actinic keratosis is present, the more likely it will transform into squamous cell carcinoma; therefore, it should be treated as early as possible. Therapy includes cryosurgery with liquid nitrogen, electrosurgery, CO_2 laser, topical 5-Fluorouracil, chemical peels, and dermabrasion. In the treatment of these lesions, only dermabrasion has been found to be prophylactic as well as therapeutic.

Methods.— A retrospective review was conducted of 23 patients with at least 2 years of good clinical follow-up after full face or partial face dermabrasion for the treatment of actinic keratoses. Patients ranged in age from 33 to 76 years. Results are available for up to 10 years after the procedure. Seventeen patients had dermabrasion of the full face, 2 of the forehead and scalp only; 3 of the nose, and 1 of the upper lip.

Results.—One year after dermabrasion, 22 of 23 patients had no actinic keratoses (96%). At 2-year follow-up, 19 (83%) had no actinic keratoses. Of the 19 patients followed for 3 years, 15 (79%) had no actinic keratoses. Of the 14 followed for 4 years, 9 (64%) had no actinic keratoses. Of the 13 followed for 5 years, 7 (54%) had no actinic keratoses. The appearance of one actinic keratoses occurred an average of 4 years after dermabrasion. In the perinasal area, dermabrasion did not prevent the appearance of basal cell carcinomas.

Conclusion.—Dermabrasion is the only modality that treats actinic keratoses and provides long-term prophylaxis. The technique is more complicated than other modalities, but it is ideal for those with multiple actinic keratoses and severe photodamage who require frequent treatment.

▶ This is a very important article for those of us who deal with actinic damage and skin cancer. Frequently, we recommend many modalities for the treatment of multiple actinic keratoses (AKs). This information allows us to be in a better position to assess long-term efficacy of our treatment options, and makes it clearer that to prevent new AKs we must attain greater controlled destruction than that which is afforded by medium-depth peels, cryosurgery, or 5-FU. This is also important information to pass along to insurance carriers because it will make it clearer to them that this is probably one of the most cost-effective methods of treating multiple actinic keratoses in predisposed individuals.

D.J. Papadopoulos, M.D.

A Comparison of Wire Brush and Diamond Fraise Superficial Dermabrasion for Photoaged Skin: A Clinical, Immunohistologic, and Biochemical Study
Nelson BR, Metz RD, Majmudar G, et al (Univ of Michigan, Ann Arbor; Univ of Manchester, England)
J Am Acad Dermatol 34:235–243, 1996   4–30

Introduction.—No prospective controlled investigations have studied whether the diamond fraise (DF) or the wire brush (WB) dermabrasion technique results in less scarring and erythema, requires shorter recovery time, and is most effective. The DF approach causes a thermal–friction injury, and WB causes microlaceration. Clinical, immunohistologic, and biological changes were compared in patients undergoing dermabrasion with DF and WB.

Methods.—Eight men (mean age, 68 years) underwent dermabrasion to the level of the papillary dermis for clinically severe facial photoaging. The procedure was performed on the lower part of the face in 5 patients and on the forehead in 3 patients. Four patients in group 1 underwent dermabrasion to the right side of the face with DF and to the left side of the face with WB. The treatment sites were reversed in the 4 patients in group 2. Facial photographs were taken at baseline and 12 weeks after dermabrasion. Three blinded clinicians graded improvement. Before dermabrasion and 3 and 12 weeks after treatment, 3 full-thickness 4-mm biopsy specimens were taken from sun-exposed facial skin from both sides of the face. One of the specimens was bisected so that half could be used for histologic

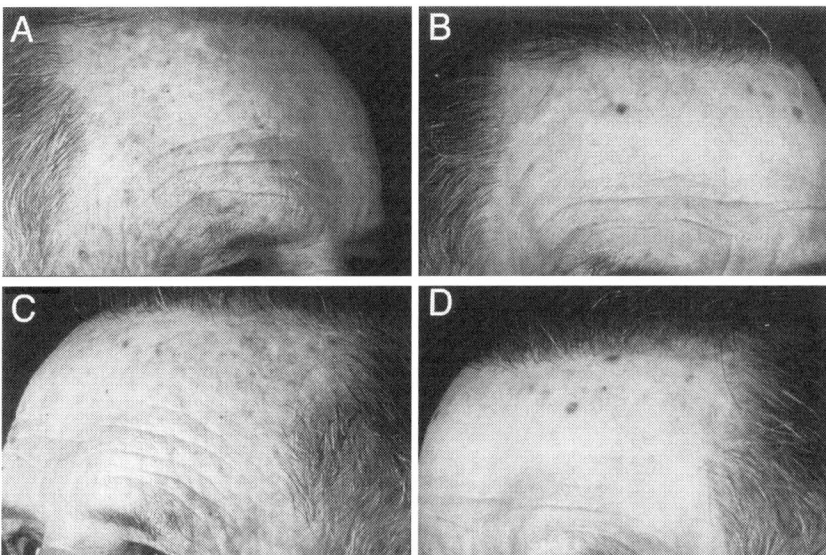

FIGURE 1.—Clinical improvement after dermabrasion. **A** and **C**, before dermabrasion; **B** and **D**, significant reduction in actinic lentigines, actinic keratoses, and wrinkles 12 weeks after dermabrasion with DF (*B*) and WB (*D*). (Courtesy of Nelson, BR, Metz RD, Majudar G, et al: A comparison of wire brush and diamond fraise superficial dermabrasion for photoaged skin: a clinical, immunohistologic, and biochemical study. *J Am Acad Dermatol* 34:235–243, 1996.)

examination and the other half could be used for immunohistologic evaluation. The second and third specimens were used for Western blot analysis and radioimmunoassay, respectively.

Results.—Twelve weeks after dermabrasion, both the DF and WB techniques produced moderate to marked improvement in actinic lentigines, actinic keratoses, and wrinkles (Fig 1). Milia was significantly less severe with DF than with WB. Erythema or inflammation was less severe with DF than with WB, but the difference was not significant. Similar increases occurred in papillary dermal staining of collagen, and similar decreases were seen in actinically altered elastic fibers consistent with solar elastosis in both approaches. Both dermabrasion techniques showed a significant increase in extracellular fibroblast procollagen type I staining at 3 weeks. Both techniques were associated with a modest decrease toward baseline at 12 weeks. Increases in type I procollagen was noted on immunohistochemical staining for both methods. Type III procollagen expression did not change from baseline with either approach. Western blot analysis indicated that levels of pN collagen I and pN collagen III were significantly greater than baseline for both DF and WB dermabrasion at 3- and 12-week follow-up. Transforming growth factor-β1 extracellular staining significantly increased with DF and WB at 3 weeks.

Conclusion.—Superficial dermabrasion with DF and WP produced similar results in the treatment of photoaged skin. Both types of dermabrasion elicited significant increases in type I pN-collagen, type III pN-collagen, and transforming growth factor-β1 in the papillary dermis.

► In this age of laser resurfacing, we must not forget that superficial dermabrasion is a time-tested, proven, and effective treatment for actinic keratoses and for rhytides. It is my opinion that in the hands of experienced practitioners, this treatment is as effective as CO_2 laser resurfacing. I prefer the diamond fraise, but those who have been trained with the wire brush usually obtain wonderful results. Milia, a minor complication, can occur with both treatments.

D.J. Papadopoulos, M.D.

Histologic Study of Dermabrasion and Chemical Peel in an Animal Model After Pretreatment With Retin-A
Vagotis FL, Brundage SR (Grand Rapids, Mich)
Aesthetic Plast Surg 19:243–246, 1995   4–31

Introduction.—A derivative of vitamin A, Retin-A has been prescribed for various forms of acne with patients reporting smoother skin and improvement of fine wrinkling. To eradicate fine wrinkling, chemical and mechanical means are used, both involving stripping of the superficial layers. The combination of Retin-A with dermabrasion and chemical peel has not been studied. In an animal model in which animals were pretreated with topical Retin-A, histologic changes were evaluated after dermabrasion and chemical peel.

Methods.—Guinea pig skin and human skin are similar in architecture, which is why guinea pigs were used in this study. Of the 12 guinea pigs used, 6 were pretreated with topical Retin-A and 6 served as controls. All of the pigs had dermabrasion and chemical peel, and the wounded areas were submitted to biopsy and evaluated for the clinical progression of healing.

Results.—Guinea pigs pretreated with Retin-A healed much more quickly than the control animals. In the Retin-A group, all of the guinea pigs had healed within 2 weeks, whereas in the control group, 75% of the wounded areas had healed. At 6 weeks, all were completely healed. After 1 month, there were an average of 7 to 8 cell layers in the epidermis of the Retin-A group, whereas the control group had 4 or 5 cell layers at this time.

Conclusion.—A statistically significant increase in epidermal regeneration was seen in the guinea pigs pretreated with Retin-A. Accelerated healing may result in pretreating patients with Retin-A before undergoing chemical peel or dermabrasion. More clinical research with Retin-A should be conducted.

► If we can extrapolate these results and apply them to humans, it certainly supports the pretreatment of our patients with Retin-A, not only for preparation and possible avoidance of posttreatment hyperpigmentation, but also for quicker healing. It would be interesting to see what the histologic picture would be in humans.

D.J. Papadopoulos, M.D.

Vitiligo: Repigmentation With Dermabrasion and Thin Split-Thickness Skin Graft
Agrawal K, Agrawal A (Jawaharlal Inst, Pondicherry, India)
Dermatol Surg 21:295–300, 1995   4–32

Background.—Vitiligo is a common benign condition that causes social problems in dark-skinned races. None of the treatments available is completely dependable. The success and complications of split-thickness skin grafting (STSG) were reported.

Methods.—Twenty-one patients with a total of 32 localized, stable, refractory vitiligo patches were included in the study. Treatment consisted of dermabrasion and thin STSG. Follow-up of all but 3 patients ranged from 1 to 6 years.

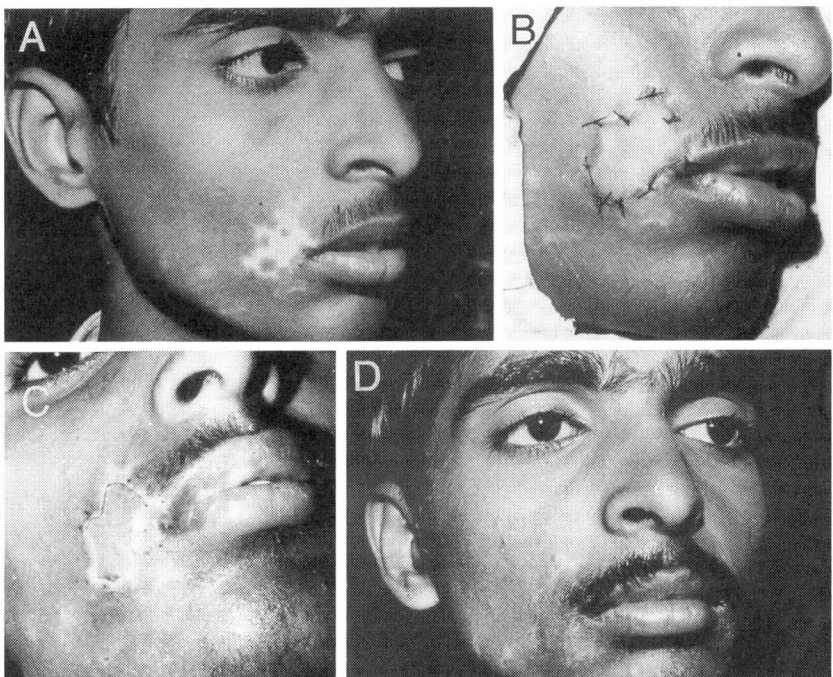

FIGURE 1.—**A,** preoperative vitiligo over right angle of mouth. **B,** Thiersch's split-thickness skin grafting sutured in place. **C,** primary dressing on seventh postoperative day with a hypopigmented halo around the skin graft. **D,** follow-up after 4 years. (Reprinted by permission of the publisher from Agrawal K, Agrawal A: Vitiligo: Repigmentation with dermabrasion and thin split-thickness skin graft. *Dermatol Surg* 21:295–300, copyright 1995 by Elsevier Science Inc.)

Findings.—Twenty-seven patches had a graft take of 100%, and 5, 90% to 95%. In 22 patches, 100% repigmentation was achieved. Repigmentation was 90% to 95% in the remaining 10 patches. Satisfactory color match was achieved in 4 to 9 months. Only minor complications occurred, none of which affected outcomes (Fig 1).

Conclusions.—Split-thickness skin grafting is a simple outpatient procedure that results in excellent color match in the long term. This procedure can be performed on any part of the body, including hair-bearing areas.

▶ Excellent results for a difficult problem. Milia and wrinkles in the graft can be alleviated by proper stretching of the graft. An alternative to 4-0 silk might be 5-0 or 6-0 nylon or prolean sutures and, for wider areas, basting sutures. This is a decent solution to a very difficult problem.

D.J. Papadopoulos, M.D.

Dermabrasion Using an Ultrasonic Surgical Aspirator

Ito Y, Kondo S, Sumiya N, et al (Showa Univ, Yokohama, Japan)
Plast Reconstr Surg 97:1034–1039, 1996   4–33

Introduction.—A motor-driven grinder is most often used for most dermabrasion techniques; however, it is inappropriate for the eyelid, ear, and mucous membranes. An ultrasonic surgical aspirator may be more appropriate for these areas because it is easier, more accurate, and provides faster healing and comparable, if not better, results. An ultrasonic surgical aspirator can be used to treat seborrheic keratoses, lentigo senilis, ephelides, and nevus spilus. In combination with cryosurgery, the device has been used to treat divided nevus and nevus of Ota.

Technique.—The US-1000 ultrasonic aspirator, manufactured by Miwa Company, Ltd., was used. First, a local or general anesthetic is administered. The operator holds the handpiece like a pen, presses the tip onto the epidermal surface of the lesion, and moves the tip around in continuous circular, brushlike motions. Petechiae will be observed in seconds. Calibrated over a range of 0 to 1,000, the device is set depending on the thickness and hardness of the affected areas. Ointment should be applied to the area when treatment is completed.

Case Studies.—One 46-year-old woman had lentigo senilis on the lower lip for 2 years. Six months after dermabrasion was performed, the hyperpigmented areas had totally disappeared (Fig 5). A 63-year-old man had a seborrheic keratosis for 10 years. Twenty-six months after dermabrasion, the keratosis still had not reappeared. A 26-year-old woman had congenital nevus spilus on the eyelids. Six months after dermabrasion, a portion of the lesion still remained, but no scarring occurred.

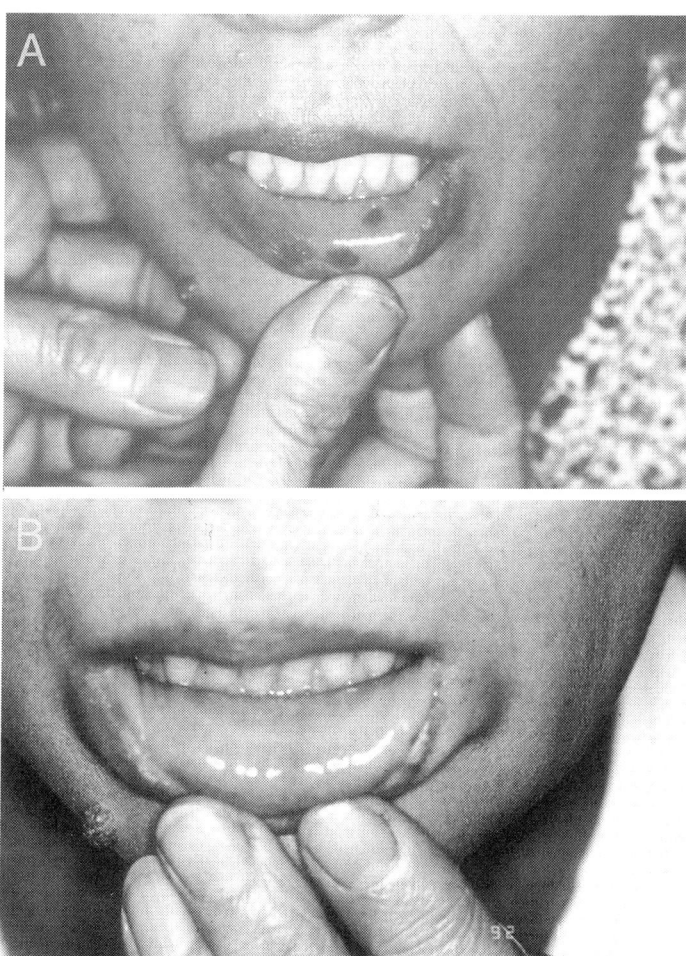

FIGURE 5.—A 46-year-old woman. **above,** preoperative appearance of the lentigo senilis located on the mucous membrane of the lower lip. **Below,** appearance approximately 6 months after procedure. No scarring or recurrence was present. (Courtesy of Ito Y, Kondo S, Sumiya N, et al: Dermabrasion using an ultrasonic surgical aspirator. *Plast Reconstr Surg* 97:1034–1039, 1996.)

Conclusion.—When used to perform dermabrasion, the ultrasonic surgical aspirator has been proven to be safe and effective with several advantages over the conventional grinder.

▶ This interesting device was used in over 300 patients, and especially in hard-to-reach anatomic areas. If one considers that this group from Yokohama only had 4 long-term complications in this very difficult-to-treat population of patients, these results are truly remarkable. I would have liked to see their results in the treatment of patients with nevus of Ota, which they mention "more than measures up to those achieved with Q-Switched ruby laser."

D.J. Papadopoulos, M.D.

Obagi's Modified Trichloroacetic Acid (TCA)-Controlled Variable-Depth Peel: A Study of Clinical Signs Correlating With Histological Findings

Johnson JB, Ichinose H, Obagi ZE, et al (Louisiana State Univ, New Orleans; Pendleton Mem Methodist Hosp, New Orleans, La; Stanford Univ, Calif)
Ann Plast Surg 36:225–237, 1996   4–34

Background.—Trichloroacetic acid (TCA) has been used increasingly in chemosurgical superficial dermatologic peels. Obagi has developed a modified TCA solution designed to slow the procedure and has identified clinical signs that indicate the depth of solution penetration. At the 50:1 level, epidermal sliding is observed. A uniform solid white frosting appears at the 50:2 level. At the 50:3 level, all background pink disappears and the skin appears grayish. The validity of these clinical signs was investigated through the use of sequential biopsy findings.

Methods.—Twenty patients underwent at least 4 weeks of skin preparation with intensive application of Retin-A tretinoin, hydroquinone, and lactic acid before they underwent the chemical peel with a solution of 41.7% TCA in a 10% glycerin diluent. The mechanisms of the acute signs were investigated in 4 patients with 3-mm punch biopsies taken 5 minutes after the clinical sign appeared. The biopsy material was examined with light microscopy and with electron microscopy in 2 patients. The longer term correlation between histological findings and clinical signs of the depth of peel was evaluated with punch biopsies obtained at 48 hours and 6 weeks after the chemical peel in 4 patients. In the remaining 12 patients, the thickness of the new dermis was assessed through the use of punch biopsy material obtained before and 6 weeks after chemical peel to a 50:2 level.

Results.—Histologic specimens of tissue at the acute 50:1 level revealed only mild changes with a thinner stratum corneum. Electron microscopy revealed nuclear leaching of the epidermal cells with chromatin concentration on the nuclear membranes. There was irregular cytoplasmic organelle coagulation and intercellular space edema. There was also nuclear leaching and shrunken mesenchymal cells in the papillary dermis. Specimens of the acute 50:2 level demonstrated complete loss of the stratum corneum and near-total loss of the stratum granulosum. Ultrastructural changes included more severe cytoplasmic organelle coagulation, intercellular swelling, and coagulative shrinkage of mesenchymal cells. The specimens of the acute 50:3 level revealed condensed squamous epithelium with nuclei arranged in parallel. Coagulation extended to the deep vascular dermal plexus. Collagen fibers had interfibrillar granules and microvesicular swelling.

The dermal changes were progressive, as shown by the biopsies at 48 hours and 6 weeks. By 6 weeks, chemical peel at the 50:2 level resulted in a new layer of fibrillar collagen in a laminar pattern that replaced the upper reticular dermis. This new dermal layer was almost the full thickness of the reticular layer in patients who underwent 50:3-level peel. After a 50:2-level peel, the new dermis accounted for an average of 33% of the full thickness of the dermis.

Conclusions.—The validity of Obagi's clinical signs was supported by the histologic and electron microscopic findings.

▶ Having known Zein Obagi from our residency days in San Diego, he has long been criticized for the lack of histologic correlation related to his proprietary peel. I would have liked to have seen his work in the dermatology journals, but I recognize his warmer reception by plastic surgeons. The comment, "Future publications will deal with the complications of TCA dermatologic chemosurgery in detail," makes me wonder about an orchestrated series. Perhaps I should have taken that position Zein offered me years ago; then again.

H.T. Greenway, M.D.

Management of Alopecia

Nontufted Incisional Slit Grafting

Hugeneck J, Kokott R, Wagner K-H, et al (Vienna)
J Dermatol Surg Oncol 21:718–723, 1994   4–35

Background.—Traditional methods of incisional grafting involve compression from the side when the grafts are placed in the incision. This can result in a tufted appearance. A nontufted incisional slit grafting technique was described (Fig 1).

> *Technique.*—In dissecting the graft, the primary ellipse is placed on a cutting surface with the hair-bearing surface facing up. The surgeon cuts it perpendicular to its longitudinal plane into secondary strips that are placed on their sides and cut into thin, flat slit grafts. The shape approximates the shape of the recipient incisional sites. The surgeon diligently trims away all excess fat and tissue from the sides and bottom to further decrease graft size. Because the epidermal surface of these grafts can contain excess tissue that expands into a mushroom-like shape (Fig 4), the surgeon trims the epidermis from each graft with a single cut at an oblique angle to reduce the surface area and achieve a uniform shape to the top of each graft (Fig 6).

Outcomes.—This technique enabled more than 2,000 very small grafts to be placed in a single session (Fig 9). Bleeding was minimal. Healing occurred so quickly that the grafts were barely visible by 10 days. There was no scarring, pitting, or tufting.

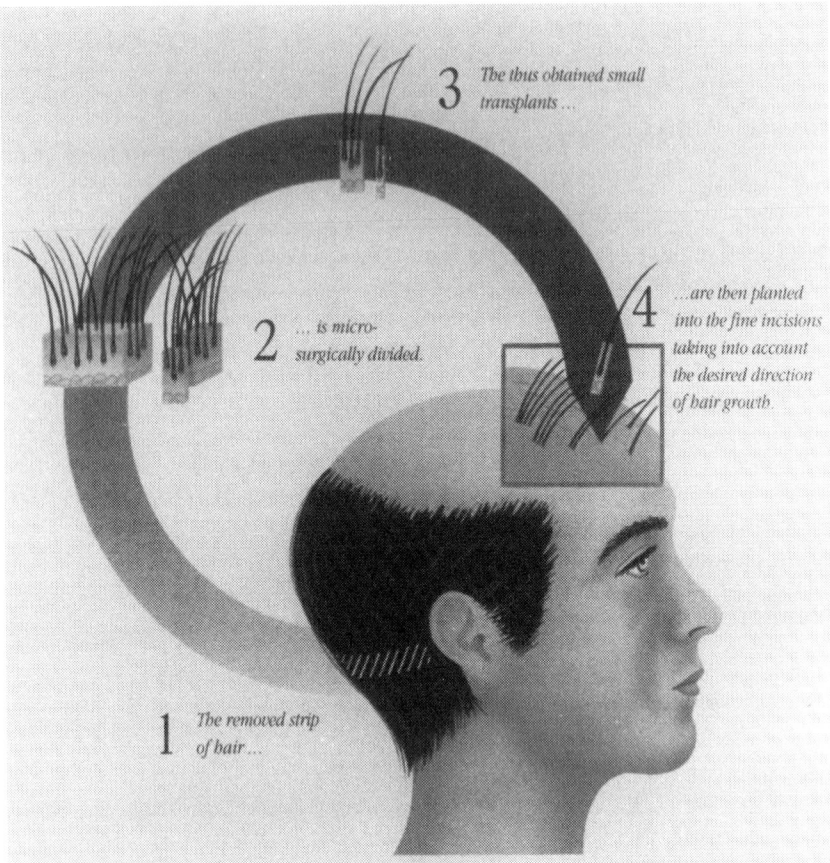

FIGURE 1.—The 4 steps of the nontufted incisional slit grafting technique. (Reprinted by permission of Elsevier Science, Inc. from Hugeneck J, Kokott R, Wagner K-H, et al: Nontufted incisional slit grafting. *J Dermatol Surg Oncol* 21:718–723, copyright 1994 by American Society for Dermatologic Surgery, Inc.)

Conclusions.—This donor hair dissection method produces very small flat grafts the same shape as the recipient sites. Because there is no graft compression, the tufted appearance is minimized. Pleasing results can be obtained in patients with extreme baldness and a relatively small fringe of hair through a very economic redistribution of donor hair.

▶ The photographic material presented in this article is excellent, with excellent results depicted, and the authors are to be commended for their fine work. Personally, I think that the old practice of making recipient sites smaller than the graft size should be abandoned because, in my experience, this only leads to cobblestoning for larger graft sizes and tufting when slits are used. I think that trimming the epidermis is unnecessary, especially for smaller grafts. I am an opponent of mega-session grafting, as I believe that the injury sustained by the scalp during this procedure probably has a

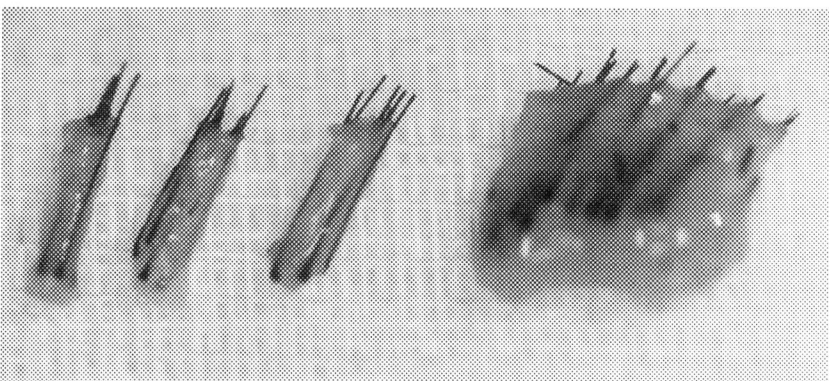

FIGURE 4.—Grafts before trimming with epidermal surface expanding into mushroom-like shape. This, along with excess tissue from the sides, must be cut away. (Reprinted by permission of Elsevier Science, Inc. from Hugeneck J, Kokott R, Wagner K-H, et al: Nontufted incisional slit grafting. *J Dermatol Surg Oncol* 21:718–723, copyright 1994 by American Society for Dermatologic Surgery, Inc.)

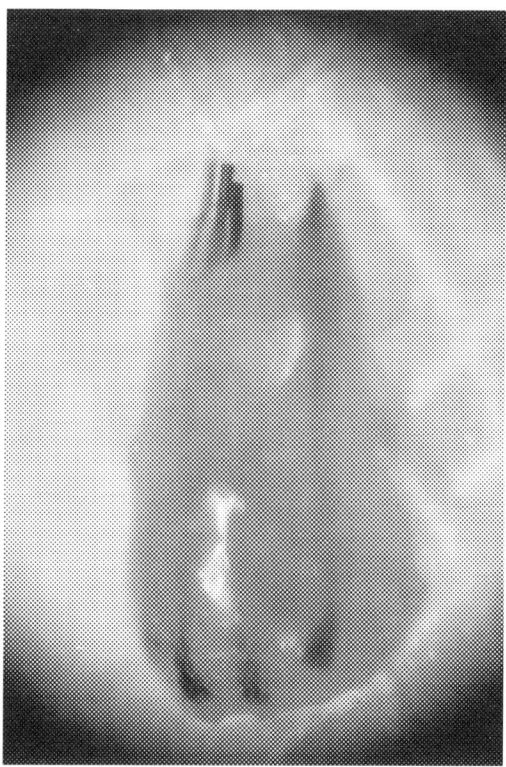

FIGURE 6.—Close-up of a graft where the epidermis is removed. (Reprinted by permission of Elsevier Science, Inc. from Hugeneck J, Kokott R, Wagner K-H, et al: Nontufted incisional slit grafting. *J Dermatol Surg Oncol* 21:718–723, copyright 1994 by American Society for Dermatologic Surgery, Inc.)

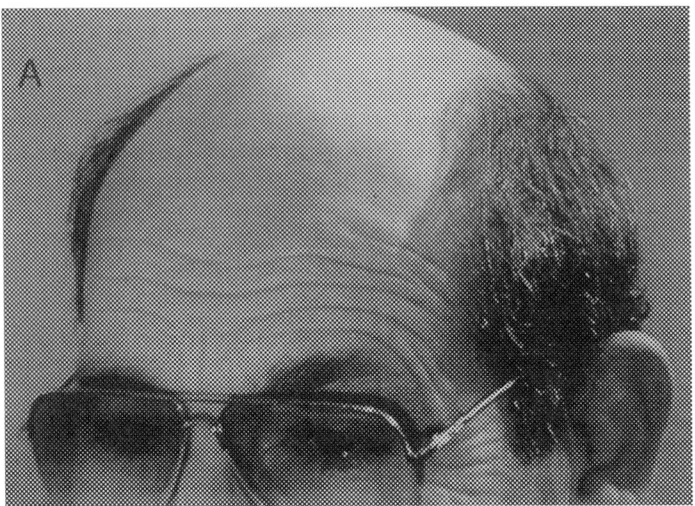

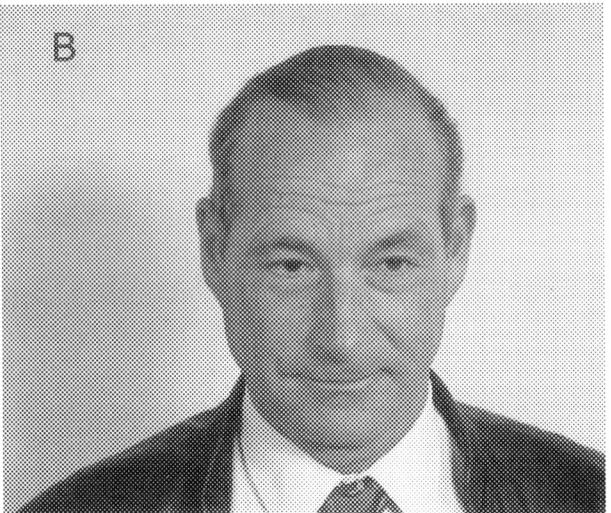

FIGURE 9.—**A,** 55-year-old patient with extensive male pattern baldness. **B,** same patient after 1 session with 1,200 grafts using the nontufted incisional slit graft technique. (Reprinted by permission of Elsevier Science, Inc. from Hugeneck J, Kokott R, Wagner K-H, et al: Nontufted incisional slit grafting. *J Dermatol Surg Oncol* 21:718–723, copyright 1994 by American Society for Dermatologic Surgery, Inc.)

detrimental effect on graft survival. The authors state that in 4 hours they can perform 1,000–1,400 grafts with 4 technicians. They do not tell us how many physicians are involved. Lastly, transplanting Norwood-type 6 patients is very much dependent on their age and with a clear understanding by the patient, inasmuch as male pattern baldness is a continuing process, that they may ultimately lose their grafts over time.

D.J. Papadopoulos, M.D.

Pursuing the Perfect Strip: Harvesting Donor Strips With Minimal Hair Transection

Arnold J (California Med Clinic, San Jose)
Int J Aesthetic Restor Surg 3:148–153, 1995   4–36

Background.—Hair transplantation is simplified by excising donor tissue in long narrow strips. In cutting donor strips, the unintentional transection of hair within the strips must be minimized. A technique designed to avoid accidental damage to the donor hair was described (Table 1).

Technique.—The surgeon decides on a path to cut across the donor area. The hair is then trimmed to a 3-mm length with an electric beard trimmer. The donor area is anesthetized and hemostasis is obtained. The surgeon then injects the maximum amount of tumescent solution along the donor path. The area of tumescence is several millimeters wider than the gang of blades, so that both upper and lower blades will cut through the fully tumid scalp. A subcutaneous injection of the tumescent solution raises the scalp 10 to 15 mm above the skull and larger blood vessels near the skull (Fig 2). The surgeon also injects tumescent solution intradermally to partially erect the hair. The scalp is very firm and blanched with maximum tumescence. The surgeon begins to cut without delay once maximal tumescence is achieved, holding the multiblade knife like a pen (Figs 1 and 3). When the knife penetrates the dermis, the surgeon begins a series of short cutting strokes using finger motions. At the end of each advancing cut, the surgeon pauses to inspect the work and reposition his or her hand for the next

---

TABLE 1.—Key Procedural Elements in Pursuing Perfect Strips

---

1. Trim donor hair no shorter than 3 mm.
2. Ensure good hemostasis with epinephrine in both anesthesia and tumescent solutions.
3. Inject maximal tumescence both subcutaneously and intradermally.
4. Hold the multi-blade knife by the fingers rather than the hand.
5. Advance the knife in short one or two cm cutting strokes generated by the fingers, with the arm and elbow held absolutely stationary.
6. Change the angle of the knife by rotating the wrist to maintain constant alignment with the hair.
7. Before each cutting stroke, visually check for parallel alignment of the knife blade and donor hair.
8. After each cutting stroke, visually examine the cut surface of the strips for signs of transected hairs.

(Courtesy of Arnold J: Pursuing the perfect strip: Harvesting donor strips with minimal hair transection. *Int J Aesthetic Restor Surg* 3:148–153, 1995.)

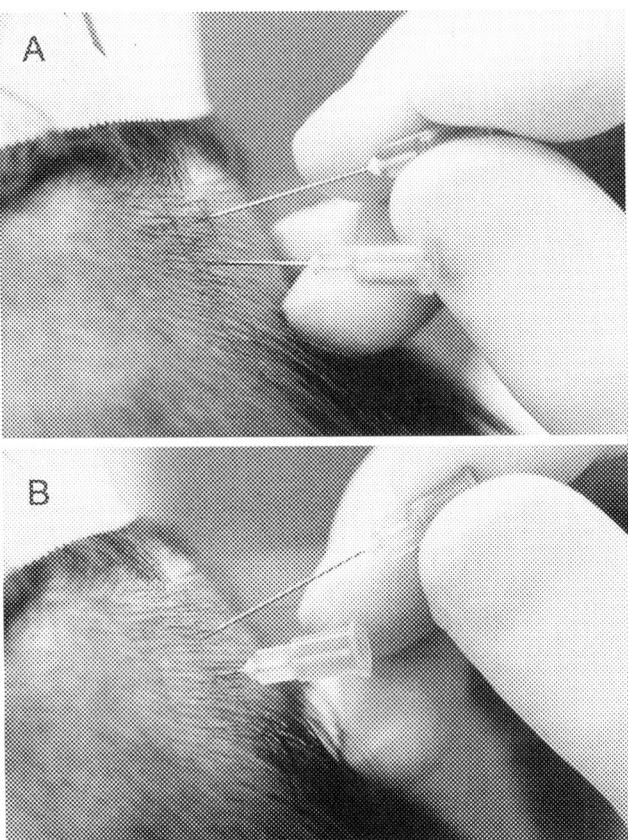

FIGURE 2.—**A**, a 1-inch needle pressed through the scalp to the skull demonstrates the thickness of the scalp prior to tumescence. A second identical needle held above is shown for comparison. **B**, with the subcutaneous tissue and the dermis fully tumid, the scalp is raised 10 to 15 mm. This distance separates the larger blood vessels near the skull from the tips of the knife blades during the cutting process. (Courtesy of Arnold J: Pursuing the perfect strip: Harvesting donor strips with minimal hair transection. *Int J Aesthetic Restor Surg* 3:148–153, 1995.)

advancing cut. This cycle is repeated as many times as necessary until the desired length of donor strips is obtained.

Conclusions.—Cutting perfect strips for hair transplantation is a seemingly impossible task. With careful attention to detail, the technique described will consistently yield donor strips of excellent quality in most patients.

▶ A technique article from an individual who typifies excellent organization, planning, and technique in hair restoration surgery. Required reading for novices who are planning to do strip harvesting.

D.J. Papadopoulos, M.D.

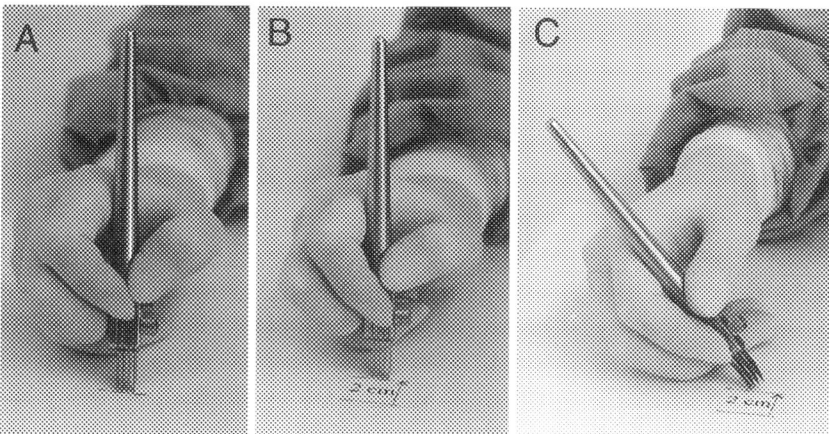

FIGURE 1.—A, the multiblade knife is held by the fingers, similar to holding a pen in an upright position. B, with the hand and arm stationary, the finger alone advances the blades. C, the angle of the knife can be controlled accurately by rotating the wrist. (Courtesy of Arnold J: Pursuing the perfect strip: Harvesting donor strips with minimal hair transection. *Int J Aesthetic Restor Surg* 3:148–153, 1995.)

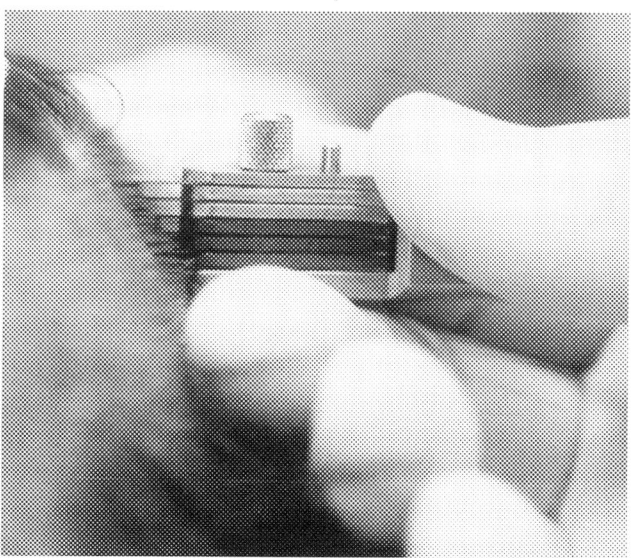

FIGURE 3.—The blades of the knife are aligned parallel with the donor hair. (Courtesy of Arnold J: Pursuing the perfect strip: Harvesting donor strips with minimal hair transection. *Int J Aesthetic Restor Surg* 3:148–153, 1995.)

Practice and Theory of Current Hair Transplantation Techniques: Applications for Hair Transplantation in Females

Cotterill PC (Toronto)
Int J Aesthetic Restor Surg 3:115–118, 1995   4–37

Background.—Current advances in hair transplantation techniques are of benefit to women as well as men. One experience with hair transplantation in 236 women was discussed.

Hair Transplantation in Women.—Physicians must ensure that their patients have realistic expectations in advance about the degree of thickening possible. For example, in 1 patient with diffuse female pattern

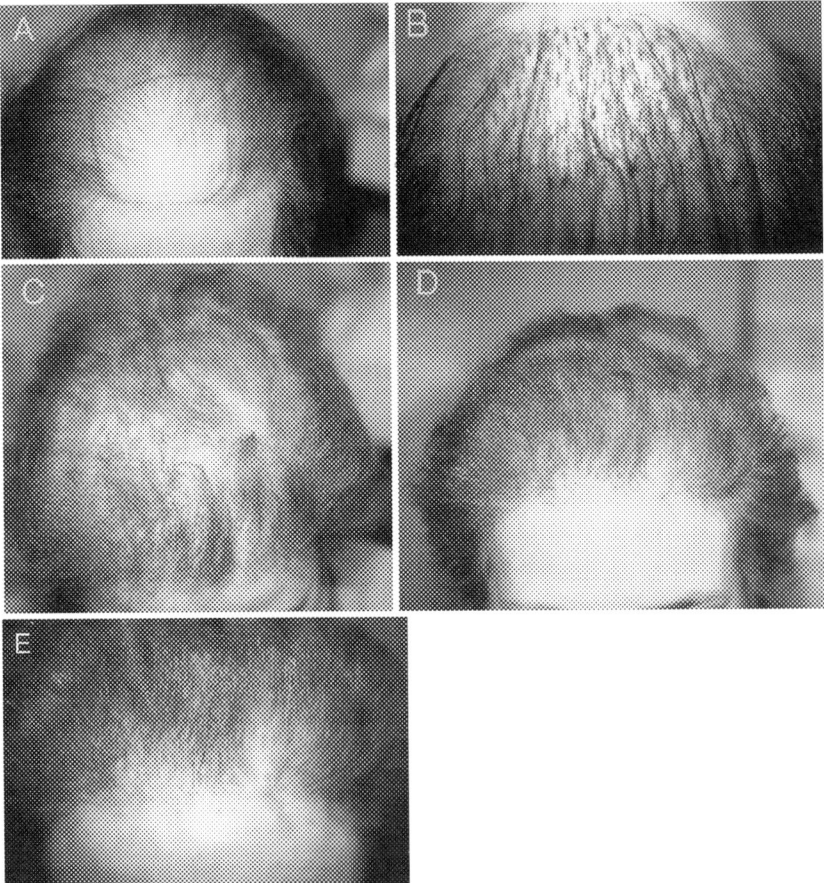

FIGURE 1.—**A**, before first session. Area to be treated outlined with black grease pencil. **B**, intraoperatively. Microsites at hairline, slit sites posterior to microsites, to augment density of existing hair. **C** and **D**, 8 months after 2 sessions. **E**, close up of hairline after 2 sessions. (Courtesy of Cotterill PC: Practice and theory of current hair transplantation techniques: Applications for hair transplantation in females. *Int J Aesthetic Restor Surg* 3:115–118, 1995.)

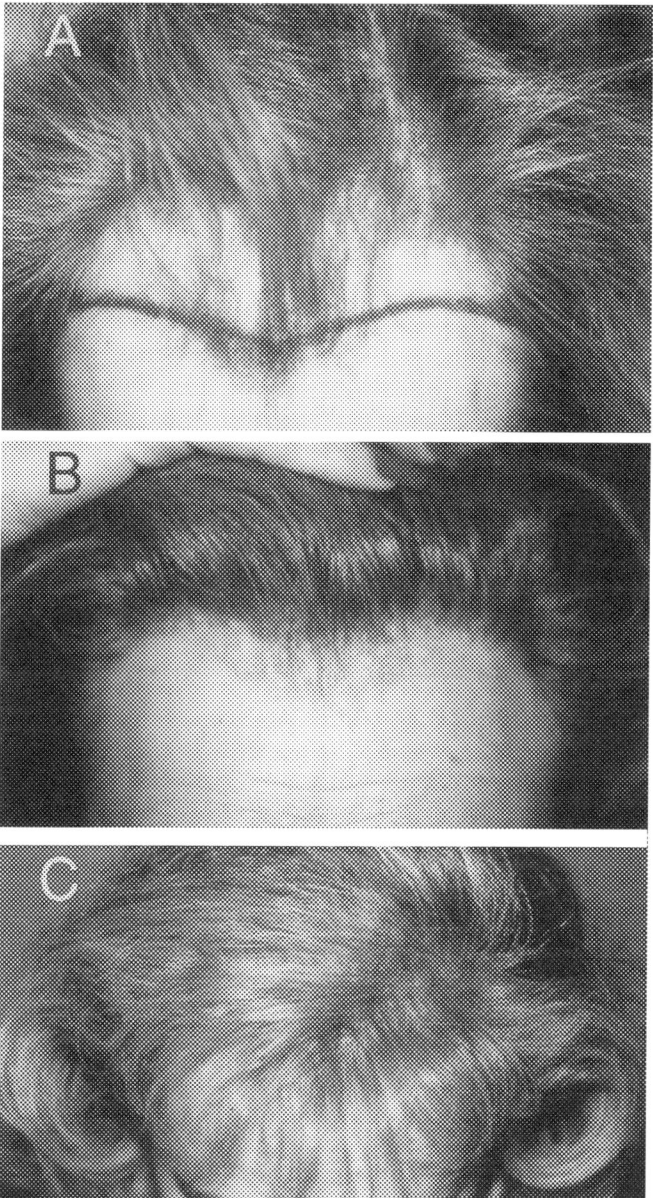

FIGURE 2.—A, before first session. The female pattern hairline is drawn on with black grease pencil to reconstitute a more feminine appearance. Note difference between this and the shape of male pattern hairline. **B,** new hairline after 2 sessions. **C,** hair as normally styled after 2 sessions. (Courtesy of Cotterill PC: Practice and theory of current hair transplantation techniques: Applications for hair transplantation in females. *Int J Aesthetic Restor Surg* 3:115–118, 1995.)

androgenetic alopecia affecting most of the scalp, it was not possible to treat the entire scalp or restore the previous density of the hair. The goal for this patient was to thicken the hair in an area posterior to the frontal hairline so that she would have more hair to style. This goal was achieved using micro and slit grafts, and the patient was very happy with the outcome (Fig 1). In another patient with loss of hair of the frontal temporal recessions and hairline similar to that seen in male pattern androgenetic alopecia, the goal was to create a more feminine, rounded hairline that filled in the temporal area rather than reconstituting a frontal temporal recession (Fig 2). Overall, 30% of the women treated had nonandrogenetic alopecia. The treatment of postrhytidectomy scars and thinning resulting from rhytidectomy can be accomplished in 1 to 3 sessions. When transplanting rhytidectomy scars, grafts will heal and grow well with 4- to 6-month intervals between sessions.

Conclusions.—Many women are now able to enjoy the benefits of added hair. Proper patient evaluation and selection are important, as are realistic expectations of outcomes.

▶ This is a good look at a patient population that is frequently neglected or forgotten by most hair restoration surgeons. Often, after proper evaluation, women are better candidates than men for hair restoration. I agree with the author that women do very well with minigrafts and slits, and because of styling and length advantages, even larger grafts are tolerated well.

D.J. Papadopoulos, M.D.

Laser Hair Transplantation II
Unger WP (Univ of Toronto)
Dermatol Surg 21:759–765, 1995
4–38

Objective.—The outcome of hair transplantation using large numbers of grafts in laser-prepared sites was investigated.

Background.—In 1994, results of studies on the use of ultrapulse CO_2 lasers for hair transplantation showed that hair growth in small grafts placed in laser-prepared sites was more diffuse and natural looking than hair growth in grafts placed in scalpel-prepared slits; hair counts were also higher compared with scalpel-prepared slits. These results could not necessarily be expected from larger numbers of grafts.

Methods.—Grafts were placed only in alopecic areas. When hair growth in a given number of grafts was good after 5 months, the number of study grafts was increased in subsequent patients. Various laser lenses and settings were tried. Direct observation and photographs were used to evaluate results.

Results.—The good results seen with small numbers of grafts were also seen in larger numbers of grafts. Hair dispersion and density were remark-

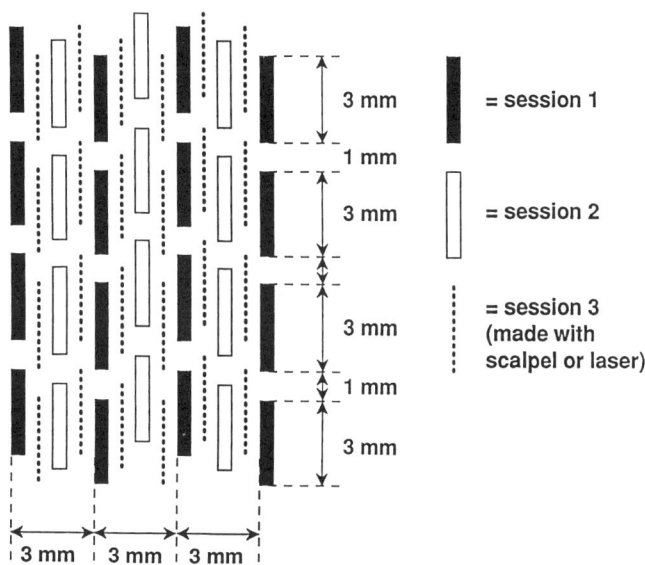

3 mm   ▮ = session 1

1 mm

3 mm   ▯ = session 2

3 mm   ⦙ = session 3
                    (made with
                    scalpel or laser)

1 mm

3 mm

| 3 mm | 3 mm | 3 mm |

FIGURE 5.—Spacing of laser slits. Note that a laser slit produced with a 0.2-mm spot in focus results in a wound that gapes to approximately 0.5 mm. Length of slits shown are 3 mm, but they could be any length that corresponds to the length of the grafts used. Distance between adjacent slits made during the same session is 3 mm. This would allow nearly complete filling of the site in 3 sessions if that were the objective. For the present, scalpel slits are used for the third session to provide a margin of safety to protect adjacent transplanted hair from possible laser thermal damage, and because complete filling in some areas, such as the hairline zone, is often not the objective. (Reprinted by permission of the publisher from Unger WP: Laser hair transplantation II. *Dermatol Surg* 21:759–765, copyright 1995 by Elsevier Science Inc.)

ably natural looking after a single session. There can be a 2- to 6-week longer delay of hair growth in laser-prepared sites compared with conventional grafting.

Discussion.—Certainly, CO_2 lasers may have a role in hair restorative procedures. One disadvantage of this procedure is the longer delay of hair growth compared with conventional grafting. Other advantages and disadvantages are discussed in detail. The benefits of this technique are more evident as hair characteristics become less advantageous for transplantation. A scanner that will soon be available will produce consistent speed and ideal graft spacing and positioning and may eliminate the most serious disadvantages. Placing adjacent laser slits 3 mm apart and either 1 mm anterior or posterior to the neighboring slit made during the same session allows virtual filling of a site in 3 sessions (Fig 5).

▶ The UltraPulse CO_2 laser is a wonderful tool that we have used in our clinic for rhinophyma, acne scars, chickenpox scars, actinic cheilitis, and actinic keratoses. The author here reports on 3 cases in which the UltraPulse CO_2 laser was used to create recipient slits; he compares hair growth in these areas to the opposite control site where cold steel was used. The maximum number of recipients created was 175, with good results obtained. I am currently of the opinion that this tool would not assist me in achieving a superior result within a shorter time frame. We await the scanner and more studies concerning long-term growth, and the evaluation of potential injury of previously placed grafts during latter sessions as a result of thermal spill. This has the potential of being a significant tool in our approach to these particular patients, but clearly much work needs to be done.

D.J. Papadopoulos, M.D.

The Isolated Frontal Forelock

Marritt E, Dzubow L (Univ of Colorado, Denver; Univ of Pennsylvania, Philadelphia)
Dermatol Surg 21:523–538, 1995   4–39

Objective.—An approach to hair restoration that is natural, requires minimal maintenance, enhances appearance, and does not deconstruct with progression of alopecia was described.

Background.—Although the end result of hair restoration should last with time, the effect of time on hair restoration has received little attention. Hair restoration that does not account for the effects of time may deconstruct and result in a very negative aesthetic outcome for the patient. A responsible restorative procedure should be done with hope for the best but must always account for dramatic, progressive loss of hair. The isolated frontal forelock is such a procedure. With limited alopecia progression, the patient will have continuous waves of hair from front to back and side to side. With more dramatic alopecia progression, the patient will have an isolated frontal forelock at the absolute minimum.

Case 1.—Man, 63, with dark brown hair, light skin, and early salt and pepper hair changes underwent transplantation in which the forelock was connected to the superior margin of the fringe. Graft placement into the superior border of the temporal fringe elevated and attached it to the lateral border of the forelock and eliminated the lateral alleys (Fig 3). This was possible because the donor fringe was judged to be stable because of the patient's age, and because a small, predictable amount of donor hair was used to elevate the superior temporal fringe. If this patient had been 20 years younger, grafting of the lateral alleys would not have been attempted.

Case 2.—Man, 50, with excellent hair color, texture, and skin camouflaging combinations, underwent transplantation of the anterior aspect of the forelock (Fig 4) and the upper aspect of the crown/vertex. This allowed the hair to fall downward over the inferior untransplanted lower vertex. All sessions were transplanted with quadrisected 5.0 mm into 2.0 mm. In a patient with

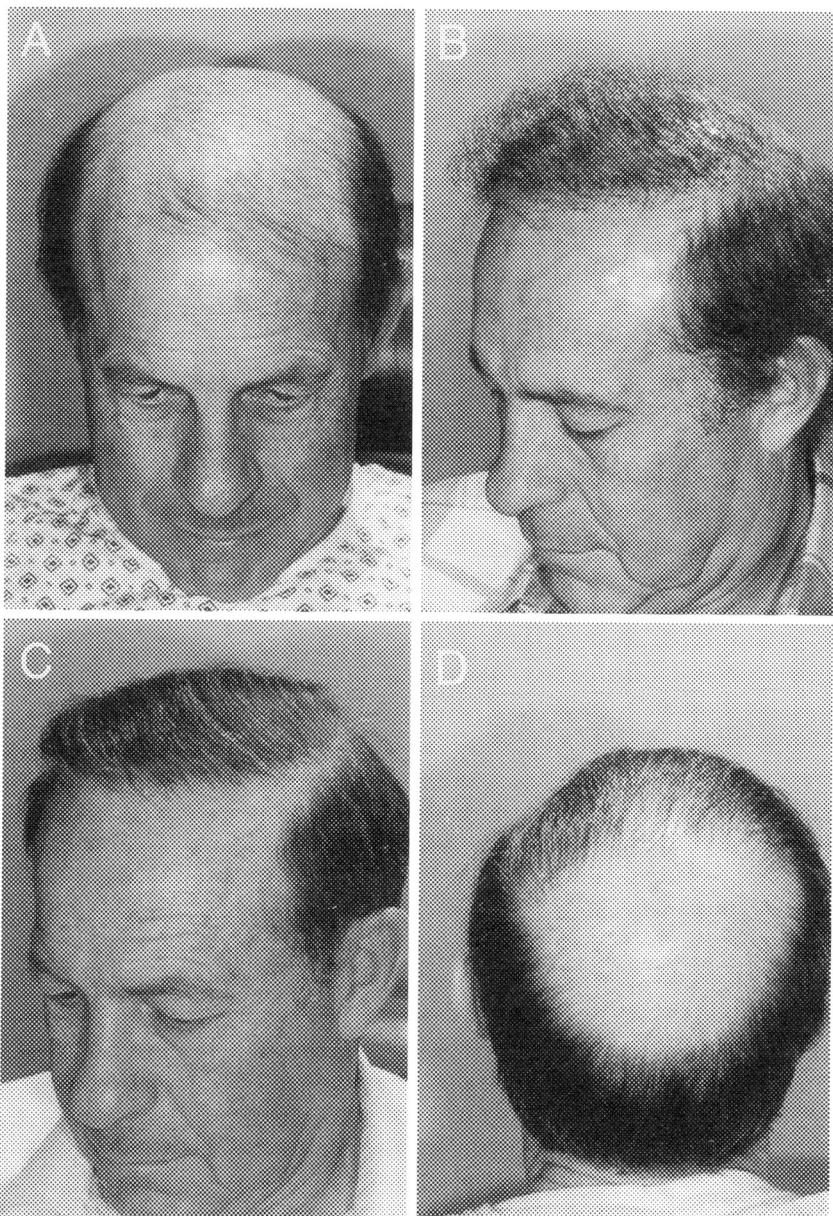

FIGURE 3.—A, preoperative view of case 1, a 63-year-old individual; **B,** graft placement into the superior border of the temporal fringe, elevating it, and attaching it to the lateral border of the forelock, eliminating the lateral alleys; **C,** frontal postoperative view showing density of constructed forelock and connection to temporal fringe; **D,** posterior postoperative view demonstrating remaining bald vertex. (Reprinted by permission of the publisher from Marritt E, Dzubow L: The isolated frontal forelock. *Dermatol Surg* 21:523–538, copyright 1995 by Elsevier Science Inc.)

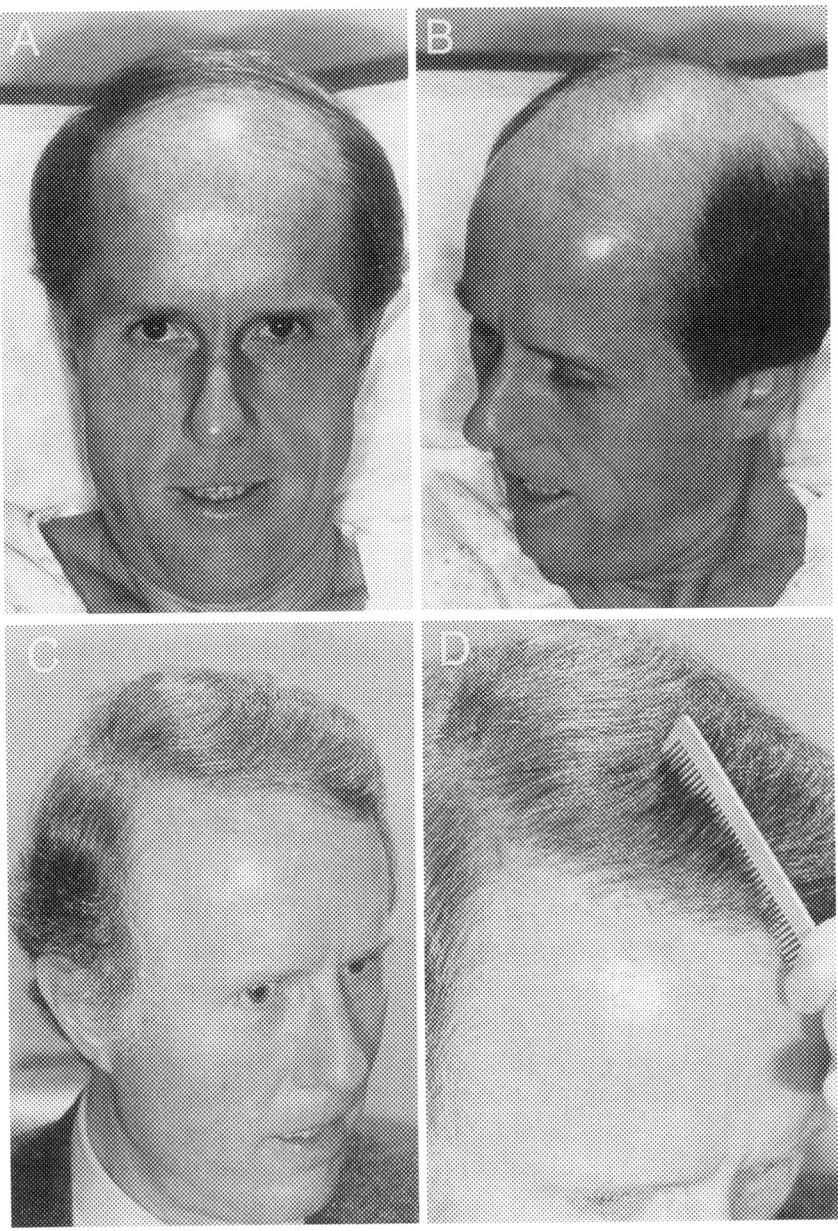

(Continued)

FIGURE 4 (cont.)

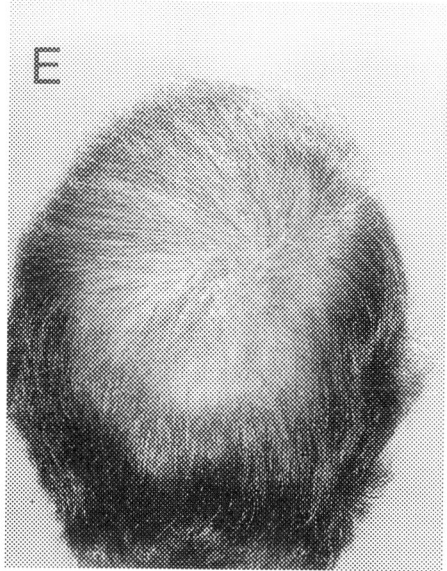

FIGURE 4.—A, preoperative view of case 2, a 50-year-old individual; B, oblique view. Note how this angle reveals a much more accurate and extensive degree of baldness than the frontal view alone; C, postoperative frontal view. No attempt is made to "chase the fringe"; D, close up view of C with hairline exposed for critical examination. Only the serendipitous combination of red hair and ruddy complexion permits such luxuriant frontal density and the added bonus of thinning hair in the crown; E, postoperative view demonstrating the effect of 400 minigrafts transplanted into the vertex. (Reprinted by permission of the publisher from Marritt E, Dzubow L: The isolated frontal forelock. *Dermatol Surg* 21:523–538, copyright 1995 by Elsevier Science Inc.)

the same pattern but who was 10 to 20 years younger, no crown/ vertex transplant would have been done because of possible future hair loss.

Discussion.—The isolated frontal forelock is a viable hair restorative alternative that preserves natural looks and good appearance regardless of the degree of future hair loss. The 5 cases described are alternative approaches to more traditional and aggressive procedures that might fail because of attempting too much with too little. At first consultation, all of these patients believed that baldness was bad and hair was good. Postoperatively, the same patients were reoriented and concluded that looking unnatural or deformed now or years from now is much worse than being bald. Considerations in the design of a reconstructed forelock are discussed in detail.

▶ A truly insightful article for those of us who are advising our patients about what they can expect after hair transplantation. This is a judicious and reasonable approach. It is important for us to advise our patients that their hair loss will continue despite transplanting hair and, as a result, we must convince them that the creation of the frontal forelock is probably a way to anticipate this further hair loss with a "look" that will persist for a long time. Dr. Marritt's article and views concerning hair transplantation and surgery have served me well in the preparation of my patients in terms of what their expectation should be. This article puts us in a position to offer a reasonable solution to some of our patients.

D.J. Papadopoulos, M.D.

Planning for Maximum Coverage in Surgical Hair Restoration
Unger WP (Toronto)
Dermatol Surg 22:161–174, 1996
4–40

Introduction.—Male pattern baldness has a relentless progression; however, not everyone progresses to type VII baldness, and 78% of men do not reach type VI or VII baldness by their 7th decade (Tables 1 and 2). New methods, such as micrografts, minigrafts, and donor area harvesting, have improved results. Generally treatment consists of creating an isolated frontal forelock and concentrating on the anterior third of the scalp or aiming for total coverage. Most physicians tend to recommend concentrating on the anterior third of the scalp, which may be a disservice to many men.

Techniques.—Total excision techniques for the donor area are a new improvement in hair transplanting and involve the excision of a single ellipse or 2 narrow longitudinal zones of donor tissue which are sectioned into grafts. A study of 328 men, 65 years or older, suggested that a permanent donor area is one that contains at least 8 hairs per 4-mm circle and has a height of 70 mm in the occipital area, 80 mm in the parietal area, and 50 mm in the temporal area (Fig 7). Minigrafting is defined as transplanting grafts that contain 1 to 6 hairs each; its main advantage is

TABLE 1.—Incidence of MPB in 1,000 Men by Type and Age

Type	18–29	30–39	40–49	Age (Years) 50–59	60–69	70–79	≥80
I	110 (60%)	60 (36%)	55 (33%)	45 (28%)	29 (19%)	18 (17%)	12 (16%)
II	52 (28%)	43 (26%)	38 (22%)	32 (20%)	24 (16%)	20 (19%)	11 (14%)
III*	14 (6%)	30 (18%)	37 (20%)	34 (23%)	22 (15%)	16 (16%)	12 (16%)
		(3V)	(15V)	(15V)	(10V)	(7V)	(8V)
IV	4 (3%)	16 (10%)	15 (10%)	21 (9%)	17 (12%)	13 (13%)	9 (12%)
V	3 (2%)	10 (6%)	13 (8%)	15 (10%)	22 (15%)	13 (13%)	9 (12%)
VI	2 (1%)	4 (3%)	7 (4%)	10 (7%)	19 (13%)	11 (11%)	10 (13%)
VII	0	2 (1%)	5 (3%)	4 (3%)	16 (10%)	11 (11%)	14 (17%)
Total	185 (100%)	165 (100%)	165 (100%)	156 (100%)	149 (100%)	102 (100%)	77 (100%)

*Numbers in parentheses under type III represent III vertex individuals.
Abbreviation: MPB, male pattern baldness.
(Reprinted with permission from: Hair Transplantation, 3rd ed. Unger W. ed. New York: Marcel Dekker Inc., 1995:42.)
(Reprinted by permission of the publisher from Unger WP: Planning for maximum coverage in surgical hair restoration. *Dermatol Surg* 22:161–174, Copyright 1996 by Elsevier Science Inc.)

TABLE 2.—Age and Degree of MPB

	Age (Years)			
Type	65–69 (%)*	60–74 (%)†	75–79 (%)‡	≥80 (%)§
I	2 (3.6)	5 (6.2)	4 (5.5)	2 (1.7)
II	9 (16.4)	7 (8.6)	7 (9.6)	12 (10.1)
III	4 (7.3)	15 (18.5)	18 (24.7)	11 (9.2)
IV	10 (18.2)	16 (19.8)	8 (11.0)	10 (8.4)
V	6 (10.9)	7 (8.6)	10 (3.7)	16 (13.4)
VI	13 (23.6)	19 (23.5)	16 (21.9)	37 (31.1)
VII	11 (20.0)	12 (14.8)	10 (3.7)	31 (26.1)
Total	55 (100)	81 (100)	73 (100)	119 (100)

*If one excludes types I and III, 33 of remaining 44 (75%) have types III-IV.
†If one excludes types I and II, 57 of remaining 69 (82.6%) have types III-VI.
‡If one excludes types I and II, 52 of remaining 62 (83%) have types III-VI.
§If one excludes types I and II, 74 of remaining 105 (70.5%) have types III-VI.
Abbreviation: MPB, male pattern baldness.
(Reprinted with permission from: Hair Transplantation, 3rd ed. Unger W. ed. New York: Marcel Dekker Inc., 1995:185.)
(Reprinted by permission of the publisher from Unger WP: Planning for maximum coverage in surgical hair restoration. *Dermatol Surg* 22:161–174, Copyright 1996 by Elsevier Science Inc.)

that it minimizes a clumsy unnatural appearance when hair density is low, avoiding the pluggy look. Micrografts are those that contain 1 to 2 hairs and are inserted into needle holes.

Alopecia Reduction.—Objections to this technique are that it causes stretchback, abnormal alteration of hair direction, decreased rim hair den-

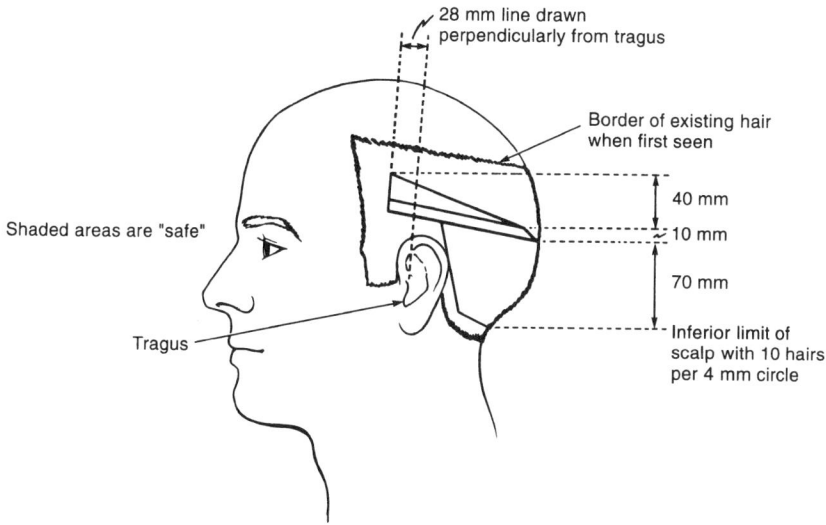

FIGURE 7.—Unger's safe donor site for 80% of patients under the age of 80 years, as determined from a study of 328 men aged 65 years and older. (Reprinted with permission from: Hair Transplantation, 3rd ed. Unger W. ed. New York: Marcel Dekker Inc., 1995:184.) (Reprinted by permission of the publisher from Unger WP: Planning for maximum coverage in surgical hair restoration. *Dermatol Surg* 22:161–174, copyright 1996 by Elsevier Science Inc.)

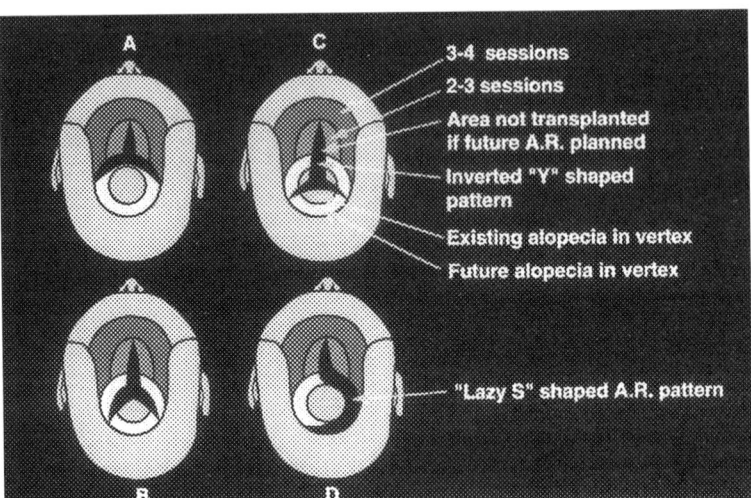

FIGURE 8.—Schematic drawing with general planning of transplanting (hair) density and incorporation of alopecia reduction into planning. (Reprinted with permission from: Hair Transplantation, 3rd ed. Unger W. ed. New York: Marcel Dekker Inc., 1995:112.) (Reprinted by permission of the publisher from Unger WP: Planning for maximum coverage in surgical hair restoration. *Dermatol Surg* 22:161–174, copyright 1996 by Elsevier Science Inc.)

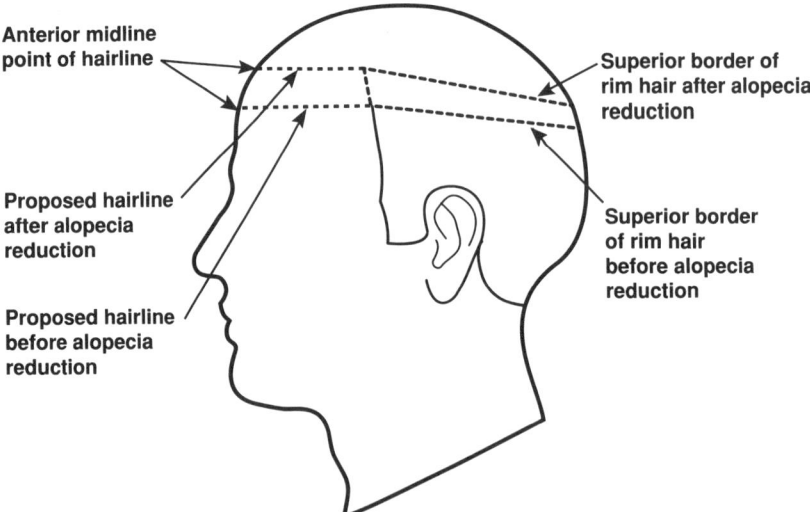

FIGURE 9.—Alopecia reduction raises the anterior-superior points of the temporal area (the starting and end points of the new hairline) so that the most anterior midline point of the hairline can also be placed more superiorly, while still maintaining a hairline that runs more or less parallel to the ground when viewed laterally. (Reprinted with permission from: Hair Transplantation, 3rd ed. Unger W. ed. New York: Marcel Dekker Inc., 1995:113.) (Reprinted by permission of the publisher from Unger WP: Planning for maximum coverage in surgical hair restoration. *Dermatol Surg* 22:161–174, copyright 1996 by Elsevier Science Inc.)

sity, poor scars, and accelerated progression of baldness. Poor scars can be avoided with a "Mercedes" pattern in which the anterior arm can be varied in length to avoid the presence of scars in nontransplanted areas or the "Lazy S" pattern (Fig 8). Advantages of this technique are that it makes the alopecic area smaller, optimizing the donor area ratio; raises the superior border of the rim hair, providing a natural look; eliminates new gaps between transplanted areas; and elevates the anterior- superior-most temporal points, reducing the width and length of baldness to be treated (Fig 9).

Conclusion.—The area of alopecia should not be closed, but reduced to about 5 cm, which would avoid most of the problems caused by altered hair direction and scarring and excessive thinning of rim density. While the debate continues between concentrating on the anterior third of the scalp or the entire scalp, surgeons have many new techniques to consider.

▶ The debate will continue over the recommendation of a frontal forelock to every patient or to total coverage in many patients, as proposed by Dr. Unger in this article. I advise my patients that I would like to create a frontal forelock first to "frame" their face and proceed from there. Whether we can achieve total coverage or not will depend on progression over time. This means that I make it clear that we need to establish a long-term relationship first and that we will go through the journey of hair restoration surgery with a goal of improving and maintaining a desirable look.

D.J. Papadopoulos, M.D.

A Scalp Garment for Prestretching Prior to Alopecia-Reducing Procedures
Brandy DA (Univ of Pittsburgh, Pa)
Dermatol Surg 21:232–234, 1995   4–41

Introduction.—Patients are often asked to perform scalp stretching exercises before scalp reduction surgery related to alopecia. Previous studies have shown that vigorous massaging enhances mechanical creep or progressive elongation of tissue that occurs when one tugs the skin with skin hooks. Biological creep occurs when there is continued stretching beyond maximum mechanical creep, resulting in breakage of collagen fibers. When skin is prestretched over a distance, the force necessary to keep it stretched decreases, resulting in closed wounds that have less tension. A scalp stretching device can improve scalp laxity before such surgery, replacing the need for the vigorous preoperative exercises, which are physically fatiguing.

Methods.—The principle of cyclic loading and biological creep was used in developing the scalp stretching device, which is used for a month before surgery. The device consists of a foam band with 3 Velcro straps and two 6-inch-wide elastic bands with Velcro at each end. Patients applied the

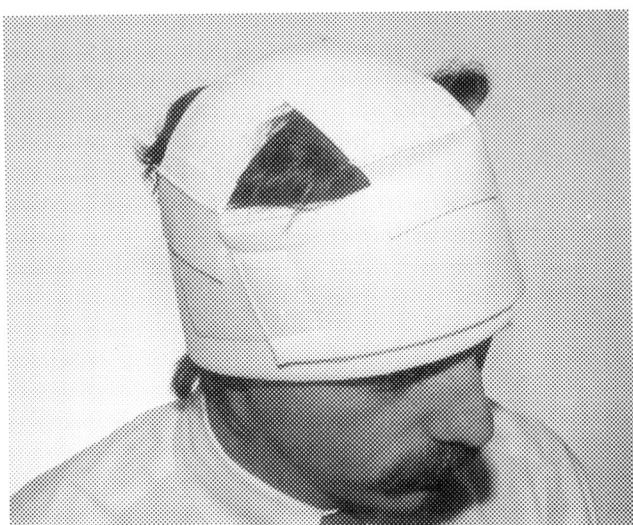

FIGURE 5.—The full garment is applied. Note that the lower border of the garment is just below the ear lobes. Reprinted by permission of the publisher from Brandy DA: A scalp garment for prestretching prior to alopecia-reducing procedures. *Dermatol Surg* 21:232–234, copyright 1995 by Elsevier Science Inc.)

device at home for 30 minutes each day for 30 days before their alopecia-reducing procedure. The garment should be uncomfortable, if properly placed (Fig 5).

Results.—The device is easily used by patients and accomplishes the same amount of laxity in a scalp that prestretching exercises formerly achieved. Patients often became fatigued after performing the previously required vigorous scalp massages, resulting in lower compliance. The new device increases compliance and the amount of alopecia removed.

Conclusion.—Using the scalp stretching device before an alopecia-reducing surgery increases the laxity of the scalp without the need for vigorous massaging. The inexpensive device can be combined with presuturing and other prestretching modalities.

▶ Interesting device for preoperative preparation of the patient about to undergo scalp surgery. I say "scalp surgery" because it could easily be used for preoperative preparation of many scalp excisional procedures in addition to alopecia reduction. Whether it is this device or preoperative massage that one uses is academic at this point in time.

D.J. Papadopoulos, M.D.

Circumferential Scalp Reduction With a Suture-in-Place Silastic-Dacron Extender

Brandy DA (Univ of Pittsburgh, Pa)
Dermatol Surg 22:137–147, 1996

4–42

Introduction.—For those surgeons who want to avoid extensive scalp-lifting, circumferential scalp reduction, defined as minimal stretch-back and decreased slot formation, combined with a suture-in-place Silastic-Dacron extender is a viable alternative. The time interval between surgeries is shortened to 1 month by using the Silastic-Dacron extender. Without the extender, the procedure is normally repeated every 3 months until closure is accomplished with a bitemporal scalp reduction (Fig 2). Scalp mobility is greatly increased with the circumferential incision's deep undermining medial and lateral to the occipital neurovascular bundles (Fig 3).

Methods.—First, a circumferential scalp reduction is performed using the same circumferential excision of extensive scalp-lifting, except that the undermining proceeds to the nuchal ridge rather than the hairline of the nape (Fig 1). This is followed by a tunnel under the central bald peninsula.

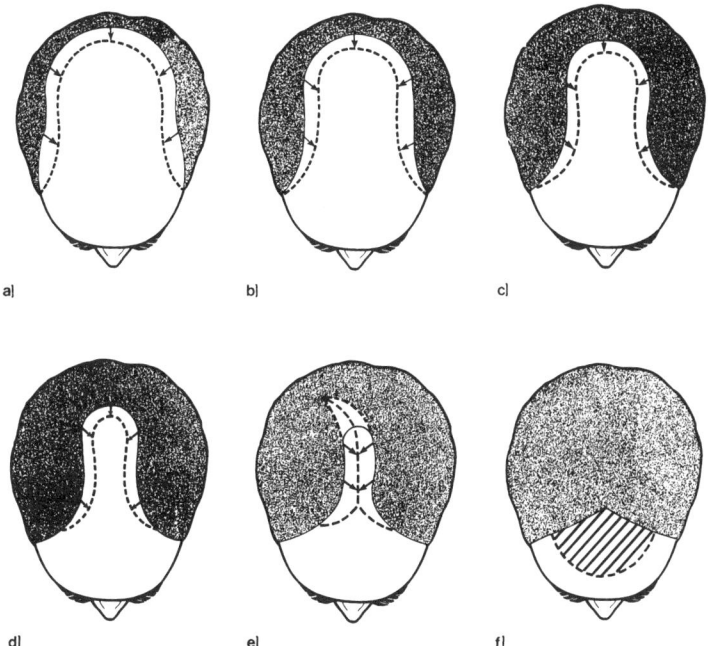

FIGURE 2.—An extensively bald (type 6) patient will usually require 3 to 5 circumferential scalp reductions (when extra maneuvers are not performed) for closure to be accomplished. This procedure is used when nape hair is sparse or the patient wishes to forgo scalp-lifting. (Reprinted by permission of the publisher from Brandy DA: Circumferential scalp reduction with a suture-in-place silastic-dacron extender. *Dermatol Surg* 22:137–147, copyright 1996 by Elsevier Science Inc.)

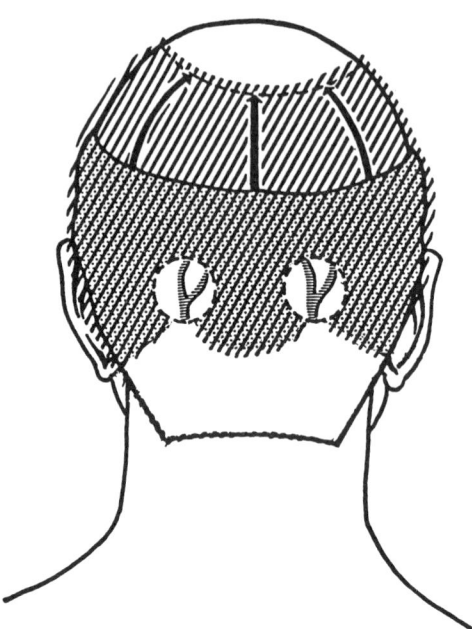

FIGURE 3.—The circumferential incision allows deeper undermining medial and lateral to the occipital neurovascular bundles. This extra undermining significantly increases scalp mobility. (Reprinted by permission of the publisher from Brandy DA: Circumferential scalp reduction with a suture-in-place silastic-dacron extender. *Dermatol Surg* 22:137–147, copyright 1996 by Elsevier Science Inc.)

Through the tunnel, a 4-cm-wide Silastic-Dacron strip is passed and sutured to the lateral edges of the galea under tension (Figs 21 and 25).

Results.—By combining a suture-in-place Silastic-Dacron extender with circumferential scalp reduction, the results are similar to scalp-lifting. However, not as much upward movement into the crown is accomplished and more procedures are required. The Silastic-Dacron extender eliminated stretch-back and improved scalp laxity. Slot formation was prevented by elevating the posterior scalp. Because the incisions are adjacent to hair, they are easier to camouflage after surgery. More bald skin can be removed because the surgeon has greater visibility in cutting the occipitalis and postauricular muscles. Small insignificant seromas have been observed, and 1 large seroma resulted in 1 patient out of more than 100.

Conclusion.—Patients with extensive baldness can benefit from suture-in-place Silastic-Dacron extender used in combination with circumferential scalp reduction. Slot formation is decreased and stretch-back is virtually eliminated. The time interval between surgeries is shorted to a month. During the early stage of the learning curve, the strip is a little difficult to suture. A circumferential scalp reduction is slightly more difficult than a midline scalp reduction.

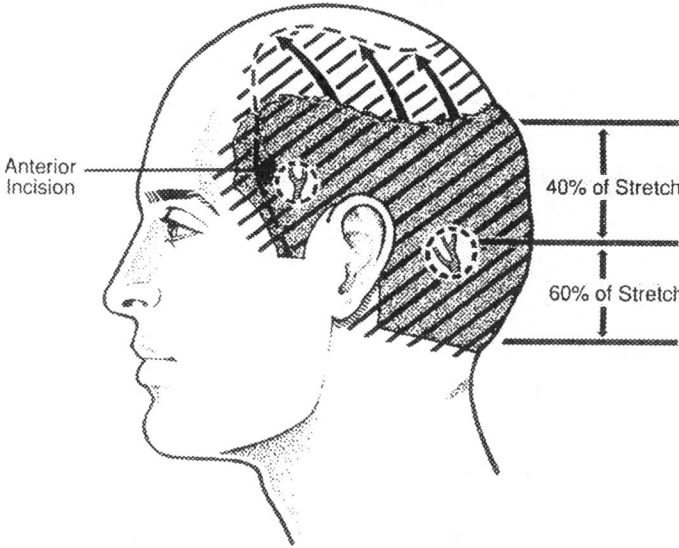

FIGURE 1.—The extra undermining of extensive scalp-lifting gives 60% added stretch when compared with undermining to the nuchal ridge. (Reprinted by permission of the publisher from Brandy DA: Circumferential scalp reduction with a suture-in-place silastic-dacron extender. *Dermatol Surg* 22:137–147, copyright 1996 by Elsevier Science Inc.)

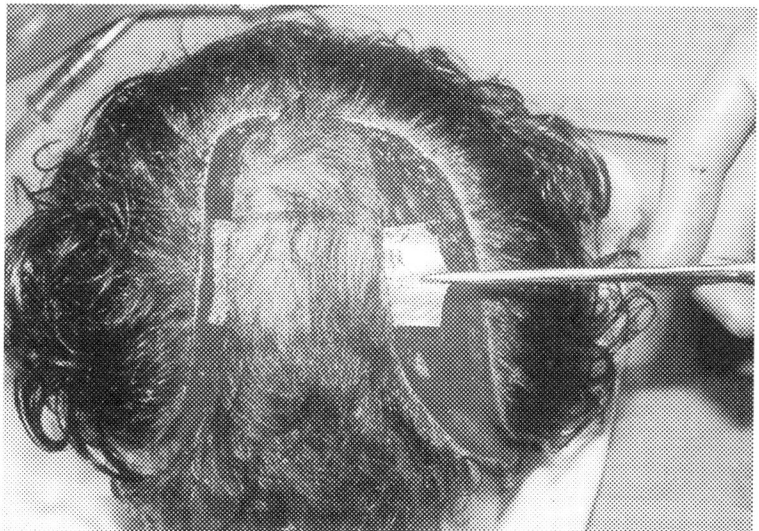

FIGURE 21.—After suturing the Silastic-Dacron extender to the right galeal edge with 2 O-PDS II sutures, the Silastic-Dacron strip is stretched through the preformed tunnel so that the opposite galeal surface is reached. (Reprinted by permission of the publisher from Brandy DA: Circumferential scalp reduction with a suture-in-place silastic-dacron extender. *Dermatol Surg* 22:137–147, copyright 1996 by Elsevier Science Inc.)

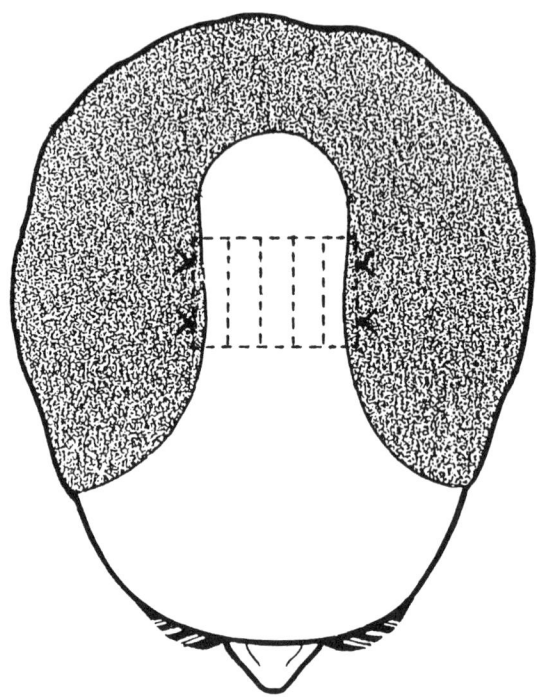

FIGURE 25.—Schematic demonstrating the final result. A Silastic-Dacron extender on tension under the central bald peninsula. (Reprinted by permission of the publisher from Brandy DA: Circumferential scalp reduction with a suture-in-place silastic-dacron extender. *Dermatol Surg* 22:137–147, copyright 1996 by Elsevier Science Inc.)

▶ Required reading for those who use extenders and who perform extensive scalp reduction/scalp lifting procedures. The area of the occipital neurovascular bundle is "tiger country," i.e., if you cut it, check your pulse and think about calling your spiritual counselor. Nevertheless, this is impressive and yields remarkable results. Dr. Brandy is to be commended, not only for this work, but for the body of work that he has contributed to the field of hair restoration surgery.

D.J. Papadopoulos, M.D.

The Burow's Triangle Scalp Reduction: A New and Improved Technique for Paramedian Scalp Reduction
Cohen BH (Univ of Miami, Fla)
Dermatol Surg 21:705–710, 1995   4–43

Introduction.—Compared with the median, or midline-sagittal, incision for scalp reduction, the paramedian incision offers some important advantages. Among other benefits, it can be used before or after frontal hairline transplantation, it offers greater overall length, and it elevates the midline posterior hair-bearing fringe. The author has developed a modified technique of paramedian incision that further extends these advntages. The new technique—called Burow's triangle scalp reduction because the tissue movement is like that of a Burow's triangle advancement flap—was described, including an experience with 20 patients.

> *Technique.*—The new technique consists of a bilateral paramedian design. The surgical design is a 3-limbed, Z-shaped incision with two, 90-degree angles. Anterior and posterior paramedian incisions are made along either side of the hairless scalp. These 2 incisions are then joined by a straight, transcoronal incision. The incision can be tailored to the individual patient, depending on the extent of alopecia and on whether a frontal hairline has been or will be created (Figs 1–3). Wide subgaleal undermining is per-

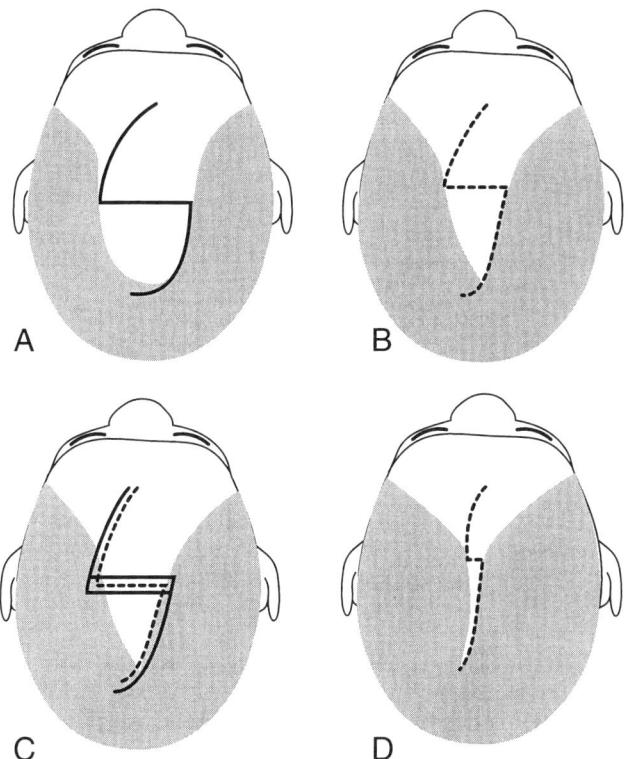

FIGURE 1.—(A) Suggested design for patients with extensive alopecia in whom a frontal hairline will be created. Final scar extends into area to be transplanted. (IU indicates incision; *dotted line* indicates scar.) (B) Scar after first procedure. (C) Suggested design for second procedure. Note that incision is placed lateral to the paramedian scars. The transcoronal scar is excised. (D) Scar after second procedure. (Reprinted by permission of the publisher from Cohen BH: The Burow's triangle scalp reduction: A new and improved technique for paramedian scalp reduction. *Dermatol Surg* 21:705–710, copyright 1995 by Elsevier Science Inc.)

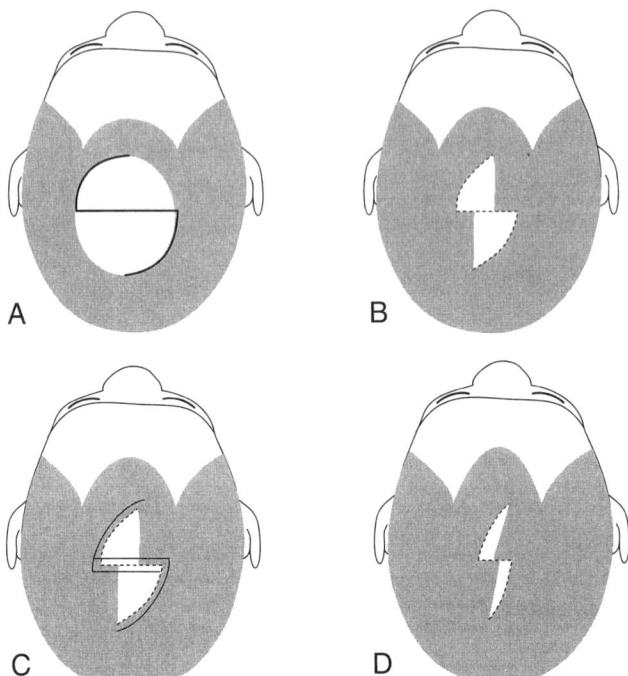

FIGURE 2.—(A) Suggested design for patients with extensive alopecia in whom a frontal hairline exists or has been created. (B) Scar after first procedure. Two triangular areas of alopecia result. The width of the frontal hairline is narrowed and bowed. (C) Suggested design for second procedure. Note that incision is placed lateral to the paramedian scars. The transcoronal scar is excised. (D) Scar after second procedure. The width of the frontal hairline is further narrowed and bowed. (Reprinted by permission of the publisher from Cohen BH: The Burow's triangle scalp reduction: A new and improved technique for paramedian scalp reduction. *Dermatol Surg* 21:705–710, copyright 1995 by Elsevier Science Inc.)

formed to raise 2 triangular flaps, which are then reflected back on their hinges. The flaps are firmly tensioned in opposite directions with towel clamps so that they pass each other along the central limb. Two Burow's triangles are excised, and the incisions are sutured closed. If a second procedure is indicated, the incision can be made lateral to the anterior and posterior limb scars.

Results.—The Burow's triangle scalp reduction has been used in 20 patients with male pattern alopecia. This technique maximized visual access with better tissue mobilization and easy handling. The scars showed little widening, because the direction of the tension-bearing vector was parallel to the transcoronal incision. No corrective procedures were needed, because no posterior "slots" or "troughs" were created. As calculated by the reduction in length of the central limb, 3 to 7 cm of tissue was excised. The posterior fringe was elevated by 2 to 3 cm. There were no surgical complications, including tip necrosis or flap loss.

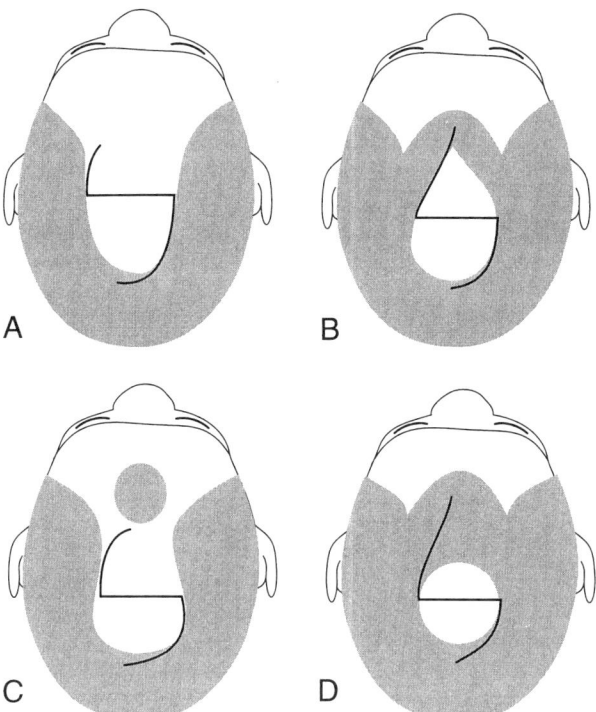

FIGURE 3.—(A) Suggested design for patients with extensive alopecia in whom a frontal hairline might be delayed. Final scar does not extend into frontal area (see Figure 1 for alternative design). (B–D) Suggested designs for patients with partial alopecia. (Reprinted by permission of the publisher from Cohen BH: The Burow's triangle scalp reduction: A new and improved technique for paramedian scalp reduction. *Dermatol Surg* 21:705–710, copyright 1995 by Elsevier Science Inc.)

Conclusions.—The Burow's triangle scalp reduction offers some important advantages for paramedian scalp reduction. The bilateral paramedian design offers a fine-scar, easier tissue handling, creation of a nonvertical posterior scar, elevation of the posterior hair-bearing fringe, and creation of a broken-line rather than a straight-line scar.

▶ A nice technique to include in our armamentarium during hair restoration surgery. This is a simple flap with instant results that can be performed in a number of situations. Long-term results will give us a clue as to how much stretch-back occurs. Nevertheless, this is simple and effective.

D.J. Papadopoulos, M.D.

Scalp Flaps in the Treatment of Baldness: Long-Term Results

Epstein JS, Kabaker SS (Univ of Miami, Fla; Univ of California, San Francisco)
Dermatol Surg 22:45–50, 1996   4–44

Introduction.—Scalp flaps have been used for managing androgenic or male pattern baldness for over 20 years. The two most common flaps are the temporoparieto-occipital (TPO) flap, which creates an entire frontal hairline and preserves a second flap to treat alopecic scalp posteriorly (Fig 1), and the shorter temporoparietal flap, which is not as useful for more extensive baldness. More than 300 procedures using these flaps in treating male pattern baldness are reviewed.

Surgical Procedure.—The proximal one-third of the TPO flap is 30 mm in width and incorporates the superficial temporal artery, while the distal two thirds, measuring 35-40 mm in width, creates the frontal hairline. One point of the flap edge is 4 cm cephalad to the anterior aspect of the helix and the other is within the hairline, 4 cm distal to the first point (Fig 2). The TOP flap is twice delayed with a 1-week interval. The third step, in 2 weeks, is to rotate the flap. The temporoparietal flap is shorter and narrower.

Results.—There were 255 TOP flaps performed and 59 temporoparietal flaps performed over a 20-year period. A review was conducted of 20 patients with 31 flaps who had scalp flap surgery 10 or more years ago. The most common indication for secondary procedures was progressive hair loss behind the flap. Other procedures were donor site scar revisions and frontal micrografting. Most patients were unavailable for follow-up, and it is probable that most had no problems. With the exception of 3 patients, the flaps maintained the initially obtained coverage. The most frequent complication was donor-site scarring. Although the shorter flaps

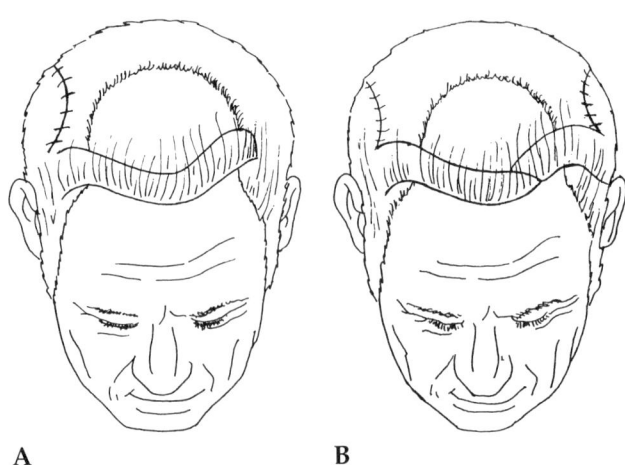

A   **B**

FIGURE 1.—Scalp flaps for frontal hairline restoration. **A**, single temporoparieto-occipital flap; **B**, two temporoparietal flaps. (Reprinted by permission of the publisher from Epstein JS, Kabaker SS: Scalp flaps in the treatment of baldness: Long-term results. *Dermatol Surg* 22:45–50, copyright 1996 by Elsevier Science Inc.)

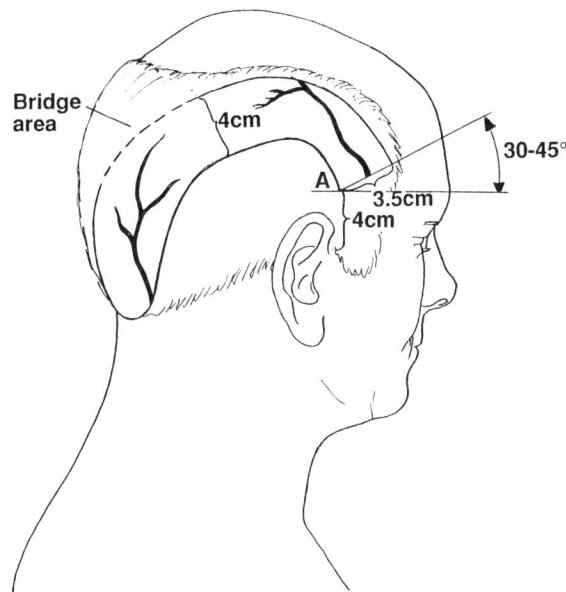

FIGURE 2.—Design of temporoparieto-occipital flap. Dotted bridge area is site of second delay. (Reprinted by permission of the publisher from Epstein JS, Kabaker SS: Scalp flaps in the treatment of baldness: Long-term results. *Dermatol Surg* 22:45–50, copyright 1996 by Elsevier Science Inc.)

are as technically demanding as the longer flaps, their yield is significantly less. One hundred percent of the population had further hair loss, the extent of which varied among patients.

Conclusion.—In the management of male pattern baldness, scalp flaps have a proven role, providing a dense hairline in a short period of time.

▶ As with any technique used for hair restoration surgery, this one is largely based on appropriate patient selection and informing the patient about long-term results. This article, although limited in its scope and by the non-consecutive nature of patient presentation, gives us a glimpse at what can be expected in selected patients over a longer period of time.

D.J. Papadopoulos, M.D.

The Feasibility of Targeted Selective Gene Therapy of the Hair Follicle
Li L, Hoffman RM (AntiCancer Inc, San Diego, Calif)
Nature Med 1:705–706, 1995
4–45

Background.—Hair loss from aging or chemotherapy is distressing. Treatment of the hair follicle involves the selective targeting of specific cells of the hair follicle. The authors have developed the histoculture of intact hair-growing skin on sponge-gel matrices, recently demonstrating that liposomes in histocultured skin can selectively target hair follicles to deliver small and large molecules. The method of entrapping DNA in liposomes for use in gene therapy was introduced 20 years ago. The selective targeting of the *lacZ* reporter gene into mouse hair follicles after topical application of the gene entrapped in liposomes was described.

Methods and Findings.—Liposome-*lacZ* was applied topically to pre-shaved 5- to 6-week-old BALB/c mice. Blue staining of the X-gal substrate indicated *lacZ* expression in the hair-forming hair matrix cells in the hair follicle bulbs and bulge area below the opening of the sebaceous gland, which is believed to contain the follicle stem cells. The transfection frequency was high. There were no other cells transfected with *lacZ* outside the follicle in the dermis or epidermis. Expression of *lacZ* in the hair matrix cells was extensive. There was also evidence of transfection of what may be follicle stem cells. Gene transfer did not occur with the topical application of the naked *lacZ* gene. Mice not treated with liposome-*lacZ* showed no *lacZ* staining.

Conclusions.—Genes can be targeted selectively to the most important cells of the hair follicle. The selectivity of gene targeting by topical liposome application suggests that targeting hair matrix cells and possibly follicle stem cells to restore hair color are feasible by delivery and expression of the tyrosinase gene and with genes to restore hair growth.

▶ This is very exciting work and we all look forward to that day when we may deliver compounds of specific capabilities to matrix or stem cell regions of the hair follicles. What also might be of future significance is our ability to deliver molecules at these specific sites that would assist us in the clonal proliferation of the donor area used in hair transplantation.

D.J. Papadopoulos, M.D.

Improvement in Androgenetic Alopecia (Stage V) Using Topical Minoxidil in a Retinoid Vehicle and Oral Finasteride
Walsh DS, Dunn CL, James WD, et al (Walter Reed Army Med Ctr, Washington, DC)
Arch Dermatol 131:1373–1375, 1995   4–46

Introduction.—The only therapy currently approved by the U.S. Food and Drug Administration is for the treatment of androgenetic alopecia, topical minoxidil. The combination of minoxidil and oral 5α-reductase inhibitor finasteride has been shown to be more effective in preventing progression and onset of alopecia than either agent used alone.

> *Case Study.*—Male, 32 years of age, with frontoparietal and vertex balding at stage V came for therapy. He wanted only medical treatment, or hair regrowth without surgery. He participated in a 6- to 12-month trial of topical minoxidil in an optimized retinoid vehicle applied twice per day and 5 mg of finasteride taken orally each day. The topical solution consisted of minoxidil tablets dis-

solved in distilled water, polyethylene glycol, and absolute ethanol in a concentration of 3.75% grams per deciliter and combined with 0.05% tretinoin for a final concentration of 3% minoxidil and 0.01% tretinoin. Each application consisted of 1 mL of solution applied to the scalp gently.

Results.—After 3 months of therapy, increased terminal hair growth on the scalp was seen, particularly over the crown and vertex. After 5 months of therapy, marked improvement was seen in the crown and vertex. After 8 months, growth in the extreme frontal area was seen and more growth continued in the crown, vertex, and parietal areas. The patient stopped taking oral finasteride after 8 months, but continued topical therapy with minoxidil and tretinoin for 4 months with continued gradual improvement. In 12 months, his baldness status improved from stage V to stage III.

Discussion.—Minoxidil alone usually results in a response in the area of the vertex. A combination of topical minoxidil and tretinoin and oral finasteride resulted in an effective combination therapy and should be considered for those patients with mild to moderate androgenetic alopecia. Finasteride results in untoward effects in fewer than 5% of patients, usually relating to impotence and decreased libido, but there is concern that this drug could mask the detection of prostate cancer.

▶ Very impressive results for this simple regimen. I would be interested in knowing what the effect of this regimen would be on postmenopausal women and on older male hair transplant recipients.

D.J. Papadopoulos, M.D.

Sclerotherapy

Guidelines of Care for Sclerotherapy Treatment of Varicose and Telangiectatic Leg Veins
Drake LA, Dinehart SM, Goltz RW, et al (Academy of Dermatology, Schaumburg, Ill)
J Am Acad Dermatol 34:523–528, 1996   4–47

Introduction.—Guidelines for sclerotherapy treatment of varicose and telangiectatic leg veins address the quality of dermatologic care and discuss its scope, providing additional information to facilitate the understanding of those outside the profession.

Scope.—Sclerotherapy involves the injection of aqueous solutions into varicose veins. The resulting damage to the endothelial lining causes the vein to be absorbed into the surrounding tissue relieving the itching, throbbing, swelling, cramping, aching, fatigue, and lancinating pain experienced by many patients. Patients with large varicose veins have a higher risk of thrombophlebitis, deep vein thrombosis (DVT), lipodermatosclerosis, and venous ulceration.

Issue.—Physician qualifications include training and experience in sclerotherapy, a residency or board certification, and a knowledge of the anatomy and physiology of the venous system. The physician should understand how sclerosing agents act, the proper use of compression bandages and stockings, and the relation of DVT to other diseases and coagulopathies.

Diagnostic Criteria.—Patient information should include a history, a physical examination, tests of venous insufficiency, and notation of any special historic conditions such as infections, diabetes, anaphylaxis, severe asthma, use of medications that may affect clotting, allergies, inability to walk, and other risk factors associated with venous disease. Instrumental and laboratory tests should be performed as necessary.

Treatment.—Patients who are not candidates for sclerotherapy may best be treated symptomatically. Several solutions and techniques are available for treating veins depending on whether the veins are truncal, perforating, communicating/side branch, reticular, venulectases, or telangiectases. Perivascular cutaneous pigmentation, edema, flare of new telangiectasia, injection pain, urticaria, blisters, folliculitis, recurrence, and vasovagal reaction are common. Extensive cutaneous necrosis, systemic allergic reactions, superficial thrombophlebitis, distal necrosis, DVT, pulmonary emboli, nerve damage, compartmental syndrome, localized hypertrichosis, and punctate ulceration occur rarely. Medications currently being developed may decrease venular inflammation and stabilize the vein wall.

Conclusion.—These guidelines are not comprehensive, and final decisions must be made by the physician.

▶ I would encourage all inspiring sclerotherapists to take a good look at these guidelines, and to consider establishing a database concerning this topic before they begin performing this procedure. In the sclerotherapist world, there are "squirters" and there are true sclerotherapists, depending on whether the practitioner has taken the time to study the many fundamentals involved in performing this treatment regimen. In addition, preceptorship with experienced and knowledgeable colleagues is invaluable. In my own case, I owe much to Dr. Helane Fronig of the Scripps Clinic and Research Foundation and Dr. Robert Weiss of Baltimore, Maryland, who through the gifts of their time and expertise began my career in this interesting field. Clearly, this is an area where we, as dermatologists, have played and will continue to play a pivotal role for many years to come.

D.J. Papadopoulos, M.D.

Biochemical Assay of Collagen and Elastin in the Normal and Varicose Vein Wall

Venturi M, Bonavina L, Annoni F, et al (Univ of Milan, Italy; "Marigo Negri" Inst for Pharmacological Research, Milan, Italy)
J Surg Res 60:245–248, 1996   4–48

Objective.—Although alteration in collagen and elastin fibers has been found in the walls of varicose veins, the cause of the condition is not known. Because studies have shown conflicting results for both collagen and elastin content in veins, the concentrations of the collagen marker 4-L-hydroxyproline (HYP) and the elastin markers desmosine (DES) and isodesmosine (IDES) in normal and varicose, dilated and nondilated, veins were measured to find an explanation for the development of varices.

Methods.—The concentrations of HYP, DES, and IDES were determined colorimetrically in 47 dilated and 32 nondilated varicose vein segments of 20 saphenous veins obtained from 20 patients (5 males) and were compared by analysis of variance testing with 24 segments removed from 14 control patients who were undergoing graft procedures.

Results.—Valvular incompetence was found in 18 patients and in none of the controls. Dilated segments had significantly less DES and IDES than did nondilated and normal segments. Whereas collagen content was similar in normal and varicose veins, elastin content was significantly lower in dilated segments compared with normal and nondilated veins. The ratio of elastin to collagen was significantly lower in dilated segments than in normal or nondilated veins.

Conclusion.—Reduced synthesis or increased catabolism of elastin may be responsible for dilation of the vein wall. Additional studies of vein-wall smooth muscle cell metabolism should be done.

▶ This study tries to shed some light on the collagen and elastin differences in varicose and normal vein walls in the hope that it can dispel the notion that valvular incompetence is the first and most important aspect in the pathogenesis of varicose veins. This is a "which came first, the chicken or the egg" question that has been most perplexing to the phlebology community. The findings presented by the authors are interesting, but greater numbers are needed to extrapolate more information. Furthermore, having a clearer view of the biochemical makeup, in terms of collagen and elastin, of the valves themselves at different periods of time in the life of affected and disease-free individuals would be interesting and important for us.

D.J. Papadopoulos, M.D.

Symptomatology of Vein Disease

Isaacs MN (Walnut Creek, Calif)

Dermatol Surg 21:321–323, 1995   4–49

Background.—Although previous studies have shown that dilated leg veins are symptomatic, whether symptoms exist that are specific for vein disease and whether vein size alone can predict symptoms are unclear. A retrospective study evaluated the extent to which vein disease is symptomatic, which symptoms are specific for vein disease, and whether vein size alone is predictive of symptoms.

Patients and Methods.—The medical records of 289 patients were reviewed, with patients categorized as having either primarily large-vein or small-vein disease (LVD and SVD, respectively). All patients had completed a questionnaire designed to determine the presence of symptoms typically associated with leg-vein disease, such as aching/pain, heaviness, tiredness/fatigue, itching/burning, swollen ankles, leg cramps, restless legs, throbbing, and other signs. Responses were reviewed retrospectively and were compared with those obtained from age- and gender-matched controls, all of whom had completed the same symptom questionnaire and all of whom reportedly were free of vein disease.

Results.—Two-hundred four patients fulfilled the study criteria, including 123 with SVD and 81 with LVD. The control group comprised 54 individuals. Patients with any form of vein disease (SVD and LVD groups combined) had significantly more symptoms compared with controls (3.2 versus 1.6, respectively). Correlations between SVD and the combination of SVD/LVD and certain symptoms including aching/pain, extreme tiredness/fatigue, itching/burning, throbbing, and ankle swelling, were noted (Table 1). The presence of symptoms was not predicted by vein size alone.

Conclusions.—The presence of specific complaints in patients with leg symptoms suggests that vein disease is the likely causative factor, regardless of vein size. A trial of graduated compression hose or rigid compres-

TABLE 1.—Symptoms of SVD and LVD

	Controls	SVD	LVD
Mean age	41.1	43.2	45.0
F/M ratio	1.1	122/1	2.5/1
No. of subjects	54	123	81
Aching/pain	14(26%)	77(63%)	60(74%)
Heaviness	8(15%)	35(29%)	35(43%)
Tired/fatigue	14(26%)	64(52%)	45(56%)
Itching/burning	8(15%)	36(29%)	36(44%)
Ankle swelling	4(7%)	23(19%)	28(35%)
Leg cramps	15(28%)	48(39%)	28(35%)
Restless legs	8(15%)	37(30%)	28(35%)
Throbbing	3(6%)	35(29%)	32(40%)
Other	3(6%)	2(2%)	1(1%)
Mean no. of Sx's	1.43	2.90	3.62

(Reprinted by permission of the publisher from Isaacs MN: Symptomatology of vein disease. *Dermatol Surg* 21:321–323, copyright 1995 by Elsevier Science Inc.)

sion should aid in establishing a cause-and-effect relationship, with rapid and distinct symptom alleviation serving to verify a venous cause.

▶ We need more articles like this that will hopefully give us some ammunition in making sclerotherapy an accepted noncosmetic treatment of venous varicosities in smaller vessels. I personally continue to be amazed at the fact that a great number of my patients' first realization after a single treatment is that they have significantly less pain and discomfort. Unfortunately, because of increasing numbers of denials by insurance companies, we have resorted to making our patients aware that the sclerotherapy at our institution is a discretionary service that must be paid for at the time of treatment. We send supporting letters to the patients who can then pass them along to their insurance companies. Despite this, we continue to fight for the patient's right to receive this treatment with our local insurance carriers. Through articles like this and through national unified participation and mutual support, we can hopefully induce insurers to fulfill their obligations of coverage.

D.J. Papadopoulos, M.D.

The Effect of Sclerotherapy on Restless Legs Syndrome
Kanter AH (Vein Center of Orange County, Irvine, Calif)
Dermatol Surg 21:328–332, 1995   4–50

Introduction.—Restless leg syndrome (RLS) is a chronic, familial, predominantly female condition of unknown cause that occurs in about 5% to 29% of the American population. The relentless leg discomfort of this disorder compels voluntary leg movement for temporary relief. Patients who have received sclerotherapy for treatment of venous disease have reported subsequent relief of RLS symptoms. The concomitant occurrence of RLS and varicose veins was prospectively investigated in patients with and without saphenous trunk reflux seeking treatment of varicose veins. The therapeutic response of RLS to sclerotherapy was also observed.

Methods.—All patients visiting a vein treatment center for lower-extremity vein evaluation over a 2-year period answered a questionnaire on RLS symptoms. Patients underwent a phlebologic clinical evaluation that included continuous-wave Doppler ultrasonography. Patients with reflux in any saphenous trunk were considered Doppler positive (DP) and those without reflux in all saphenous trunks were classified as Doppler negative (DN). Of 1,397 patients evaluated, 312 (22%) had RLS symptoms. Of the 312 patients with symptoms, 113 (36%) underwent sclerotherapy with sodium tetradecyl sulphate.

Results.—Symptoms of RLS had lasted a mean of 8.8 years in this cohort (94% female and 6% male). Forty-six percent of patients reported a family history of RLS. Ninety-four percent of patients had daytime symptoms, 45% had nighttime symptoms, and 39% experienced symptoms during the day and night. The DN to DP ratio was 3:2 (61%

TABLE 1.—Demographic Characteristics of Patients

	All Patients with RLS		Treatment Group	
N	312		113	
Female	294	94%	104	92%
Male	18	6%	9	8%
Vein disease:				
Doppler-positive	123	39%	49	43%
Doppler-negative	189	61%	64	57%
Symptoms:				
Nighttime	139	45%	65	58%
Daytime	294	94%	107	95%
Both	121	39%	59	52%
Family history	142	46%	45	40%
Partner PLMS complaint	64	21%	20	18%
Duration of symptoms (years)	8.8 ± 8.4		8.5 ± 8.1	
	(1–45)		(1–45)	
	(N = 232)		(N = 81)	
Doppler-positive	10.9 ± 9.6		12.0 ± 9.7	
Doppler-negative	7.4 ± 7.2		6.2 ± 5.8	

*The difference in duration of symptoms in Doppler-positive and Doppler-negative vein disease was statistically significant (P = .0042 for all patients and P = .0038 for the treatment groups, by independent t-test).

Abbreviation: PLMS, periodic leg movements in sleep.

(Reprinted by permission of the publisher from Kanter AH: The effect of sclerotherapy on restless legs syndrome. Dermatol Surg 21:328–332, copyright 1995 by Elsevier Science Inc.)

compared with 39%) (Table 1). Of 113 patients who received sclerotherapy, 98% reported relief of RLS symptoms. No patients reported worsened symptoms. One and 2 treatments, respectively, were sufficient for relief in 40% and 78% of patients who responded to therapy. The mean number of treatments required for relief of symptoms was 2.2. The recurrence rate was 4% at 6 months, 8% at 12 months, and 28% at 24 months. No apparent difference in the recurrence rate was seen between patients who were DP and those who were DN. Two patients had no relief of RLS symptoms at completion of sclerotherapy.

Conclusion.—Symptoms of RLS were relatively common in middle-aged, primarily female patients seeking treatment at a vein clinic. Nearly all patients who underwent sclerotherapy for treatment of concurrent vein disease experienced rapid relief of RLS symptoms. The RLS symptoms were observed in patients with and without saphenous vein disease. Patients with symptoms of RLS should be considered for phlebologic evaluation and possible sclerotherapy treatment before receiving long-term drug therapy.

▶ In my assessment of patients with venous disease, I have found it truly amazing how many report restless leg syndrome. Patients will frequently say that before they had pain or heaviness associated with their venous varicosities, they had restless leg syndrome. Interestingly, this symptom is one of the first to be relieved with treatment. The return of the symptom may signify recurrence, and patients should be examined for it at that time.

D.J. Papadopoulos, M.D.

Continuous Wave Venous Doppler Examination for Pretreatment Diagnosis of Varicose and Telangiectatic Veins
Weiss RA, Weiss MA (Johns Hopkins Univ, Baltimore, Md)
Dermatol Surg 20:58–62, 1995   4–51

Background.—Doppler evaluation of varicosities is an important part of pretreatment diagnosis in patients with varicose and telangiectatic veins. All dermatologic practitioners involved with treating the venous system of the leg therefore should be familiar with Doppler techniques. The indications, basic principles, and guidelines for venous continuous-wave Doppler evaluation are discussed.

Indications for Doppler Assessment.—Patients with varicose veins large enough to be considered hemodynamically significant should undergo Doppler ultrasound assessment. Specifically, Doppler examination is indicated in patients with varicosities greater than 4 mm in diameter; any varicosity over 2 mm in diameter that extends throughout the calf or thigh; any varicosity that extends into the groin or popliteal fossae; and "starburst" clusters of telangiectasia, particularly when noted over the usual positions of perforating veins, such as the mid-posterior calf, medial knee, medial mid-thigh, and medial distal calf. Patients with a history of deep-vein thrombosis and/or thrombophlebitis, as well as those who have had previous venous surgery or sclerotherapy with unfavorable outcomes or recurrent varicosities, also are candidates for Doppler ultrasound.

General Principles and Evaluation Guidelines.—In veins, unlike arteries, a spontaneous flow signal is uncommon. The venous system represents a series of wide channels in which flow is decelerated, with force of flow generated by muscle contractions occurring at irregular intervals. To generate or enhance an audible signal or flow, manual compression of the calf, for example, may be required to simulate muscle contraction. When compression is released, gravitational hydrostatic pressure results in the cessation of reverse flow when competent valves are present. The sounds heard after manual compression vary according to Doppler transducer position. In a standing patient, manual compression of the calf distal to the Doppler probe over a competent vein produces a short sound of upward flow. With compression release, valves snap shut and flow sounds are promptly terminated. Compression proximal to the transducer produces a very short sound that ceases abruptly when blood flow is halted by competent valves. When incompetent valves are present, compression proximal to the Doppler probe results in a long whooshing sound as blood flows unimpeded distally through such valves. The sound continues as long as compression is maintained; with compression release, flow stops. When compression is applied distal to the transducer, normal proximal flow is audible; with release of compression, however, blood flows distally through incompetent valves. When the patient is standing or sitting in an upright position, this results in a considerably extended reflux sound that is generated by hydrostatic pressure (Fig 1).

Proximal Compression Phase

Distal Compression Phase

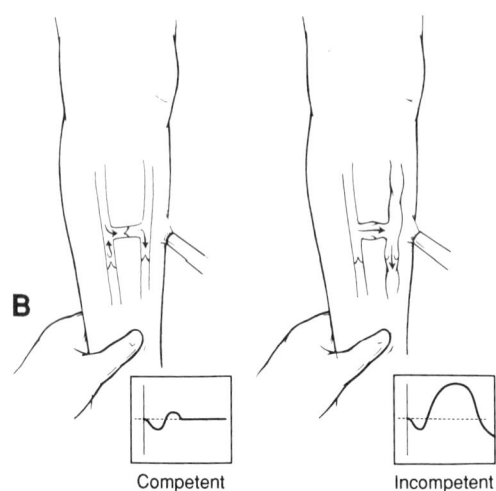

FIGURE 1.—Schematic of principles of evaluation by Doppler. (A) Proximal compression phase. During proximal compression with competent valves, a brief sound is heard (inset) that rapidly concludes as blood movement is stopped by competent valves. A long sound is heard (inset) as blood movement is detected though a wide-open incompetent valve. The sound continues as long as compression is applied. As compression is released, flow stops. (B) Distal compression phase. With competent valves, brief normal forward flow is heard. As distal compression is released, blood flows backwards under gravity but is rapidly stopped by competent valves. With incompetent valves, a brief normal upward flow is heard; however, as distal compression is released, blood flow continues backward with a prolonged sound because incompetent valves are unable to prevent continued flow propelled by hydrostatic pressure (gravity). Schematic insets show bidirectional tracings of sounds produced; flow towards the transducer is shown as positive whereas flow away from the transducer is shown as negative. (Reprinted by permission of the publisher from Weiss RA, Weiss MA: Continuous wave venous Doppler examination for pretreatment diagnosis of varicose and telangiectatic veins. *Dermatol Surg* 20:58–62, copyright 1995 by Elsevier Science Inc.) Courtesy of Goldman MP, Weiss RA, Bergan JJ: Varicose veins, diagnosis and treatment: A review. *J Am Acad Dermatol* 31:393–413, 1994.

The suggested sequence for Doppler examination is as follows. With the patient in a standing or upright seated position, the deep system at the groin is first evaluated, after which the superficial groin system is assessed. The popliteal fossa/knee, anteromedial calf, and the deep and superficial veins at the ankle next are evaluated. Multiple small perforators, resulting in smaller reticular varicosities, may also be distributed on the thighs and calves. The most frequent sites are the mid-lateral thigh and mid-lateral calf, although a great many more anatomic variations do exist. A 10-MHz Doppler transducer, applied with ultra-light pressure, can aid in identifying these perforators. Their presence may, at times, be verified by the presence of a small palpable fascial defect. Reflux determination can be useful in managing associated telangiectasia; however, reflux is not readily elicited from these sites by inexperienced practitioners.

Conclusions.—In patients with varicose and telangiectatic leg veins, sources of reverse physiologic flow (reflux) can be quickly and precisely located using continuous-wave Doppler ultrasound. Before treatment is initiated in such patients, physical examination followed by Doppler-assisted mapping of venous system physiologic anomalies should be undertaken.

▶ Take note that if you are going to get involved in a "serious" way in performing sclerotherapy, you must understand and be functional in the use of continuous-wave Doppler. This takes time and constant use in the pre- and posttreatment evaluation of sclerotherapy patients. Getting started is difficult, and a definite learning curve is involved. Articles like this one by people who are willing to share information in our literature are extremely valuable in the development of the field.

D.J. Papadopoulos, M.D.

Identification of Arteriovenous Anastomoses by Duplex Ultrasound: Implications for the Treatment of Varicose Veins
Kanter A, Gardner M, Isaacs M (Irvine, Calif)
Dermatol Surg 21:885–889, 1995   4–52

Background.—Arteriovenous anastomoses (AVA) may be involved in the etiology of varicose vein disease. Duplex ultrasound, a noninvasive technique commonly used in the diagnosis of venous disease, may help clarify the role of AVA and also may serve to guide treatment of varicose veins. In the present study, duplex ultrasound was used to evaluate the incidence and site of AVA in patients with clinically evident varicose veins caused by underlying saphenous vein reflux.

Patients and Methods.—Five-hundred ten patients from 3 private practices seen over a 12-month period were included in the study. All patients underwent evaluation of leg varicose veins using continuous-wave Doppler and were found to have junctional and/or axial reflux in one of the saphenous systems. Duplex ultrasound examinations of all saphenous vein

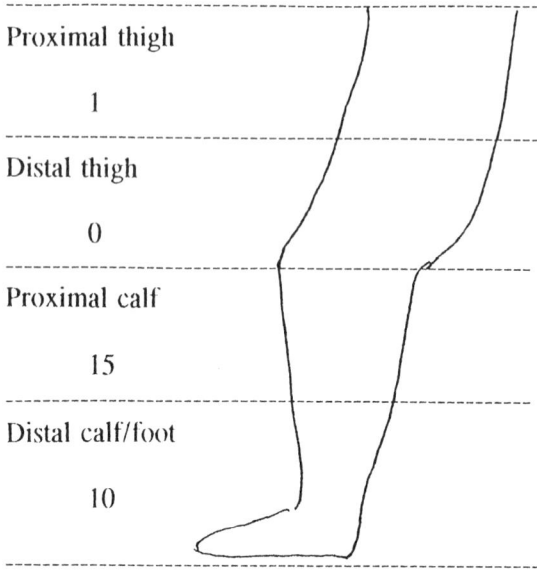

Proximal thigh

1

Distal thigh

0

Proximal calf

15

Distal calf/foot

10

FIGURE 3.—AVA location by level. (Reprinted by permission of the publisher from Kanter A, Garner M, Isaacs M: Identification of arteriovenous anastomoses by duplex ultrasound: Implications for the treatment of varicose veins. *Dermatol Surg* 21:885–889, copyright 1995 by Elsevier Science Inc.)

axes were performed with the patient in standing and supine positions. When AVA was suspected, a pulsed-Doppler was focused at its origin and followed continuously along its length. An AVA was considered present when distinct arterial waveforms underwent a progressive transition to venous waveforms along a visualized continuous vessel. Both AVA position and associated saphenous site were documented when AVA were found.

Results.—Twenty-six AVA were documented in 19 patients (4 of whom had multiple AVA) including 13 women and 6 men. Overall incidence was 3.7%. Nine of the patients had undergone previous vein stripping, whereas the remaining 10 had not. Fourteen AVA were noted in right legs and 12 in left legs. The majority of AVA (19 of 26) were found in the long saphenous system, just below the knee (Fig. 3). Three patients had venous ulcers, and in all 3 AVA were noted at the ulcer base adjacent to the medial malleolus. Most patients with AVA were between 41 and 50 years or 61 and 70 years of age (8 and 5 patients, respectively). The use of higher resolution ultrasound led to better identification of AVA.

Conclusions.—Most AVA occurring in association with saphenous vein disease are found below the knee in the long saphenous system and occasionally at the base of venous ulcers, as demonstrated by duplex ultrasound studies. Complications of sclerotherapy may be averted and treatment better guided with knowledge of AVA presence and site.

▶ How AVAs contribute to the pathophysiology of varicose veins is still an enigma. Knowing where they occur most frequently is important, and we always welcome any techniques that assist us in the detection of these structures. Inadvertent injection into varicose veins leads to necrosis which, unless it is excised, may take months to heal. Most of us cannot afford duplex machines in our offices, but with the information presented in this article and with our physical examination and continuous wave Doppler examination, we can be, hopefully, a little closer to increased detection and further evaluation before we embark on risky treatment.

D.J. Papadopoulos, M.D.

Sclerotherapy: Continuous Wave Doppler-Guided Injections
Cornu-Thenard A, de Cottreau H, Weiss RA (Hôpital Saint-Antoine, Paris; Johns Hopkins Univ, Baltimore, Md)
Dermatol Surg 21:867–870, 1995   4–53

Background.—The injection of sclerosing agents has traditionally been guided by clinical recognition and visualization of the varicose vein. Continuous wave Doppler sclerotherapy, a simple 4-step technique requiring minimally sophisticated equipment, offers more accurate sclerotherapy in instances in which varicose veins cannot be palpated in the supine position but can be felt while standing. The protocol for continuous-wave, Doppler-guided sclerosing injections, based on 3 years' experience, was described.

    Technique.—The first step of this 4-step method is identical to standard sclerotherapy procedures. Varicose veins are marked with an indelible felt-tip pen during palpation-percussion maneuvers with the patient in a standing position.

    The second step, which ensures avoidance of arterial vessels in the proposed injection site (via absence of a rhythmic arterial bruit) and also provides verification of the topography of the varicose vein, is next carried out. Verification is done by Doppler with the patient in the supine position. After coating the transducer tip with a small amount of ultrasound gel, the transducer is placed at an approximately 45-degree angle and is skimmed along the previously marked venous axis by compressing the venous segment above and below the transducer. This is accomplished using sudden to and fro movements and is continued until the movements become completely audible over a length of 1 to 3 cm. This maneuver ensures that the varicose vein to be injected and the Doppler transducer form a well-defined "vein-transducer" plane, which is essential for the next step.

    The third step involves the actual puncture-aspiration and is done while holding the transducer in one hand and the syringe in the other. With the transducer left in the "vein-transducer" plane (at an approximately 45-degree angle), the needle is placed 2 to 3 cm anteriorly to the tip of the transducer (also at an approximately

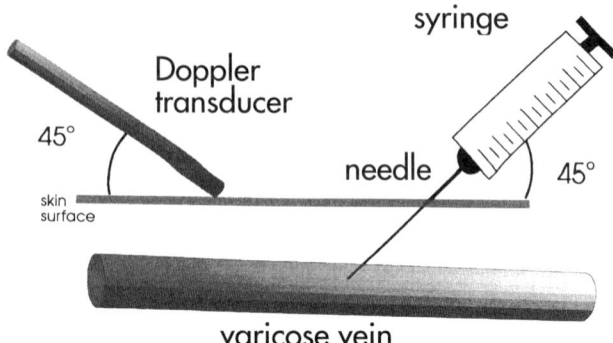

FIGURE 2.—Schematic representation of the relationship between the Doppler transducer and syringe. Continuous-wave Doppler localizes the inflow and outflow at the needle tip. The continuous wave beam and the long axis of the needle are virtually perpendicular as the needle tip passes under the Doppler transducer. The needle and Doppler transducer must be separated by several centimeters at the skin surface for proper alignment and transmission of suction and injection sounds. (Reprinted by permission of the publisher from Cornu-Thenard A, de Cottreau H, Weiss RA: Sclerotherapy: Continuous wave Doppler-guided injections. *Dermatol Surg* 21:867–870, copyright 1995 by Elsevier Science Inc.)

45-degree angle). During vein penetration, the needle tip is situated just beneath the Doppler beam, allowing any liquid movement in the vein and at this site to be detected by Doppler effect (Fig 2). Once the needle is introduced under the previously disinfected skin, aspiration pressure is applied to the syringe and the needle is slowly advanced until vein puncture occurs. A short suction noise is emitted by the Doppler amplifier once the needle penetrates the vascular lumen, as a result of blood passage in front of the transducer as it is aspirated into the needle. The lower part of the syringe slowly fills with nonpulsatile venous blood, and the fourth step, which consists of the actual injection, is then carried out.

With the needle bevel properly situated, the sclerosing agent is injected. The Doppler effect causes a liquid sound, essentially until the injection is completed. When plunger pressure is released, the characteristic sound stops. After pressure is reapplied, the typical sound once again is heard. In instances in which the injection is interrupted and the aspiration procedure is repeated, the suction noise and venous reflux should reappear.

Conclusions.—This technique is mainly indicated for patients whose varicose veins can be palpated while standing but not while in the supine position. Patients with varicose veins in the groin area, lower third of the thigh, and along the axis of the small saphenous vein also may be treated with this method. The authors have used this procedure in 220 patients (approximately 1,400 injections) and have had successful results in all but 18 instances. No serious adverse effects were noted. Accessibility, cost-effectiveness, simplicity, and the ability to confirm intravenous injection of sclerosing agents are all advantages associated with this technique, although it should not be considered a substitute for duplex ultrasound-guided injections.

▶ An interesting method for a difficult problem, which would be very valuable for those who do not possess a duplex ultrasound in their office. What is amazing here is that 1,400 injections were performed without any complications. This is a procedure for the experienced sclerotherapist who has performed a significant number of injections in larger vessels. Note that successful large-vessel sclerotherapy usually precludes that tactile and visual feedback be appreciated appropriately by the sclerotherapy. This technique makes it mandatory to appreciate auditory feedback adding to the complexity and degree of difficulty associated with the procedure.

D.J. Papadopoulos, M.D.

The Australian Polidocanol (Aethoxysklerol) Study: Results at 2 Years
Conrad P, Malouf GM, Stacey MC (Nepean Hosp, Sydney, Australia; Westmead Hosp, Sydney, Australia; Fremantle Hosp, Western Australia)
Dermatol Surg 21:334–336, 1995   4–54

Background.—Available reports suggest that polidocanol, when used as a sclerosing agent, is associated with a very low incidence of toxic reactions, skin necrosis, or pigmentation. This agent is also less painful on injection compared with sodium tetradecyl sulfate (STD) or hypertonic saline solution, because of its local anesthetic action. An ongoing study evaluating the safety and efficacy of polidocanol has been conducted over a 2-year period by 98 investigators in Australia—the results of which are reported.

Patients and Methods.—The aim of this single-arm prospective study was to evaluate the efficacy of polidocanol as a sclerosant and to record any treatment-related complications. Comparisons between investigators' experience with polidocanol and other sclerosing agents also were made. A total of 16,804 limbs of patients with either varicose veins or venule ectasias and/or spider veins (telangiectasia) were treated over a 2-year period. In patients with telangiectasias or spider veins, 0.5% to 1% polidocanol was used, whereas in those with varicose veins, 3% polidocanol was administered.

Results.—Of the 16,804 legs in this study, 6,476 had varicose veins and 10,328 had spider veins and venules. No deaths or anaphylactic reactions occurred as a result of polidocanol therapy. Very few complications were reported during the 2-year study. Those that were noted included a possible allergic reaction in 34 instances (0.2%), injection site ulceration in 32 (0.2%), significant or severe pigmentation in 30 (0.2%), superficial thrombophlebitis in 14 (0.08%), deep-vein thrombosis in 3 (0.02%), and telangiectatic matting in 7 (0.04%). Of the 65 investigators with previous experience using STD, 85% indicated that the effectiveness of polidocanol was superior to that of STD. Similarly, of the 58 investigators with previous experience using hypertonic saline, 84% felt that polidocanol was the superior agent. In terms of treatment-related complications, 90% of the investigators felt that polidocanol resulted in less frequent complication than did STD, and 80% indicated that the polidocanol-related complications were less severe. Seventy-four percent of the investigators indicated that compared with hypertonic saline, polidocanol was associated with fewer side effects; 74% reported that these were less severe.

Conclusions.—Polidocanol is an effective sclerosant and is considered by many to be a better agent than STD and hypertonic saline. Few complications are associated with use of polidocanol as a sclerosing agent for varicose veins, spider veins, and venules.

▶ Another study suggests that polidocanol is a superior agent, determined subjectively by those performing much sclerotherapy. If one looks at this data carefully, it becomes obvious that this is a subjective study for the most part by physicians who had used sodium tetradecyl sulfate (STD) or hypertonic saline in the past, but who were currently using polidocanol. My personal feeling is that we need to develop an objective model for head-to-head comparison of the effectiveness of these three agents compared to their complications. My instinct, after having used STD and hypertonic saline and having observed my European colleagues use polidocanol is that their effectiveness is probably similar and that the main complication, in which a significant difference exists upon comparison of these agents, is pain. In my opinion, pain can be reduced significantly when using hypertonic saline or STD by injecting very slowly. This is not to imply that pain can be reduced to the amount elicited by polidocanol. Polidocanol is a superior agent in this respect. We await, with hopeful anticipation, Food and Drug Administration approval of polidocanol, but we must continue to be cautious as we are with all sclerosants in the way that we embrace and use them.

D.J. Papadopoulos, M.D.

Hyaluronidase in the Prevention of Sclerotherapy-Induced Extravasation Necrosis: A Dose-Response Study
Zimmet SE (Univ of Texas, Austin)
Dermatol Surg 22:73–76, 1996   4–55

Background.—Extravasation-related necrosis can occur in patients undergoing sclerotherapy, with such events becoming more likely as the number of practitioners performing such procedures continues to grow. In a previous study, hyaluronidase was found to have a significant protective effect against necrosis after extravasation of sodium tetradecyl sulfate and 23.4% sodium chloride in rats; however, dose-response studies have not been published. A 2-part, dose-response study using hyaluronidase in the prevention of necrosis after intradermal 23.4% sodium chloride was therefore undertaken.

Methods.—During the first study, 40 female Sprague-Dawley rats weighing between 150 and 200 g were evaluated. Twenty animals were injected with either 150, 300, or 450 U of hyaluronidase (all in a volume of 3 mL) immediately after having received an intradermal injection of 0.25 mL of 23.4% hypertonic saline. The remaining 20 animals received identical intradermal injections, but subsequent treatment was withheld in this group. During the second study, 20 to 30 animals were given 0.25 mL of 23.4% sodium chloride intradermally. Some of the animals immediately received either 18.75, 37.5, 75, 150, or 900 U of hyaluronidase (all in a volume of 3 mL), whereas the remaining rats received no treatment. Both studies were randomized and blind. Animals were evaluated for subsequent necrosis 3 days after injections were delivered, and a dose-response curve was constructed.

Results.—In both studies, a statistically significant protective effect was noted in the animals treated with hyaluronidase compared with the untreated groups. Hyaluronidase given at doses of 75 U offered the best protection against necrosis. The observed protective effect was not enhanced when doses higher than 75 U were administered.

Conclusions.—The results of this rat-model study indicate that a dose of 75 U of hyaluronidase provides maximal protection against necrosis should extravasation with 23.4% sodium chloride take place. Further protection is not realized when doses higher than 75 U (up to 900 U) are given.

▶ As the number of patients treated with sclerotherapy during a physician's career increases, so does the possibility of accidental extravasation. The information provided in this article is important, because it gives us another tool to use when this unfortunate event occurs. Sclerotherapy-induced necrosis occurring after treatment by an experienced sclerotherapist is more often due to injection of the sclerosant into an arteriovenous anastomosis. With the less experienced sclerotherapist, it tends to occur as a result of extravascular injection. Hopefully in either case, the use of hyaluronidase will be helpful in reducing the incidence of this complication. Also interesting would be to see how hyaluronidase compares to procaine head-to-head in extravasation injury induced by sodium tetradecyl sulfate.

D.J. Papadopoulos, M.D.

Varicose Vein Surgery: Patient Satisfaction
Davies AH, Steffen C, Cosgrove C, et al (Derriford Hosp, Plymouth, England)
J R Coll Surg Edinb 40:298–299, 1995   4–56

Background.—Approximately one third of adult women have varicose veins, and surgical intervention for reasons ranging from ulceration to cosmesis is not uncommon in this patient population. Similar to other surgical procedures, risk of morbidity is associated with varicose vein surgery. Patient satisfaction with treatment outcome is therefore important, and was considered in the present study.

Patients and Methods.—A postal questionnaire was sent to 456 patients who had undergone varicose vein surgery over a 10-year period. The questionnaire was designed to determine patient satisfaction with overall surgical results and with communication and explanations about the procedure and to collect information pertaining to immediate postoperative complications, subsequent recurrences, persistent symptoms, and need for additional treatment. Three-hundred twenty-seven of the patients had received care through the National Health Service (NHS), whereas 129 patients were treated by surgeons in private practice (PP). Primary treatment consisted of a high tie and stripping of the long saphenous vein, with numerous avulsions carried out as needed.

Results.—Three hundred eleven patients, including 219 of the NHS and 92 of the PP patients, completed the questionnaire, yielding an overall response rate of 68%. Fifty-six percent of the NHS and 54% of the PP patients were reportedly satisfied with the overall treatment results, and 19% and 34%, respectively, indicated that they were entirely satisfied with procedure-related communications and had been free of postoperative complications. In comparison, 26% of the NHS and 13% of the PP patients reported being very dissatisfied with the procedure, and 23% and 22%, respectively, indicated that they had experienced immediate postoperative complications. Of the 60 women in the PP and the 142 women in the NHS groups, 7 and 39, respectively, were dissatisfied with their results. Of the 32 men in the former and 77 men in the latter groups, 5 and 7, respectively, reported dissatisfaction with outcome. No differences in reports of scarring, persistent ache, recurrence, or additional treatment were noted between the NHS and PP groups. More than two thirds of the patients did indicate an improvement in postoperative versus preoperative symptoms.

Conclusions.—Varicose vein surgery, although considered a safe and fairly straightforward procedure, is associated with considerable morbidity and patient dissatisfaction. The results of this study indicate that patient communication is important; patients should be advised of potential surgical outcomes and should understand that favorable results are not necessarily guaranteed.

▶ Interesting information for two reasons. First, clearly a great number of patients are not satisfied with varicose vein surgery, predominantly because of morbidity and recurrence. Second, we must inform our patients appropriately that, in the best of circumstances, whether with surgery or sclerotherapy, temporary relief rather than cure occurs in many circumstances. I personally feel that because of the type of information presented in this article and that which we constantly hear from our patients, sclerotherapy and less invasive techniques such as ambulatory phlebectomy have and will continue to play a significant role in the treatment of venous disease.

D.J. Papadopoulos, M.D.

Subject Index*

A

---

* *All entries refer to the year and page number(s) for data appearing in this and previous
editions of the* YEAR BOOK.

suctioned and surgically removed, fate
after reimplantation for soft tissue
augmentation (in rabbit), 95: 340
transplantation
guidelines for, 97: 212
long-term survival of, 97: 211
Fatty acids
in healing, 97: 2
Ferritin
levels, serum, correlation with
postsclerotherapy pigmentation,
96: 286
Fetal
skin wounds, expression of
transforming growth factor-β in (in
rabbit), 96: 5
wound repair, spectral nature of, 97: 8
Fever
after interferon–α2a for complex
hemangiomas of infancy and
childhood, 96: 171
Fibrin glue
for skin grafting of contaminated burn
wounds, 95: 227
for temporoparietal flaps, bilateral, in
male baldness, 96: 259
Fibroblast(s)
growth factor, basic
endogenous, in chronic wounds,
determination of, 96: 5
in wound fluid, skin graft donor site,
95: 1–2
wound healing and, 96: 3
hypertrophic scar, collagen synthesis
modulation by transforming
growth factor-β in, 96: 13
keloid
collagen synthesis modulation by
transforming growth factor-β in,
96: 13
growth inhibition by isotretinoin and
triamcinolone, in vitro, 96: 12
Fibrokeratoma
of nail apparatus, MRI in diagnosis of,
96: 16
Fibroma
cutaneous soft, cryo-technique for,
95: 28
Fibronectin
in basal cell carcinoma, 96: 125
in wounds covered with skin grafts,
immunohistochemistry of (in rat),
95: 216
Filler
permanent, expanded
polytetrafluoroethylene as, 96: 245

Films
as wound dressings, clinical review,
97: 13
Finasteride
minoxidil in retinoid vehicle and, for
androgenetic alopecia, 97: 258
Fine needle aspiration cytology
of cutaneous metastases, 95: 180
Fire
intraoperative, with electrocautery,
97: 71
Fistula
arteriovenous (see Arteriovenous,
fistula)
Flammacerium
for burns, 95: 16
Flank
area, upper lateral, liposuction of,
96: 233
Flap
advancement
chondrocutaneous helical rim, of
Antia and Buch, 97: 153
perialar crescentic, modified, in upper
lip reconstruction, 97: 158
postauricular cutaneous, for ear rim
defects, 97: 154
rotation-advancement, deep-plane
cervicofacial, for reconstruction of
large cheek defects, 96: 185
axial, of nasal muscle, for nasal tip
repair, 97: 148
BAT, expanded, for male pattern
baldness, 95: 362
bilobed, for nasal tip reconstruction,
96: 179
buttock, blunt suction lipectomy in,
blood circulation and viability after
(in pig), 95: 331
canthal and glabellar, island inner, for
nasal tip reconstruction, 97: 144
circulation compromised, calcitonin
gene-related peptide treatment of,
95: 215
coverage after wide excision for axillary
hidradenitis suppurativa, 95: 59
fascial, temporoparietal, in head and
neck reconstruction, 95: 195
forehead
expanded unilateral, for coverage of
opposite forehead defect, 95: 214
midline, for nasal tip reconstruction,
analysis of, 96: 179
nasal reconstruction, esthetic
refinements in, 97: 150
frontonasal, axial, refinements in,
95: 198
island

Author Index